POCKET ATLAS

Emergency
Ultrasound

POCKET ATLAS OF
Emergency Ultrasound
Second Edition

Robert F. Reardon, MD
Assistant Chief, Department of Emergency Medicine
Hennepin County Medical Center
Professor of Emergency Medicine
University of Minnesota Medical School
Minneapolis, Minnesota

Andrea Rowland-Fisher, MD
Ultrasound Fellowship Director, Department of Emergency Medicine
Hennepin County Medical Center
Assistant Professor of Emergency Medicine
University of Minnesota Medical School
Minneapolis, Minnesota

O. John Ma, MD
Professor and Chair
Department of Emergency Medicine
Oregon Health & Science University
Portland, Oregon

New York   Chicago   San Francisco   Athens   London   Madrid   Mexico City
Milan   New Delhi   Singapore   Sydney   Toronto

Pocket Atlas of Emergency Ultrasound, Second Edition.

1 2 3 4 5 6 7 8 9   DSS   22 21 20 19 18 17

ISBN 978-0-07-184898-5
MHID 0-07-184898-3

The book was set in Garamond Premier Pro by Cenveo® Publishers Services.
The editors were Brian Belval and Christie Naglieri.
The production supervisor was Catherine Saggese.
Project management was provided by Anju Joshi, Cenveo Publishers Services.
This book is printed on acid-free paper.

Library of Congress Cataloging-in-Publication Data

Names: Reardon, Robert F., author. | Rowland-Fisher, Andie, author. | Ma, O. John, author.
Title: Pocket atlas of emergency ultrasound / Robert F. Reardon, Andie Rowland-Fisher, O. John Ma.
Description: Second edition. | New York : McGraw Hill Companies, Inc., [2017] | Includes bibliographical references and index.
Identifiers: LCCN 2017002633| ISBN 9780071848985 (pbk. : alk. paper) | ISBN 0071848983 (pbk. : alk. paper)
Subjects: | MESH: Emergency Medical Services | Ultrasonography | Handbooks | Atlases
Classification: LCC RC78.7.U4 | NLM WX 39 | DDC 616.07/543—dc23 LC record available at https://na01.safelinks.protection.outlook.com/?url=https%3A%2F%2Flccn.loc.gov%2F2017002633&data=01%7C01%7Cjessica.gonzalez%40mheducation.com%7C7730d93497e74a2a361f08d44eae78bf%7Cf919b1efc0c347358fca0928ec39d8d5%7C1&sdata=joQ7Eau7i0O3%2FjmmlqhX3f0k%2BRJapccqfNbBP8c2M5M%3D&reserved=0

McGraw-Hill books are available at special quantity discounts to use as premiums and sales promotions, or for use in corporate training programs. To contact a representative please visit the Contact Us pages at www.mhprofessional.com.

This book is dedicated to students of Emergency Ultrasound who devote their time and effort to learn this invaluable skill, and to my wife Julianne and my girls Kylie, Kate, and Shea.

Robert F. Reardon, MD

To my parents, Chris and Elaine, for always believing in me and providing encouragement along the way.

Andrea Rowland-Fisher, MD

To the patients who we serve—may Emergency Ultrasound help facilitate high quality and safe patient care.

O. John Ma, MD

Contents

Preface

Pocket Atlas of Emergency Ultrasound is intended to help clinicians learn to perform and interpret point-of-care ultrasound exams. The format and content have been carefully chosen to maximize its usefulness at the bedside. *Pocket Atlas of Emergency Ultrasound* is meant to be a companion to the comprehensive textbook *Ma and Mateer's Emergency Ultrasound, Third Edition*, where readers can find important details about the clinical applications and utility of point-of-care ultrasound, as well as instructional case studies and thousands of references.

Robert F. Reardon, MD
Andrea Rowland-Fisher, MD
O. John Ma, MD

Acknowledgments

Thanks to the following authors whose work on *Ma and Mateer's Emergency Ultrasound, Third Edition* was adapted to create this book.

Alyssa M. Abbo, MD

Srikar Adhikari, MD, MS, RDMS

Frederic Adnet, MD

Gernot Aichinger, MD

Aaron E. Bair, MD, MSc

Raoul Breitkreutz, MD

Franziska Brenner, MD

Gavin R. Budhram, MD

Donald V. Byars, MD, RDMS

Marco Campo dell'Orto, MD

Liberty V. Caroon, RDMS

Michelle E. Clinton, MD

Thomas P. Cook, MD

Thomas G. Costantino, MD

Innes Crawford, MBChB, BSc

Andreas Dewitz, MD, RDMS

Jason W. Fischer, MD, MSc

J. Christian Fox, MD, RDMS

Harry J. Goett, MD

Corky Hecht, BA, RDMS, RDCS, RVT

William G. Heegaard, MD, MPH, MBA

Jamie Hess-Keenan, MD

Jeffrey D. Ho, MD

Timothy Jang, MD

Scott A. Joing, MD

Robert A. Jones, DO

Andrew W. Kirkpatrick, MD, MHSC

Thomas Kirschning, MD, DESA

Barry J. Knapp, MD, RDMS

Dietrich von Kuenssberg Jehle, MD, RDMS

Michael J. Lambert, MD

Frederic Lapostholle, MD

Andrew Laudenbach, MD

Resa E. Lewiss, MD, RDMS

Matthew Lyon, MD

Frank Madore, MD

William Manson, MD, RDMS

Ingo Marzi, MD

James R. Mateer, MD, RDMS

Paul B. McBeth, MD, MASc

Lisa D. Mills, MD

Masaaki Ogata, MD

Aman K. Parikh, MD

Michael A. Peterson, MD

Tomislav Petrovic, MD

David W. Plummer, MD

Gerhard Prause, MD

Daniel D. Price, MD

Jessica G. Resnick, MD

Chad E. Roline, MD

John S. Rose, MD

William Scruggs, MD, RDMS

Dina Seif, MD, MBA, RDMS

Fernando R. Silva, MD, MSc

Adam B. Sivitz, MD

Michael B. Stone, MD

Stuart P. Swadron, MD

Daniel L. Theodoro, MD, MSCI

Corina Tiruta, MSc

Felix Walcher, MD, PhD

Gernot Wildner, MD

Peter M. Zechner, MD

CHAPTER 1

Ultrasound Basics

► TRANSDUCERS

- Ultrasound transducers contain piezoelectric crystals that convert electrical energy to mechanical energy (sound waves) and transmit them into the body. The crystals also receive reflected sound waves and convert them back into electrical energy.

- Most ultrasound transducers produce sound waves between 2 and 10 MHz.

- Lower-frequency transducers can penetrate deeper tissues but provide poorer resolution (Figures 1-1 and 1-2).

- Higher-frequency transducers provide better resolution but cannot penetrate deeper structures (Figures 1-3 and 1-4).

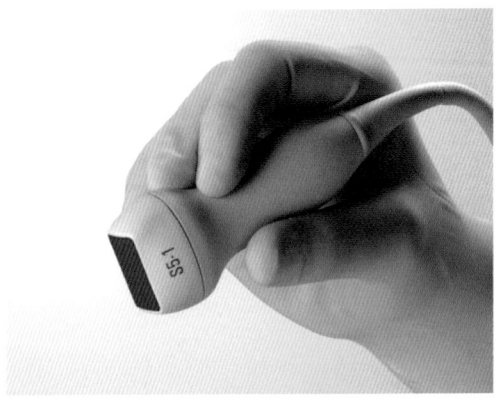

A

Figure 1-1. **A.** A phased array probe with 2.5- to 3.5-MHz frequency range is best used for cardiac imaging. (Photo contributed by SonoSite.)

(Figure 1-1B continued on next page)

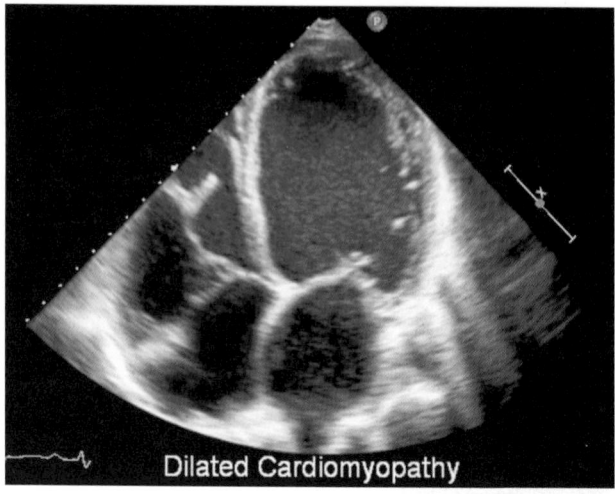

Dilated Cardiomyopathy

B

Figure 1-1. **B.** Phased array probe image. A phased array probe is also used for abdominal and pelvic imaging in larger patients. (Image contributed by Philips Healthcare.)

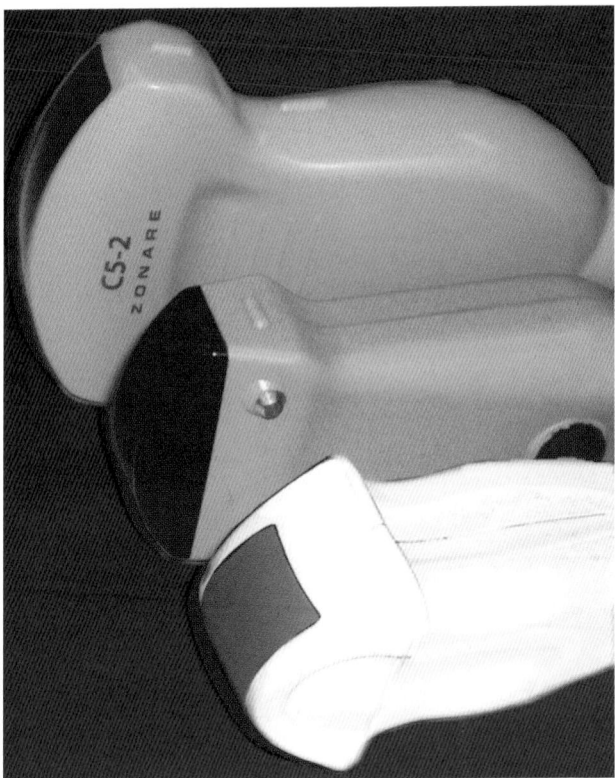

A

Figure 1-2. Lower-frequency curved array probes (3–3.5 MHz) are commonly used for abdominal and pelvic imaging in adults. Curved probes: C15, C30, C60. **A.** These three curved array probes each have different footprint sizes. Note that the smaller footprint probes have a tighter curvature. The image created by each is pie shaped.

(Figures 1-2B and C continued on next page)

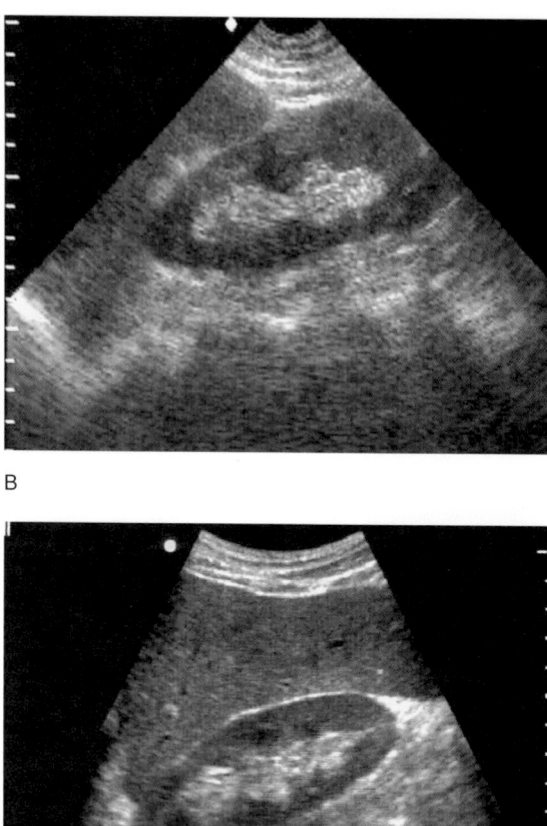

B

C

Figure 1-2. Curved array probe images. **B.** The smaller footprint probe has a much smaller near-field image allowing greater intercostal access than the larger footprint probe. **C.** Larger footprint probe.

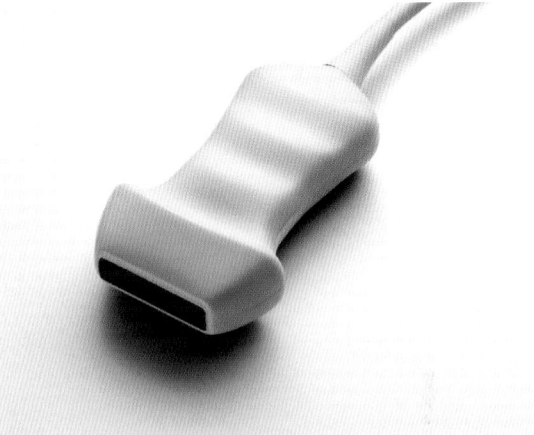

A

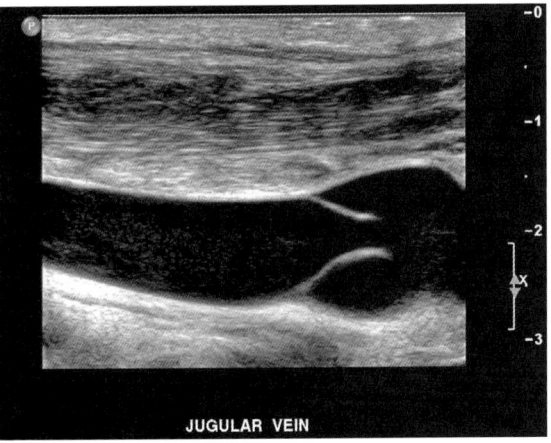

JUGULAR VEIN

B

Figure 1-3. **A.** High-frequency (7.5–10 MHz) linear array probes are best used for superficial vascular imaging. (Photo contributed by SonoSite.) **B.** These probes are also used for soft tissue imaging. (Image contributed by Philips Healthcare.)

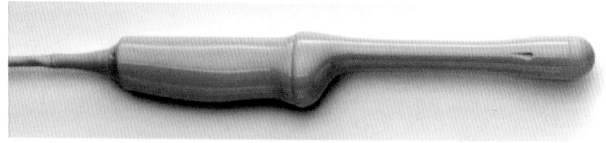

A

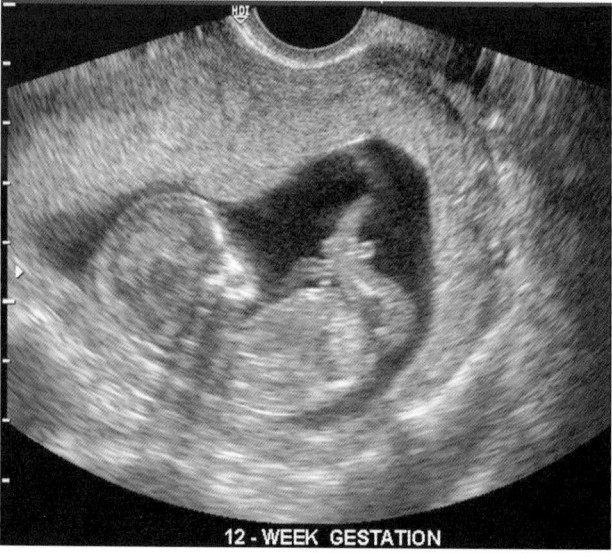

B

Figure 1-4. **A.** An endocavitary probe. (Photo contributed by SonoSite.) **B.** Endocavitary probes (5–7.5 MHz) provide high-resolution views of pelvic structures.

▶ ORIENTATION

- All transducers have an indicator mark (bump or groove) that correlates with a symbol on the display monitor.

- For abdominal and pelvic imaging, by convention, the symbol is positioned on the left side of the display, and the probe indicator is aimed toward the patient's head (longitudinal orientation) or the patient's right side (transverse orientation).

- For cardiac imaging, the symbol is positioned on the right side of the display, and the indicator is aimed toward the patient's right shoulder (long axis) or the patient's left shoulder (short axis).

▶ BASIC OPERATING INSTRUCTIONS

- **Patient data entry:** One button usually opens this field and allows identification of the patient on the ultrasound study.

- **Transducers:** Some machines can change these with the touch of a button; others require the operator to change the transducer manually.

- **Depth:** Adjustment of how far into the body the machine produces an image (Figure 1-5).

- **Zoom:** This magnifies a portion of the image on the screen (Figure 1-6).

- **Gain:** Adjustment of brightness (Figure 1-7).

- **Time gain compensation:** Adjustment of gain at different depths (Figure 1-8).

- **Freeze button:** Freezes image on the monitor.

- **Cineloop:** Most machines save a cineloop, several seconds of image in retrospect, whenever the freeze button is touched; the buttons, the trackball, or the touchpad are used to scroll backward or forward through the cineloop.

- **Enter button:** Functions like the enter button on a computer keyboard.

- **Changing frequency:** Broadband transducers can image with a variable range of frequencies. The frequency is selected by the operator and can be decreased for better penetration or increased for better resolution.

- **Image processing:** Electronic features such as tissue harmonics, spatial compounding, and speckle reduction often improve image quality (Figure 1-9), but they can also be turned off with the touch of a button if they are detrimental to image quality.

- **Focus:** The best lateral resolution is found at the focal zone, which is usually represented by an arrow on the side of the image; the focal zone (arrow) can be moved up or down with one button.

- **Presettings:** Automatic adjustments made by the ultrasound machine to optimize the image based on which body system is being imaged (eg, abdominal, obstetric, cardiac); some machines allow for different calculations based on the presettings.

- **Optimization button:** With the touch of one button, the machine automatically adjusts the gain, focus, and image processing features in an attempt to create the ideal image (Figure 1-10).

- **Measurements and calculations:** Simple measurements can be made with electronic calipers or clinically important calculations (gestational age) can be made automatically.

- **Image viewing and data storage:** Important for archiving, credentialing, teaching, and so on. (Several digital storage solutions are now available.)

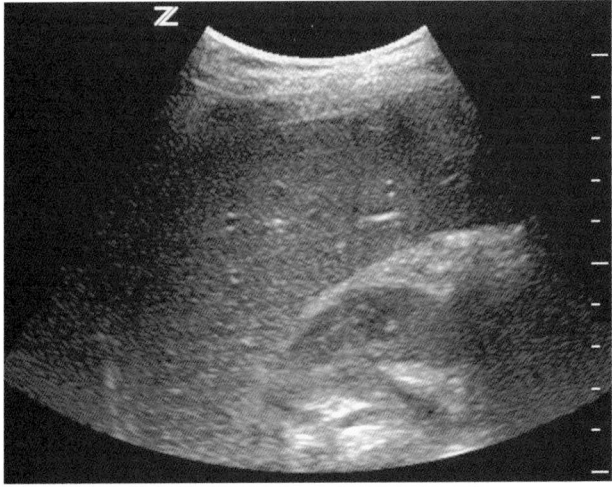

A

Figure 1-5. Depth adjustment. **A.** Note that the depth is set too shallow, leaving out important structures in the deeper field.

(Figures 1-5B and C continued on next page)

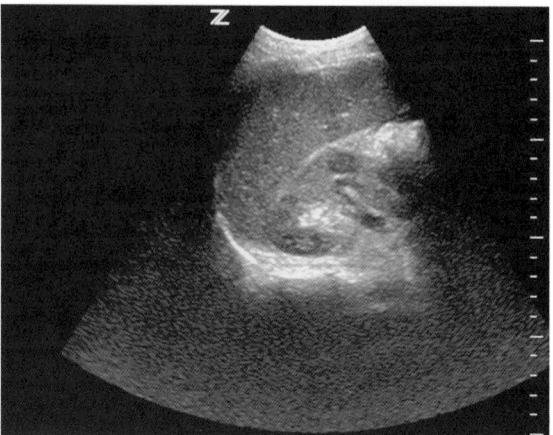

B

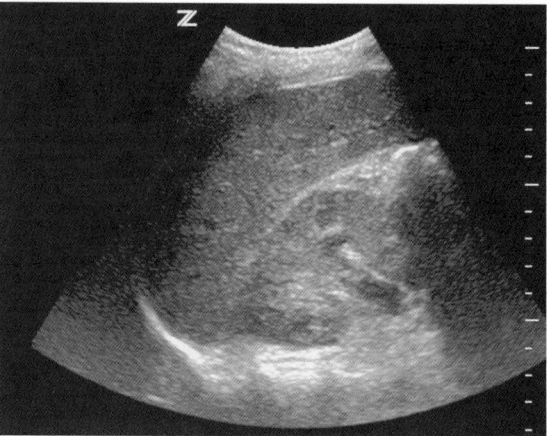

C

Figure 1-5. Depth adjustment. **B.** The depth is set too deep wasting valuable space in the far fields. **C.** The depth is set correctly providing the balance of including all important structures while using the entire display.

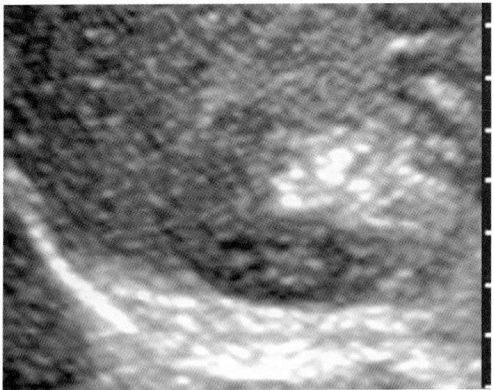

Figure 1-6. Zoom. The image of the kidney has been created from the image shown in Figure 1-5B by using the zoom function. It is magnified, but the overall resolution is not as sharp as the image created by decreasing the depth (Figure 1-5C) because there are fewer pixels creating the image.

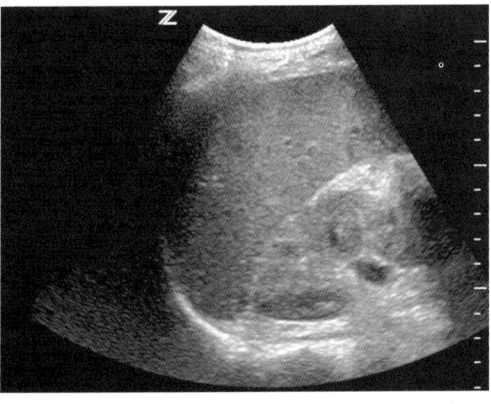

A

Figure 1-7. Gain adjustment. **A.** (Correct) The image is correctly gained.

(Figures 1-7B and C continued on next page)

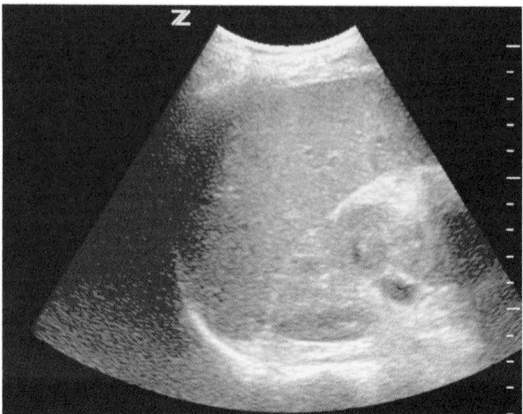

B

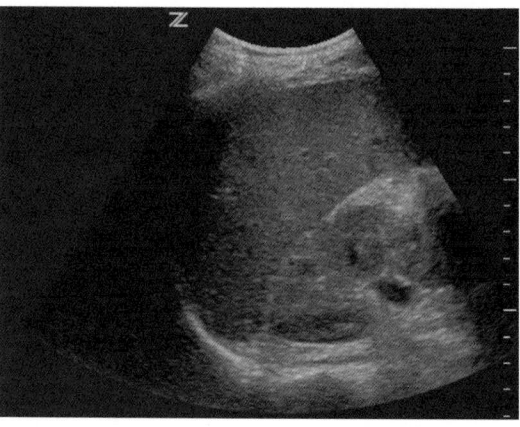

C

Figure 1-7. Gain adjustment. **B.** (Over) The image is over-gained. Compared with image **A.** echoes are found where there should be none. **C.** (Under) The image is undergained. The image is too dark, potentially making it difficult for accurate diagnosis.

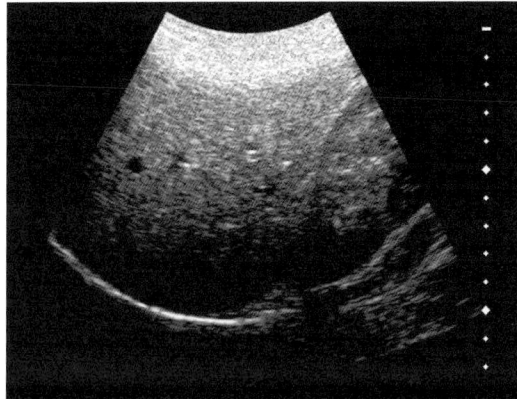

A

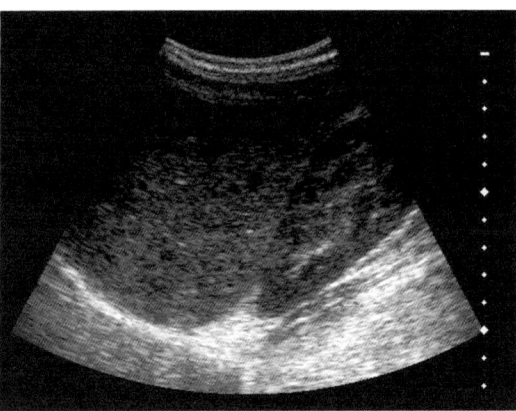

B

Figure 1-8. Time gain compensation (TGC) settings. **A.** Maladjusted far field/posterior setting does not permit visualization of posterior structures. **B.** Incorrect TGC settings. Maladjusted near field/anterior TGC setting does not permit visualization of structures positioned closer to the transducer.

(Figures 1-8C and D continued on next page)

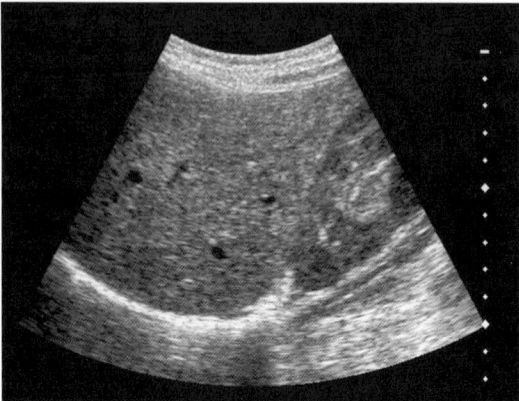

C

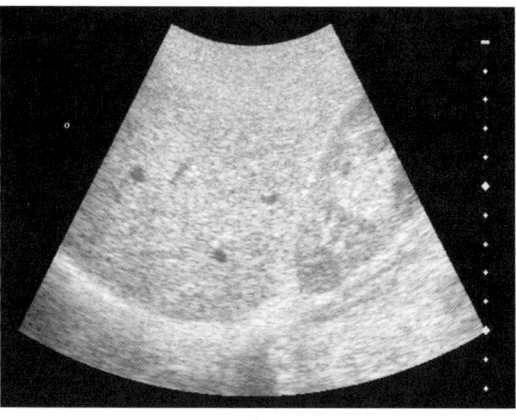

D

Figure 1-8. Time gain compensation (TGC) settings. **C.** Correct TGC and gain settings. By balancing the display of echogenic information, one can appreciate the subtleties that occur among tissues. **D.** Excessive gain settings reduce the ability to differentiate subtleties among various tissues. (Photos contributed by SonoSite.)

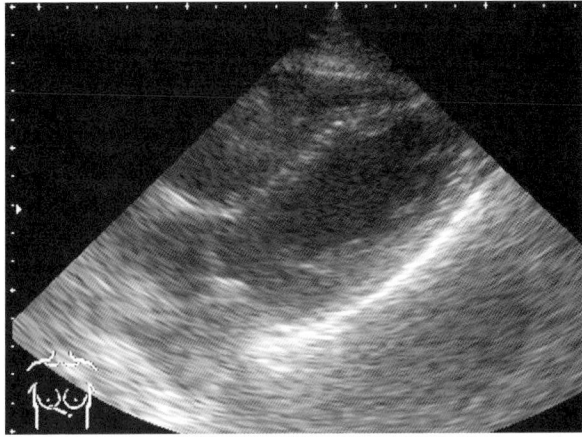

A

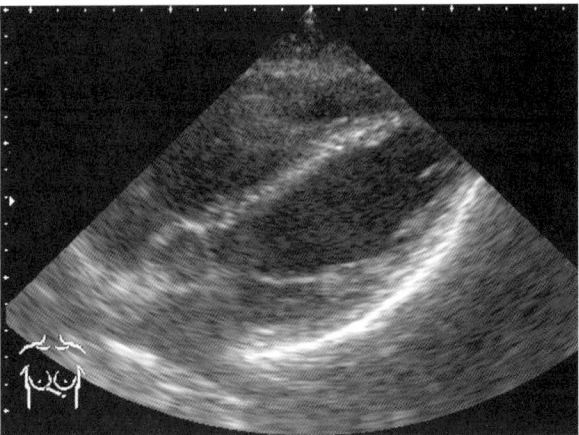

B

Figure 1-9. Harmonic imaging (subcostal cardiac view).
A. An image without harmonic imaging. **B.** The same image with harmonics. Note the improved detail of the left ventricular walls, endocardium, and mitral subvalvular and aortic valve areas.

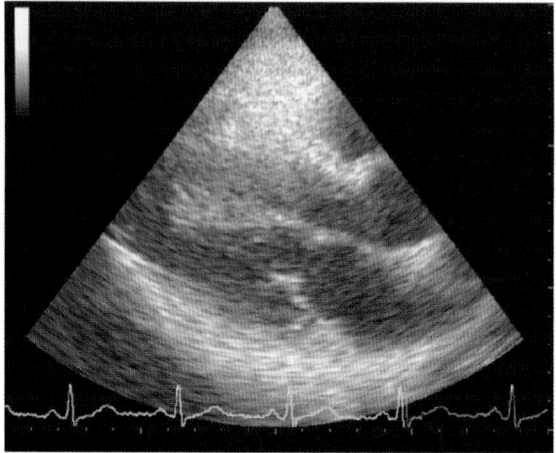

A

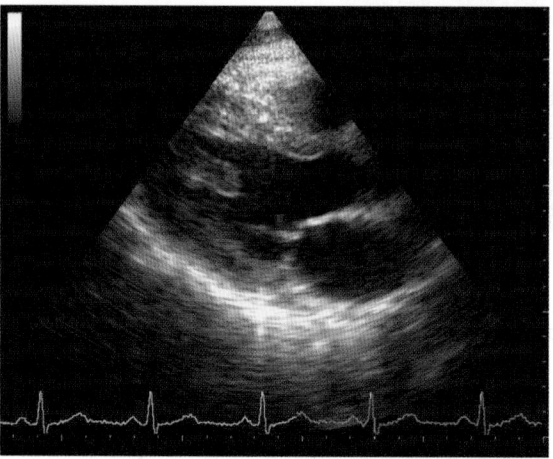

B

Figure 1-10. Image "optimization" (parasternal long-axis view). **A.** An image without "optimization." **B.** The same image with "optimization." (Photos contributed by Biosound Esaote.)

▶ BASIC DEFINITIONS

- **Resolution:** The quality of the image; the ability to differentiate the anatomical and pathological areas of interest (Figure 1-11).
- **Near field:** The part of the image closer to the transducer.
- **Far field:** The part of the image farther from the transducer.
- **Echogenicity:** The ability to create an echo (Figure 1-12).

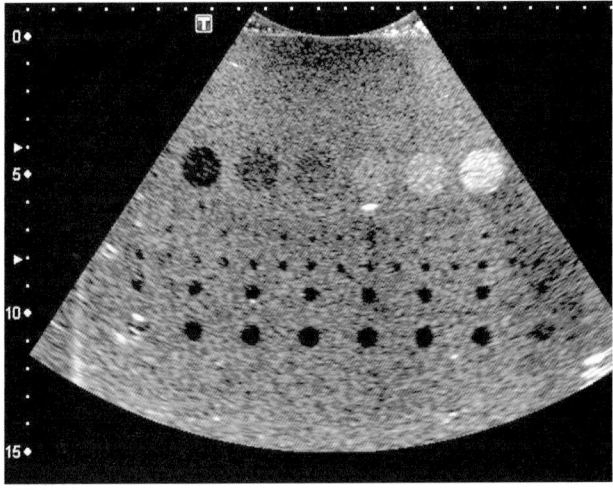

A

Figure 1-11. Axial and lateral resolution. **A.** Note how grainy and pixilated the lower-frequency (1.9 MHz) image is.

(Figure 1-11B continued on next page)

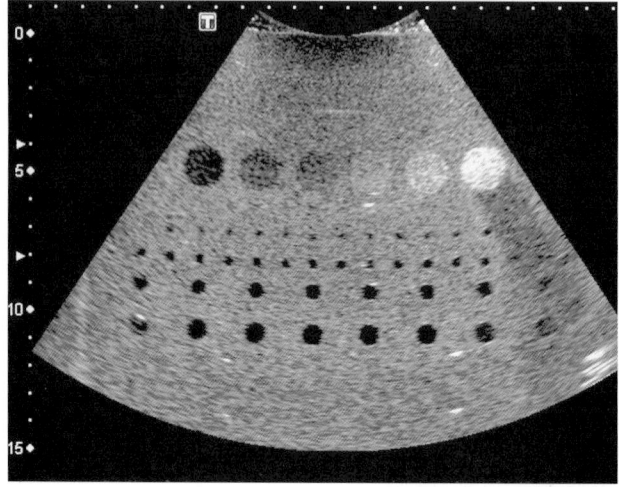

B

Figure 1-11. Axial and lateral resolution. **B.** The higher-resolution (5.0 MHz) image has smoother characteristics. Both images were obtained using a multipurpose phantom. (Model 539 Multipurpose, ATS Laboratories, Inc.)

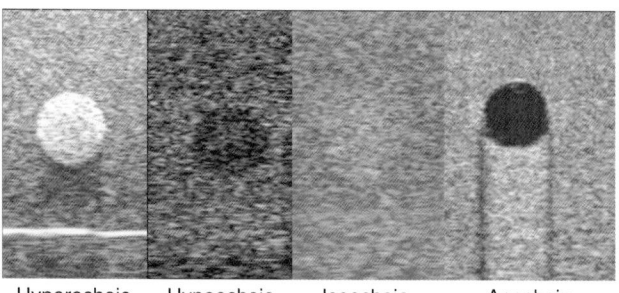

Hyperechoic   Hypoechoic   Isoechoic   Anechoic

Figure 1-12. Echogenicity refers to the amplitude or brightness display of the returning echoes and is further defined by the above subcategories. (Photos contributed by SonoSite.)

▶ IMAGE ARTIFACTS

- Shadowing (Figures 1-13 and 1-14).
- Refraction or edge shadows (Figure 1-15).
- Acoustic enhancement—helpful for differentiating liquid from solid density masses (Figure 1-16).
- Gas dispersion (Figure 1-17).
- Reverberation (Figure 1-18).
- Mirroring (Figure 1-19).
- Side lobes (Figure 1-20).

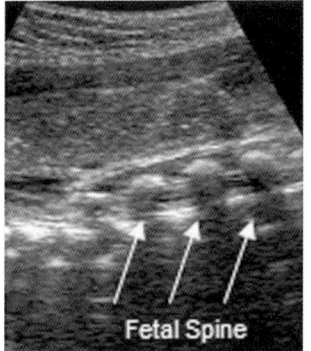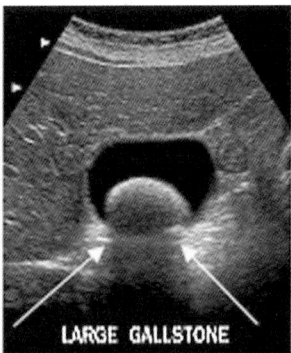

Figure 1-13. Clean shadowing from attenuation. Bone density objects such as this fetal spine and a large gallstone generally result in a darker, more homogenous ("clean") shadow (*arrows*).

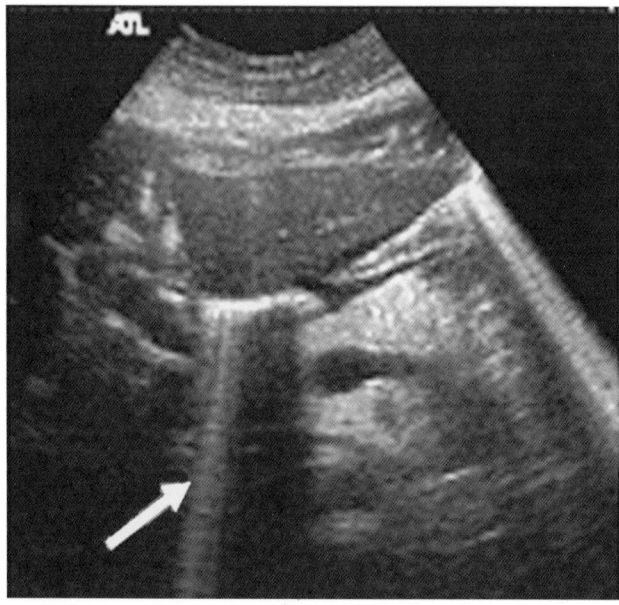

Figure 1-14. Dirty shadowing from air (*arrow*). Gas density objects such as bowel gas produce a shadow containing lighter, irregular gray level ("dirty") echoes.

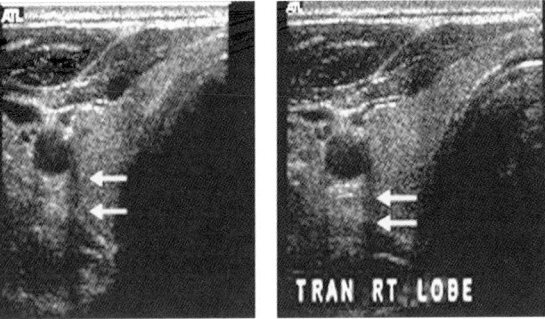

Figure 1-15. Transverse view of the thyroid. The *arrows* indicate the "edge artifact" that is seen in both images despite moving away from the density seen on the first image of the carotid artery. The sound is refracted off the side of the vessel, creating the acoustic shadow.

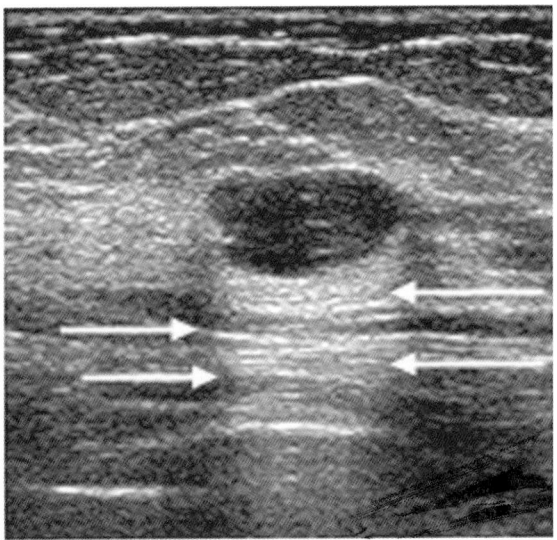

Figure 1-16. Acoustic enhancement. This artifact (*arrows*) is also referred to as "increased through transmission."

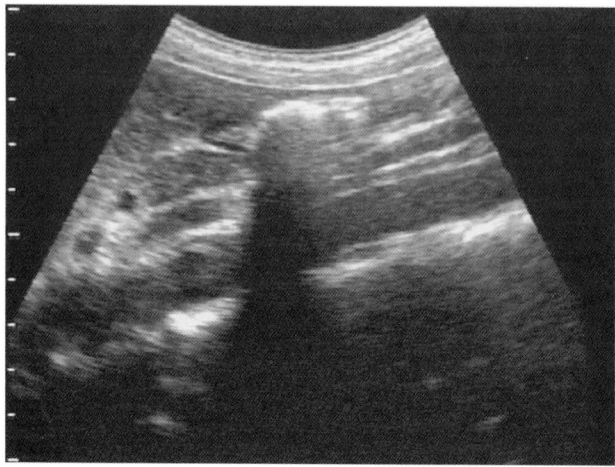

Figure 1-17. Longitudinal aorta partially obscured by bowel gas. (Photo contributed by SonoSite.)

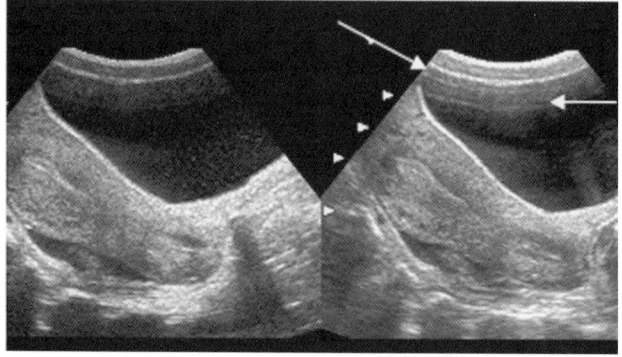

Figure 1-18. Longitudinal suprapubic view of the bladder and uterus. The *arrows* on the *right image* indicate a reverberation artifact. The time gain compensation (TGC) was adjusted on the *left image* to reduce this artifact.

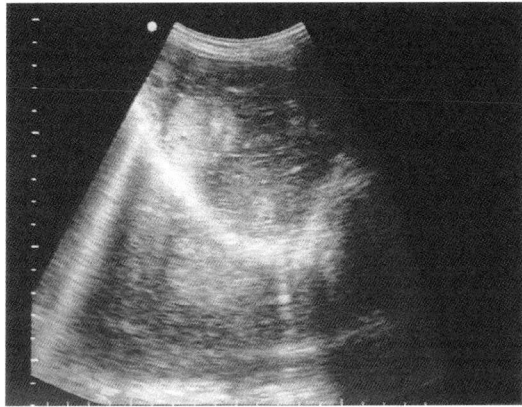

Figure 1-19. Mirror image artifact. Liver tissue and hyperechoic liver lesion are duplicated above the diaphragm. (Photo contributed by SonoSite.)

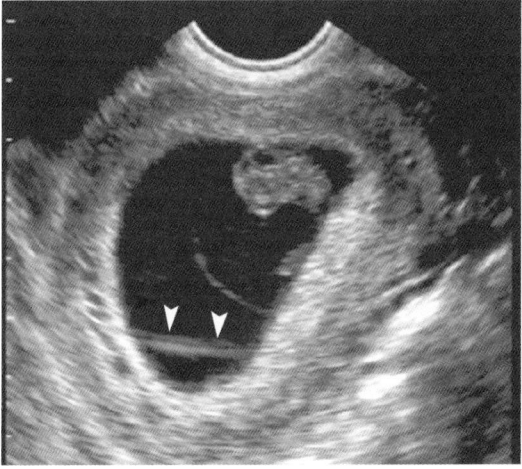

Figure 1-20. Side lobes. Endovaginal image reveals intrauterine gestation with embryonic pole and thin amniotic membrane. A side lobe artifact is demonstrated within the gestational sac (*arrowheads*). (Photo contributed by SonoSite.)

► MODES

- **B-mode:** "Brightness," two-dimensional grayscale image with up to 256 shades of gray. (Most emergency ultrasound imaging can be accomplished with B-mode alone.)

- **M-mode:** "Motion"; displays motion on the vertical axis and time on the horizontal axis (Figure 1-21).

- **Doppler modes:** Use the ultrasound frequency shift to display velocity or direction of movement.

- **Color Doppler:** It detects movement (flow) toward and away from the probe and displays the movement in different colors, usually blue and red (Figure 1-22).

- **Power Doppler:** It displays flow without regard to direction and is more sensitive to slower flow (Figure 1-23).

- **Pulsed wave Doppler (Spectral Doppler):** A type of quantitative Doppler that displays the velocity of moving structures (blood cells) on the vertical axis and time on the horizontal axis (Figure 1-24).

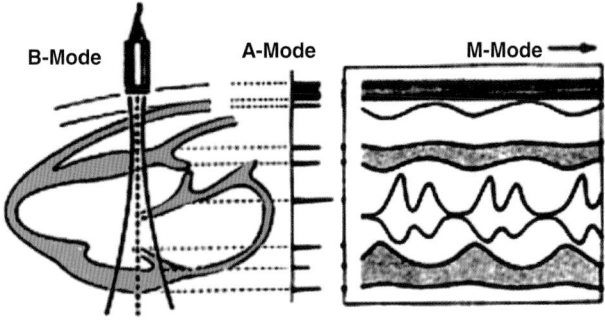

A

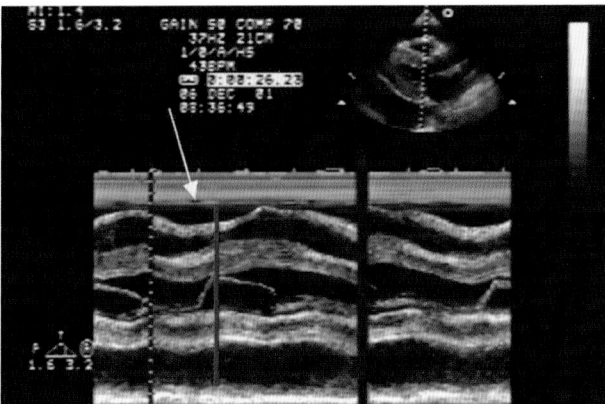

B

Figure 1-21. Comparison of modes. **A.** The image display
for each of three modes: B-mode, A-mode, and M-mode.
M-mode is useful for demonstrating fast moving structures, such
as the biphasic opening of the mitral valve during diastole in
normal sinus rhythm. **B.** M-mode ultrasound of pericardial
effusion with tamponade. The *arrow* shows that the right ventricle
collapses during early diastole (when the MV is open as indicated
by the *red timeline*).

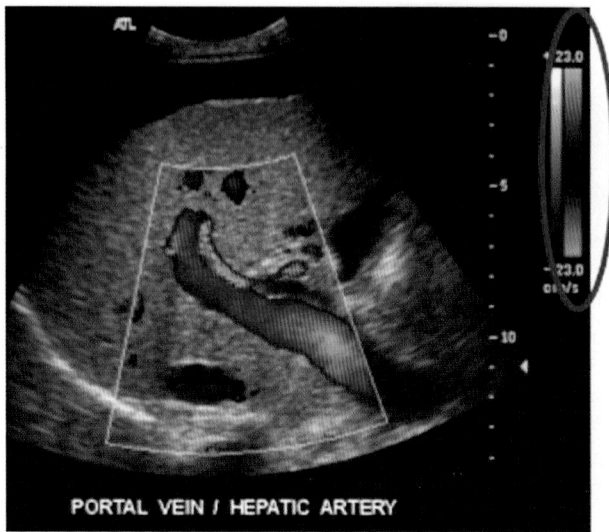

PORTAL VEIN / HEPATIC ARTERY

Figure 1-22. Color Doppler of the portal vein. The *red circle* emphasizes the color key for direction and the mean velocity of flow.

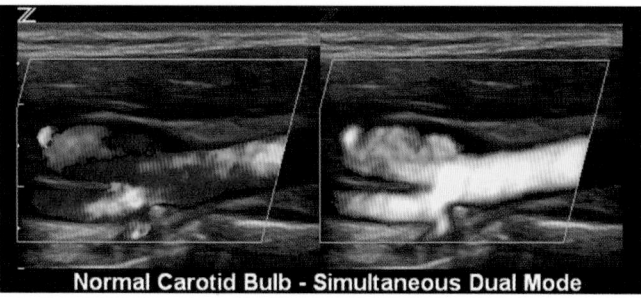

Normal Carotid Bulb - Simultaneous Dual Mode

Figure 1-23. Color Doppler versus power Doppler. The *left image* demonstrates normal flow in the carotid sinus with bidirectional color Doppler. The *right image* uses power Doppler. Note the single color for all directional flow in the power Doppler image versus the color-flow Doppler image that uses two colors to indicate flow toward and away from the probe. (Photos contributed by Zonare.)

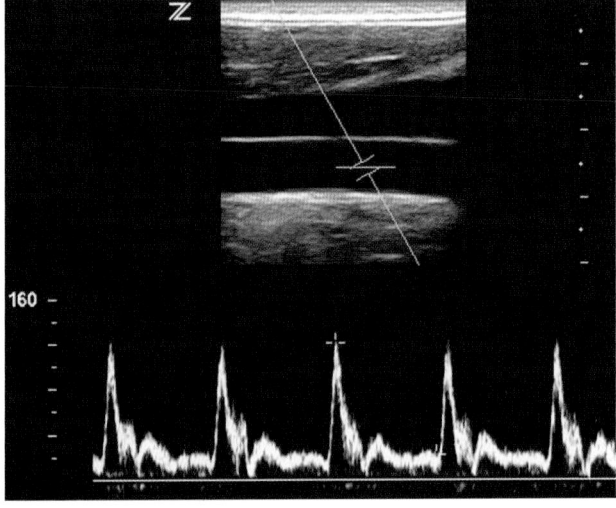

A

Figure 1-24. **A.** Duplex spectral ultrasound. Duplex ultrasound consists of either the grayscale image with color Doppler or the grayscale image with the spectral Doppler graph.

(Figure 1-24B continued on next page)

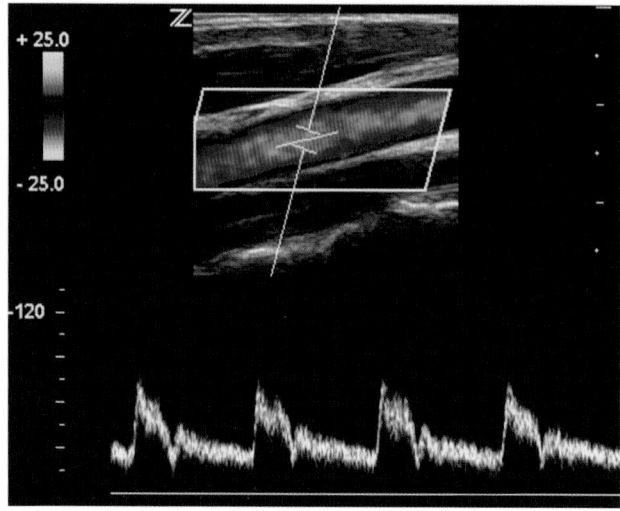

B

Figure 1-24. **B.** Triplex ultrasound. Triplex ultrasound displays consist of a grayscale image, color Doppler, and spectral Doppler graph all on the same display. (Photos contributed by Zonare.)

For more detailed information go to the comprehensive textbook Ma and Mateer's Emergency Ultrasound, 3rd edition, Chapter 2 "Equipment" by Will Scruggs, MD, and J. Christian Fox, MD; and Chapter 3 "Physics and Image Artifacts" by Corky Hecht, BA, and Jason Wilkins, MD.

CHAPTER 2
Trauma

▶ CLINICAL CONSIDERATIONS

- The focused assessment with sonography for trauma (FAST) exam is a bedside screening tool used by clinicians worldwide.
- Ultrasound is sensitive for detecting clinically significant hemoperitoneum, hemothorax, pneumothorax, and pericardial effusion.
- Ultrasound is accurate, rapid, noninvasive, repeatable, and portable and involves no nephrotoxic contrast material or radiation exposure to the patient.
- The extended FAST (EFAST) exam includes evaluation of the pleural sliding sign to rule out a pneumothorax.
- Ultrasound examinations can be performed in just a few minutes during initial trauma management.

▶ CLINICAL INDICATIONS

- Acute blunt or penetrating torso trauma
- Trauma in pregnancy
- Pediatric trauma
- Subacute torso trauma
- Undifferentiated hypotension

▶ ANATOMIC CONSIDERATIONS

- FAST images are obtained by looking through the liver, bladder, and spleen, so it is important to understand the concept of sonographic "windows."

- In the supine patient, intraperitoneal blood accumulates in the dependent areas of Morison's pouch, the left subphrenic space, both paracolic gutters, and the pelvis (Figure 2-1).

- The pelvis is the deepest intraperitoneal recess, but it is often easier to see free fluid in Morison's pouch.

- Hemothorax is easier to detect on the right side, because the liver is a better sonographic window than the spleen.

- It is usually best to obtain subxiphoid cardiac views in critically ill trauma patients.

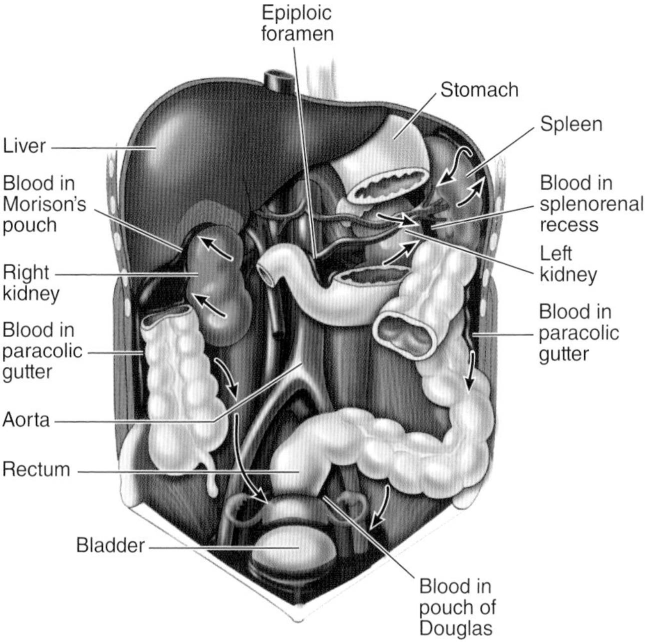

Figure 2-1. Movement patterns of free intraperitoneal fluid within the abdominal cavity. (Adapted from Mark Hoffmann, MD.)

► TECHNIQUE AND NORMAL FINDINGS

Subxiphoid Four-Chamber Cardiac View

- This is usually the best cardiac view in trauma patients (see Chap. 3).

- The probe position is in the anterior midline over the left lobe of the liver (Figure 2-2A).

- The pericardium is a hyperechoic (white) line surrounding the heart (Figure 2-2B).

- Sweep anterior to posterior to fully evaluate the pericardium.

Right Intercostal Oblique and Right Coronal Views

- Position the probe in the mid-axillary line at about the 8th to 11th rib interspace.

- Use an oblique scanning plane with the indicator pointing toward the right posterior axilla (Figures 2-3A and 2-3B).

- Move and angle cephalad to examine the right diaphragm and supraphrenic region (Figures 2-3C and 2-3D).

- Rotate the transducer to the coronal plane (probe indicator cephalad) and move caudally to evaluate the paracolic gutter and pararenal regions (Figure 2-4).

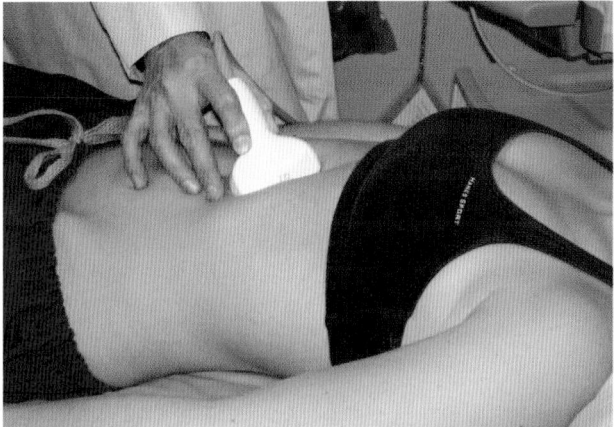

A

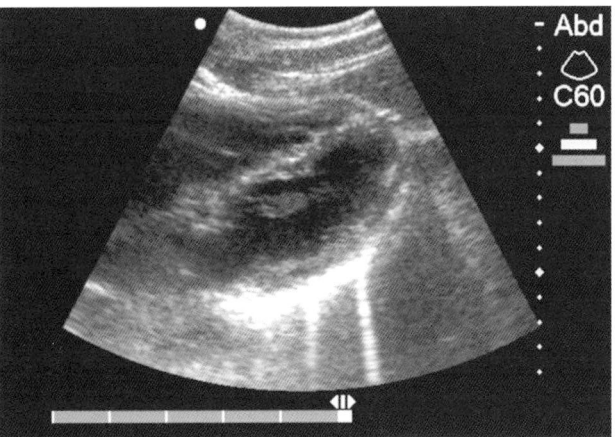

B

Figure 2-2. Subxiphoid four-chamber view of the heart. **A.** Probe position. **B.** Corresponding ultrasound image. The normal pericardium is seen as a hyperechoic (*white*) line surrounding the heart.

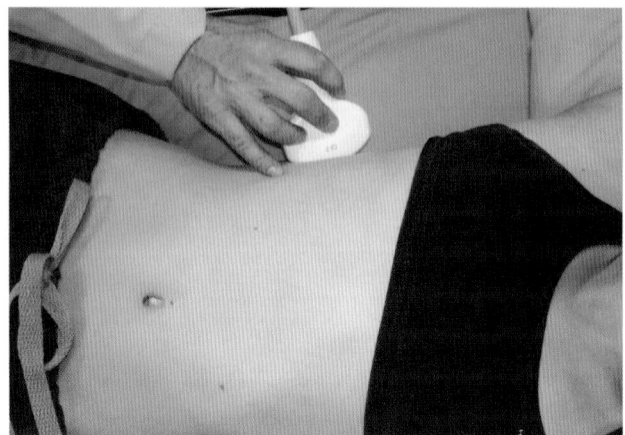

A

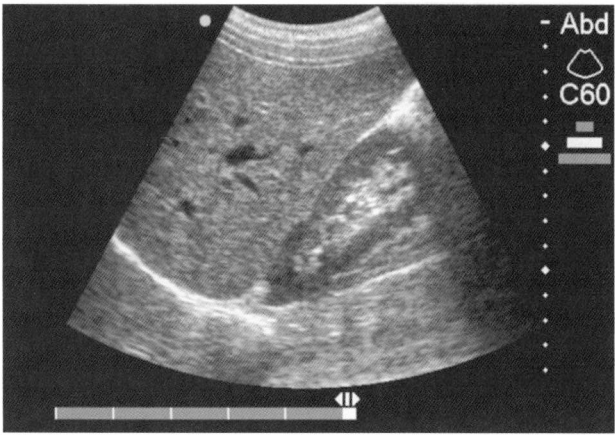

B

Figure 2-3. Right intercostal oblique view. **A.** Probe position. **B.** Corresponding ultrasound image. The liver, right kidney, and Morison's pouch are readily identified. Right intercostal oblique view.

(Figures 2-3C and D continued on next page)

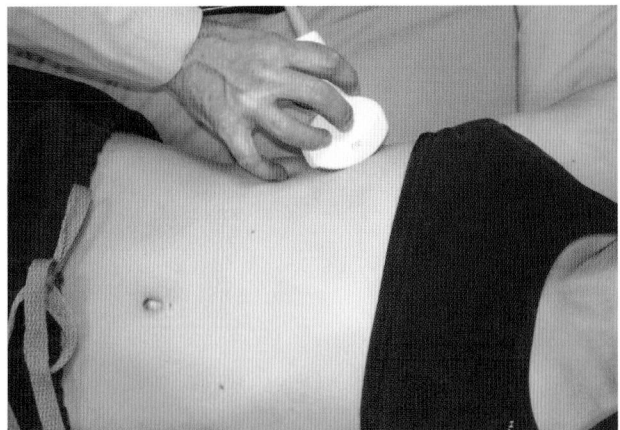

C

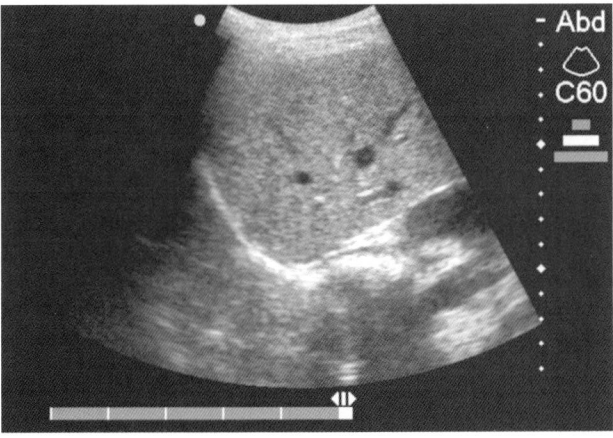

D

Figure 2-3. **C.** Probe position. **D.** Corresponding ultrasound image. The right diaphragm appears as a hyperechoic structure.

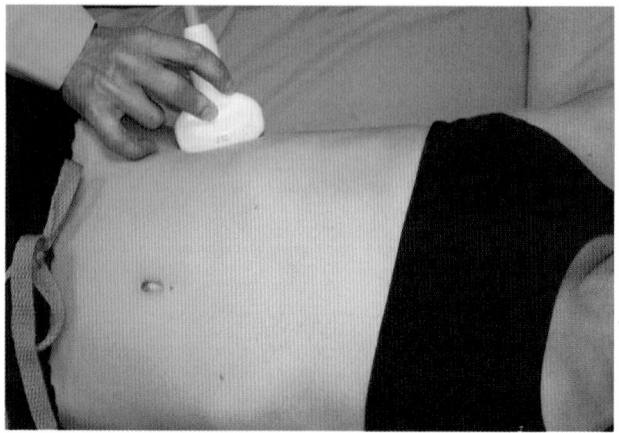

A

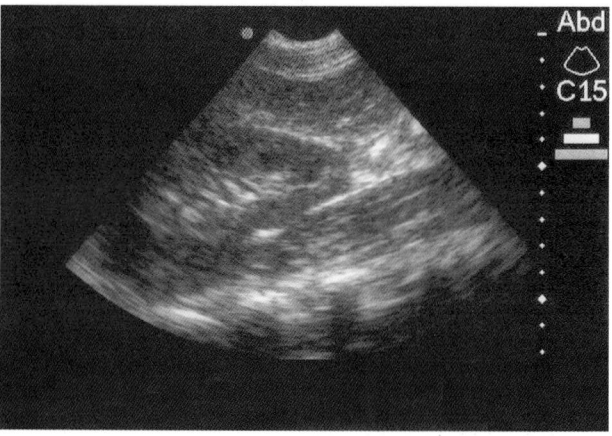

B

Figure 2-4. Right coronal view. **A.** Probe position. **B.** Corresponding ultrasound image. The right pararenal retroperitoneum and paracolic gutter areas are identified above the psoas muscle in this view.

Left Intercostal Oblique and Left Coronal Views

- Position the probe in the posterior-axillary line at about the 7th to 9th rib interspace.

- Use an oblique scanning plane with the indicator pointing toward the left posterior axilla.

- Optimize the splenic image and angle slightly cephalad to examine the left diaphragm and supraphrenic region (Figure 2-5).

- Rotate the transducer to the coronal plane (probe indicator cephalad) and move caudally to evaluate the paracolic gutter and pararenal regions (Figure 2-6).

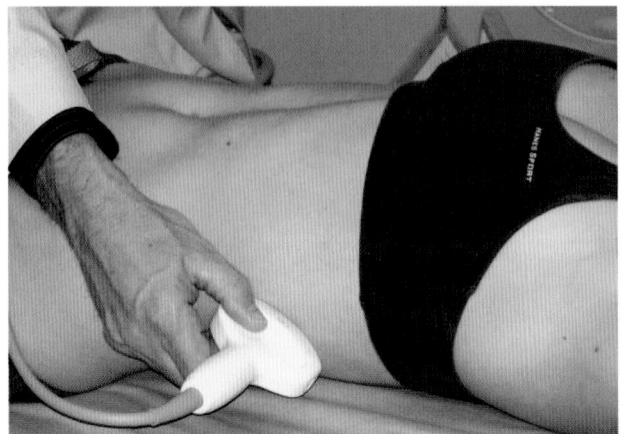

A

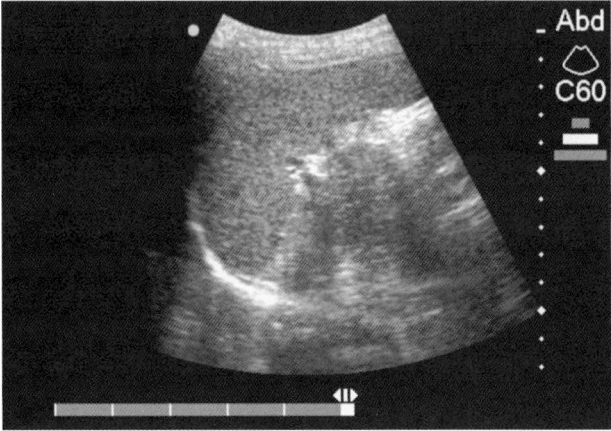

B

Figure 2-5. Left intercostal oblique view. **A.** Probe position. **B.** Corresponding ultrasound image. A longitudinal view of the spleen, a portion of the diaphragm, and surrounding areas are visualized.

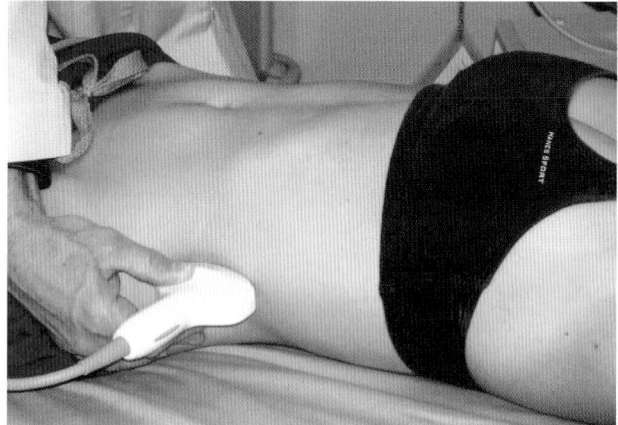

A

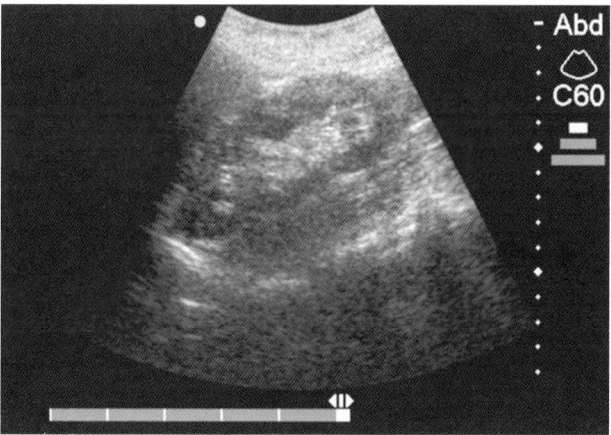

B

Figure 2-6. Left coronal view. **A.** Probe position. **B.** Corresponding ultrasound image. The left pararenal, paracolic gutter areas, and kidney are examined in this view.

Longitudinal and Transverse Pelvic Views

- Perform pelvic imaging before Foley catheter placement.

- Position the transducer in the midline just caudad to the pubic symphysis with the indicator cephalad.

- The posterior angle of the bladder and the uterus are the most important pelvic landmarks (Figures 2-7A and 2-7B).

- After the anatomy has been defined in the sagittal plane, aim the indicator to the patient's right and obtain transverse images (Figures 2-7C and 2-7D).

- A partially filled bladder can be differentiated from free fluid by emptying the bladder or by instilling 400 mL of sterile saline through a Foley catheter and repeating the exam.

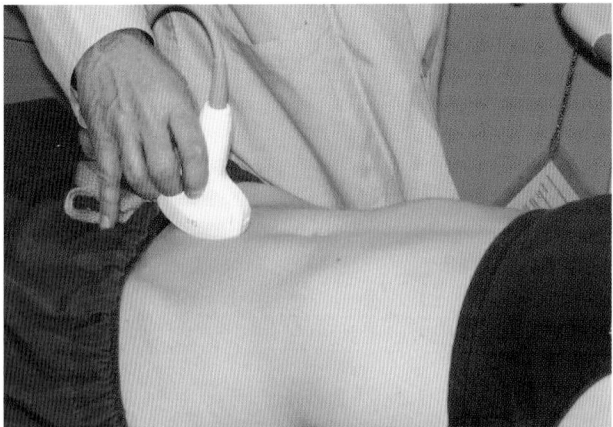

A

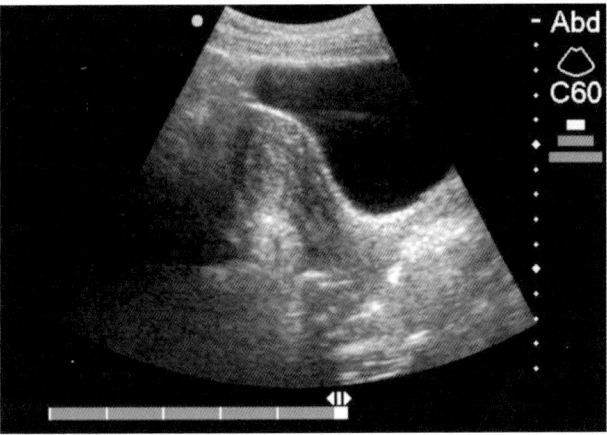

B

Figure 2-7. Pelvic longitudinal views. **A.** Probe position.
B. Corresponding ultrasound image. Ideally, these pelvic views
should be obtained before the placement of a Foley catheter.

(Figures 2-7C and D continued on next page)

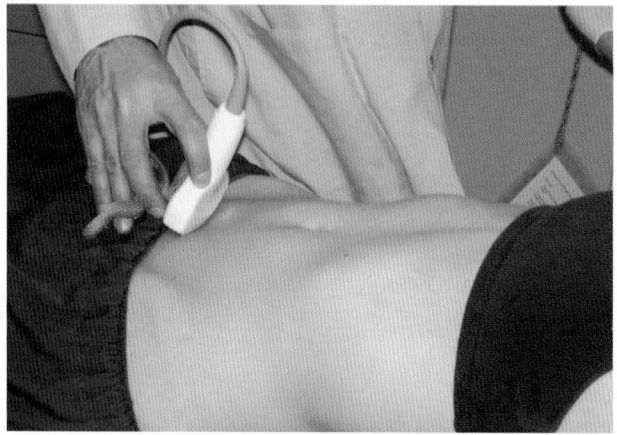

C

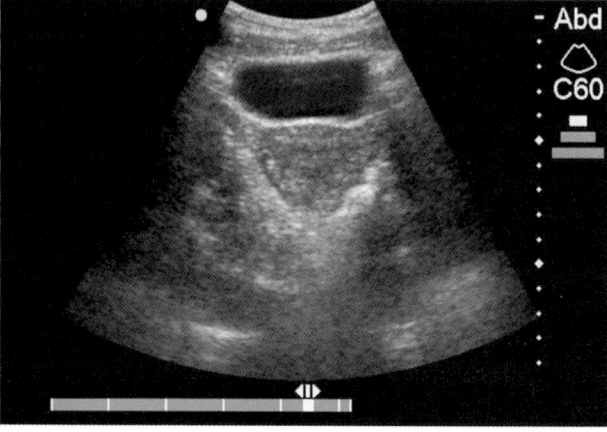

D

Figure 2-7. Pelvic transverse views. **C.** Probe position.
D. Corresponding ultrasound image. In addition to potential
fluid spaces, the bladder, prostate or uterus, and lateral walls
of the pelvis can also be inspected briefly.

Anterior Thoracic Views

- Position the transducer in the sagittal plane in the midclavicular line at the 2nd to 4th rib interspace with the indicator cephalad.
- Identify the ribs, rib shadows, and pleural interface.
- Look for respiratory motion at the pleural interface (lung sliding) and normal "comet tail" and "A-line" artifacts (Figures 2-8 and 2-9).
- Power Doppler (Figure 2-10) and M-mode analysis (Figure 2-11) may further document normal lung sliding.
- For a more comprehensive chest exam, look for the "lung point" sign by rotating the probe parallel to the ribs and sliding it laterally within successive rib interspaces (Figure 2-12).

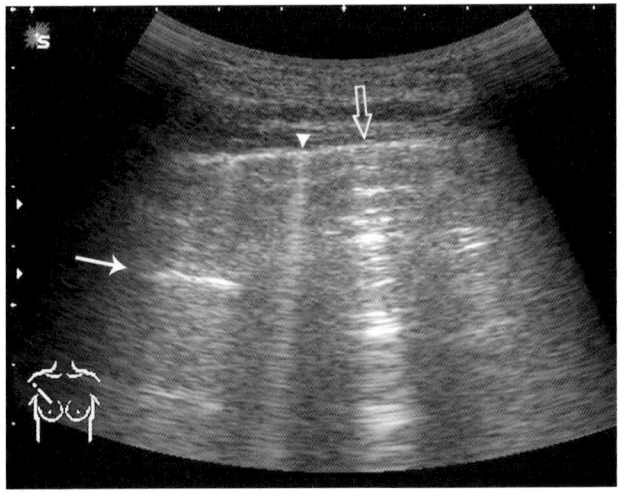

Figure 2-8. Normal lung artifacts (3.5 MHz). The A-line represents the horizontal reverberation artifact generated by the parietal pleura (*arrow*). Comet tail artifacts arise from the pleura and project to the depth of the image. They move back and forth along with the pleura in real time and may vary between a narrow (*arrowhead*) or wider (*open arrow*) appearance.

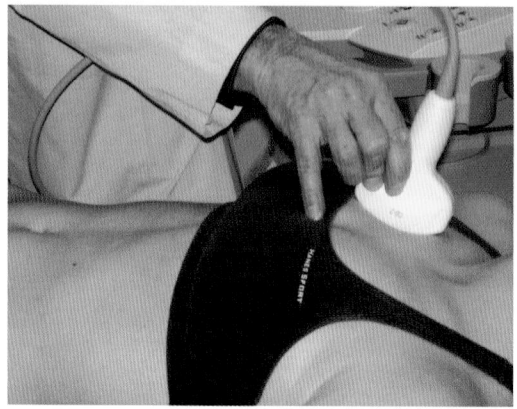

A

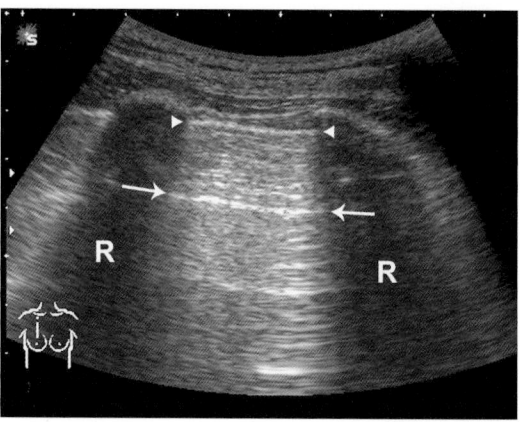

B

Figure 2-9. Longitudinal view: The "bat sign." Normal lung with 3.5-MHz, curved array probe. **A.** Probe position. **B.** Corresponding ultrasound image. This probe may allow a view of more than one rib interspace and can show normal artifacts more consistently. The A-line (*arrows*) is obvious and repeats at regular intervals.

(Figures 2-9C and D continued on next page)

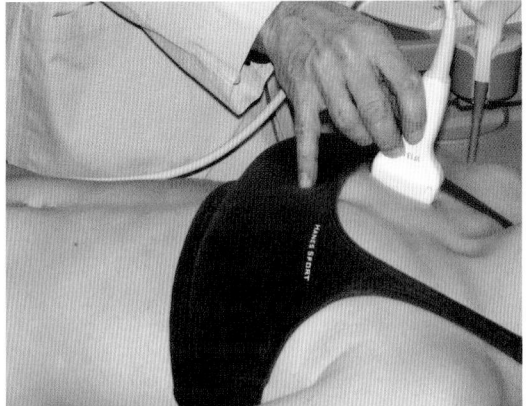

C

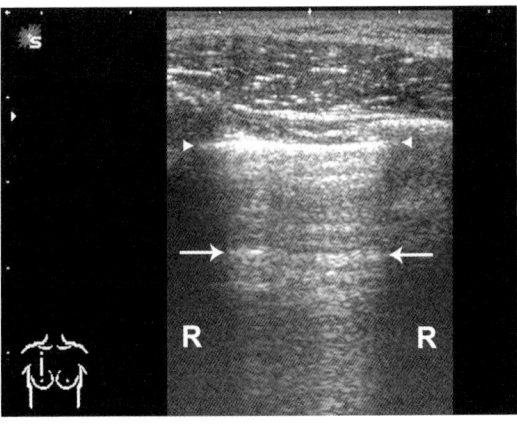

D

Figure 2-9. Normal lung with 7.5- to 10-MHz linear array probe. **C.** Probe position. **D.** Corresponding ultrasound image. This probe provides more detail of the pleural interface (*arrowheads*) and better visualization of sliding in real time. R = rib shadow.

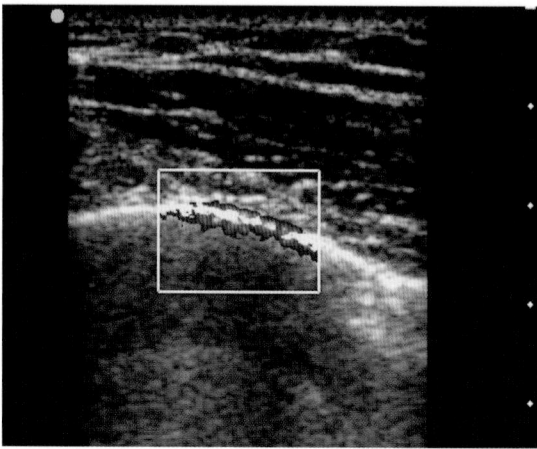

Figure 2-10. Power Doppler of the pleural interface demonstrates pleural sliding with color.

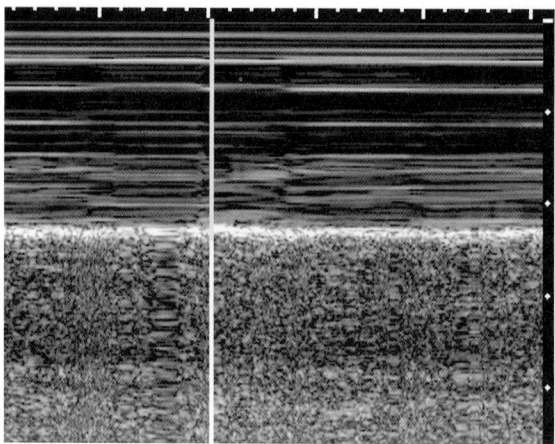

Figure 2-11. M-mode ultrasound of normal lung at 7.5 to 10 MHz ("seashore sign"). Granular artifacts below the bright pleural line represent normal pleural sliding and lung motion on M-mode.

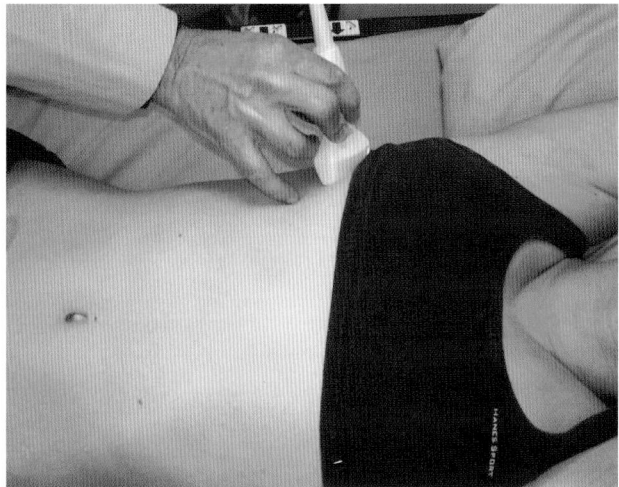

Figure 2-12. Extended lung examination. In a supine patient, the extent of a pneumothorax can be outlined by orienting the probe parallel to the ribs and sliding it laterally along successive rib interspaces.

▶ TIPS TO IMPROVE IMAGE ACQUISITION

- Aim the probe indicator cephalad for all initial EFAST views (except cardiac).

- Consider using a phased-array transducer in large and obese patients.

- Place the transducer at an acute angle and push downward to obtain better subxiphoid cardiac images and use a deep inspiratory hold (if possible) to bring the heart closer to the probe.

- Perihepatic images can be obtained from the right posterior axillary line to the anterior midline.

- Perisplenic views must be obtained from a much smaller window near the posterior axillary line.

- Avoid rib shadows by aligning the ultrasound plane with the intercostal space.

- Begin pelvic scanning in the longitudinal (sagittal) plane and use the bladder angle as a landmark.

- Decrease the depth to about 5 cm when looking for the pleural sliding sign.

▶ COMMON AND EMERGENT ABNORMALITIES

Hemopericardium

See Figure 2-13.

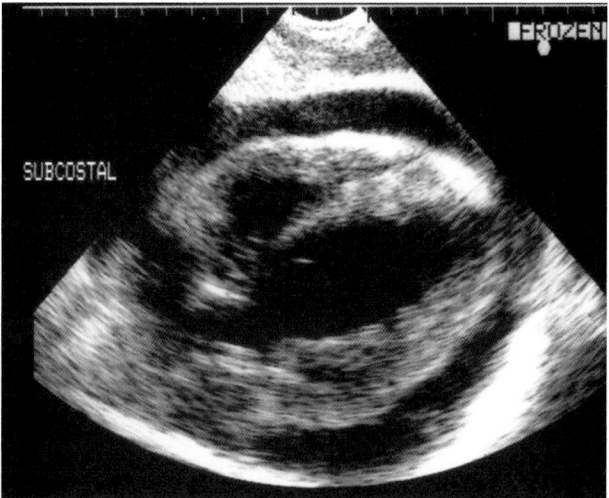

Figure 2-13. Hemopericardium. Free pericardial fluid is identified as an anechoic stripe surrounding the heart between the parietal and visceral layers of the bright hyperechoic pericardial sac.

Hemothorax

See Figure 2-14.

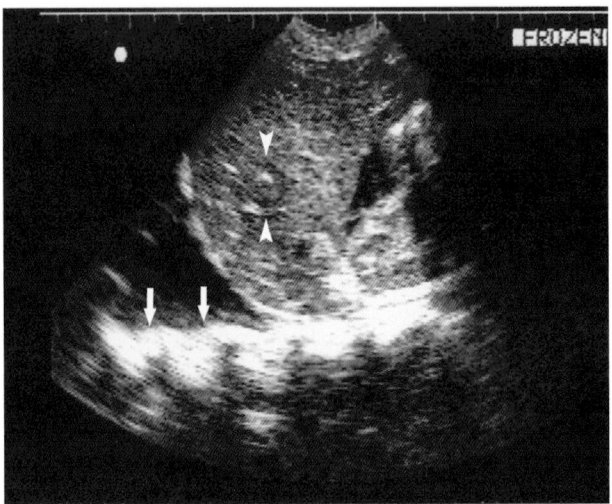

Figure 2-14. Free pleural fluid. The right diaphragm appears as a bright hyperechoic structure along the border of the liver. Free pleural fluid can be identified as an anechoic stripe superior to the diaphragm. The pleural fluid allows visualization of the lateral chest wall (*arrows*) that cannot be visualized when the air-filled lung is normally present. The patient also has a circular defect in the liver (*arrowheads*) from a bullet wound and fluid in Morison's pouch.

Hemoperitoneum

See Figures 2-15 to 2-19.

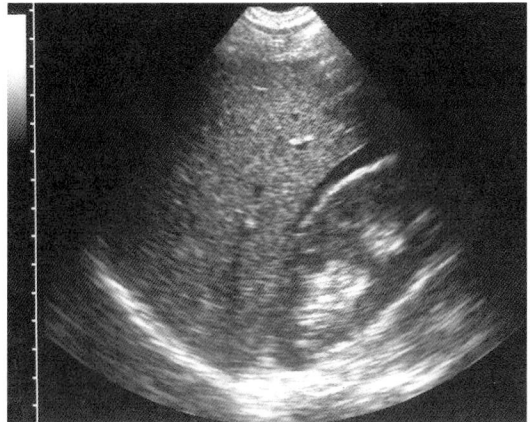

Figure 2-15. Hemoperitoneum. Free fluid in Morison's pouch.

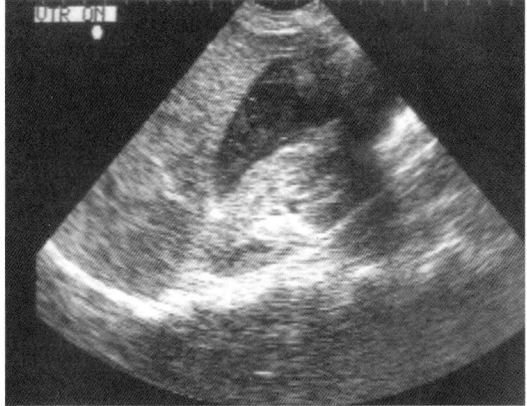

Figure 2-16. A large quantity of free intraperitoneal fluid is present in Morison's pouch. The fluid is mildly echogenic because of clotting of the blood.

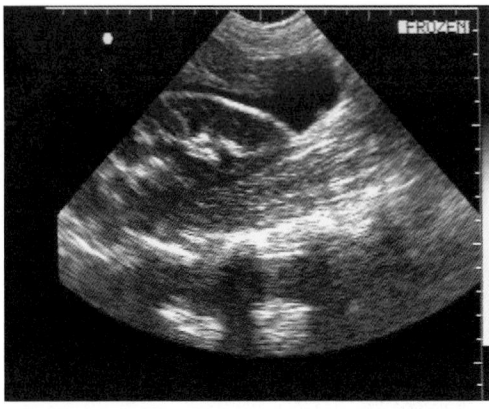

Figure 2-17. Hemoperitoneum. Free peritoneal fluid around the liver tip and in the right paracolic gutter.

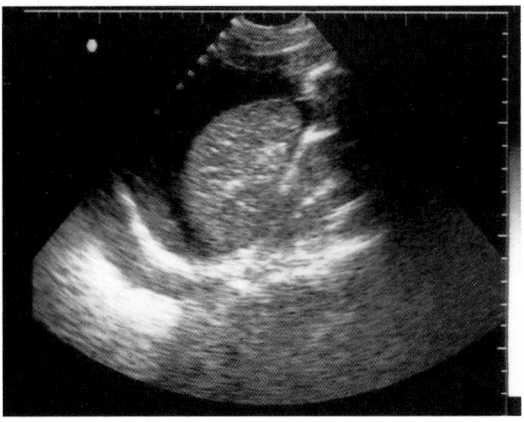

A

Figure 2-18. **A.** Left intercostal oblique views reveal the spleen surrounded by hypoechoic fluid in the subdiaphragmatic space. A small amount of clotted blood is also noted adjacent to the bright curvilinear diaphragm.

(Figure 2-18B continued on next page)

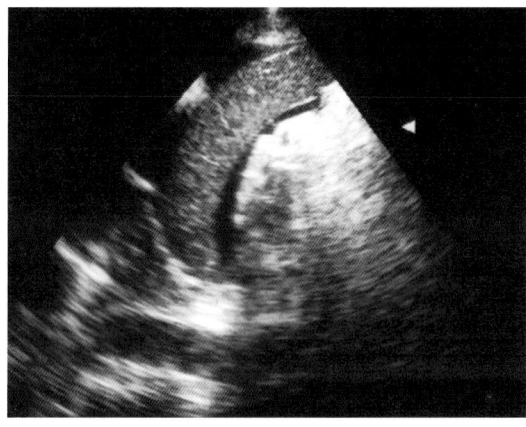

B

Figure 2-18. **B.** Free intraperitoneal fluid as an anechoic stripe in the splenorenal recess. The tubular fluid-filled object at the bottom of the image is the aorta. (Photo contributed by Lori Sens, Gulfcoast Ultrasound.)

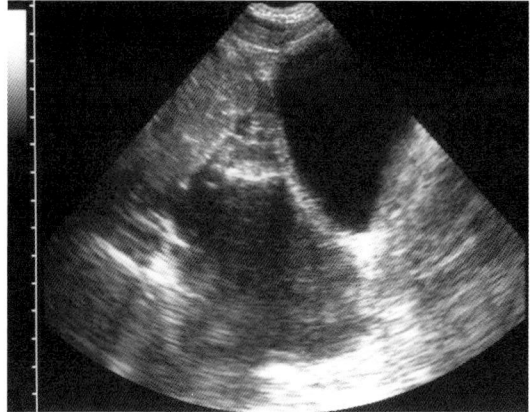

Figure 2-19. Hemoperitoneum. Longitudinal pelvic view in a male patient shows peritoneal blood in the usual location posterior and cephalad to the bladder.

Pneumothorax

See Figures 2-20 and 2-21.

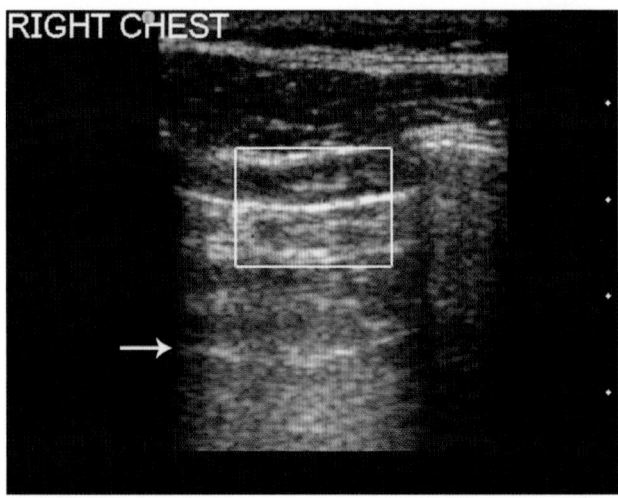

Figure 2-20. Pneumothorax (7.5–10 MHz). Power Doppler is activated and the gain adjusted correctly by comparison with the normal left hemithorax. The patient's right hemithorax showed a negative pleural sliding sign, no comet tail artifacts, and no power Doppler signal at the pleural interface. The specificity for pneumothorax is improved when an A-line is also visible (*arrow*).

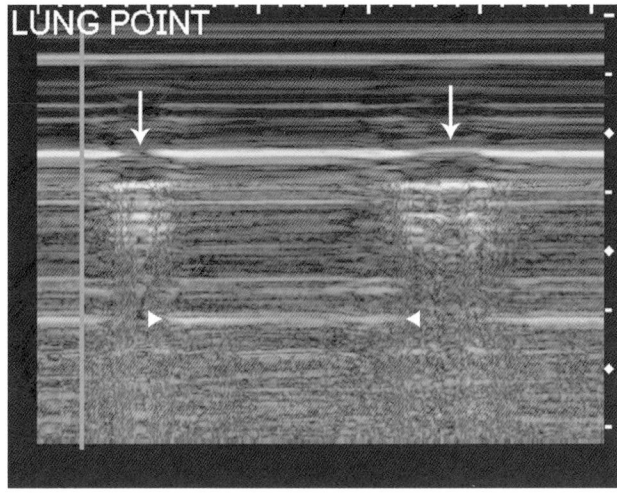

Figure 2-21. Lung point. The probe is located on the chest at the edge of a pneumothorax. During the M-mode sweep, the patient has taken two breaths, allowing normal pleural movement to be documented briefly (*arrows*) as the "seashore sign." The remainder of the M-mode sweep shows the "stratosphere sign" of pneumothorax. *Arrowheads* show the A-line.

▶ ADDITIONAL FINDINGS

See Figure 2-22.

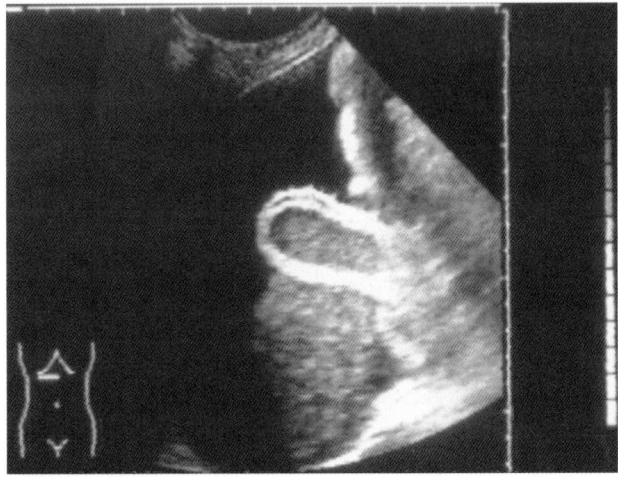

Figure 2-22. Massive free intraperitoneal fluid and thickening of the gallbladder wall. This gallbladder finding is common with chronic ascites.

▶ PITFALLS

- Overreliance on the FAST examination
- Missed pathology caused by an incomplete EFAST exam
- Technical difficulties (eg, obesity and subcutaneous air)
- Misinterpretation of images (Figures 2-23 and 2-24)
- Limitations associated with pregnancy
- Undetected injuries

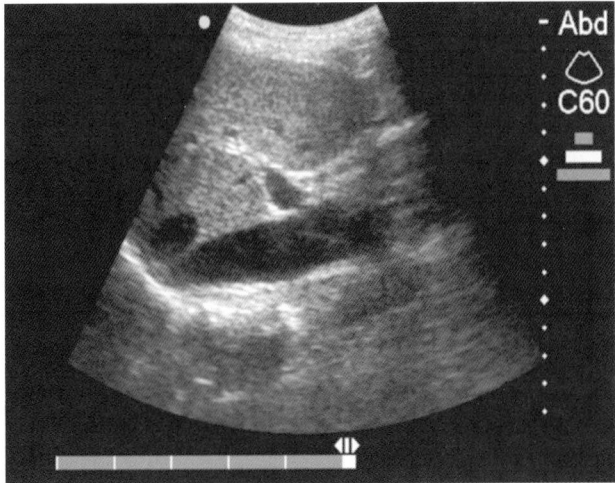

A

Figure 2-23. Fluid pitfalls. **A.** Oblique view of the liver shows fluid below that is contained within the inferior vena cava.

(Figure 2-23B continued on next page)

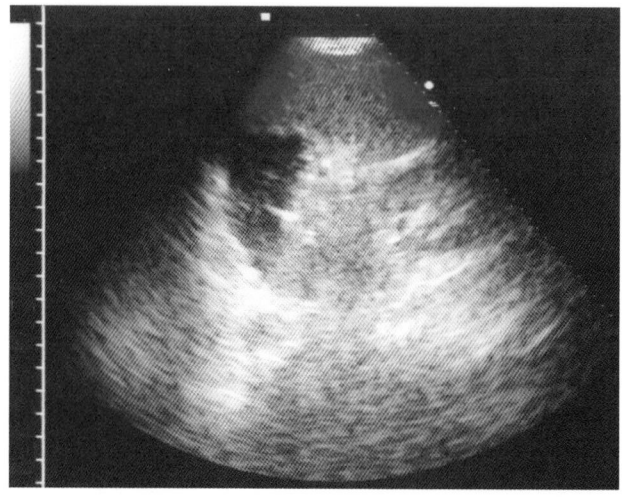

B

Figure 2-23. Fluid pitfalls. **B.** When examining the perisplenic views, fluid in the stomach (or other bowels) may be erroneously identified as free intraperitoneal fluid.

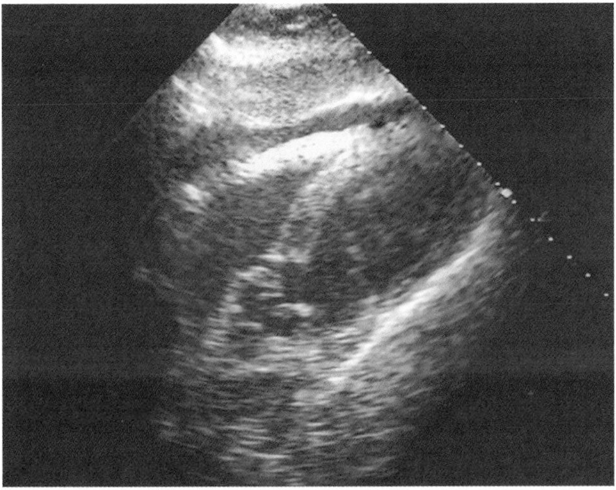

Figure 2-24. Subcostal long-axis view of the heart and pericardium. A pericardial fat pad can be hypoechoic or contain grey-level echoes. The pericardial fat pad is almost always located anterior to the right ventricle and is not present posterior to the left ventricle.

For more detailed information go to the comprehensive textbook Ma and Mateer's Emergency Ultrasound, 3rd edition, Chapter 5 "Trauma" by O. John Ma, MD, James R. Mateer, MD, and Andrew W. Kirkpatrick, MD.

CHAPTER 3
Cardiac

▶ CLINICAL CONSIDERATIONS

- Focused echocardiography is the ideal diagnostic tool for life-threatening cardiac conditions.
- Physical exam findings are unreliable for making critical diagnoses.
- Noncardiologists can use focused echocardiography safely and accurately in a variety of clinical settings.
- Focused echocardiography provides real-time information about cardiac structure and function.
- The key is to keep the exam simple and look for gross abnormalities.

▶ CLINICAL INDICATIONS

- Cardiac arrest
- Pericardial effusion
- Massive pulmonary embolism
- Assessment of left ventricular function
- Unexplained hypotension
- Estimation of central venous pressure
- External cardiac pacing
- Severe valvular dysfunction
- Proximal aortic dissection
- Myocardial infarction

▶ ANATOMIC CONSIDERATIONS

- The long axis of the heart is from the 10 o'clock to 4 o'clock positions (Figure 3-1).

- The short axis is from the 2 o'clock to 8 o'clock positions.

- The cardiac axes are slightly different in each patient.

- Ultrasound images can only be obtained where the heart touches the chest wall, so standard views are obtained at the subcostal, parasternal, and apical positions.

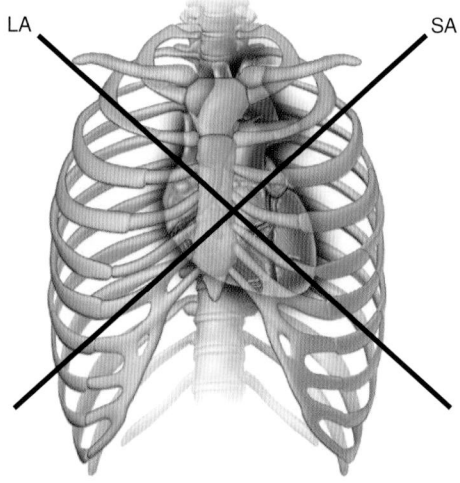

Figure 3-1. Orientation of the long (LA) and short (SA) cardiac axes relative to the torso.

► TECHNIQUE AND NORMAL FINDINGS

- The transducer orientation depends on cardiac or abdominal/pelvic preset.
- The descriptions that follow assume a cardiac preset.

Subxiphoid Four-Chamber View

- This is one of the easiest echocardiographic views (Figure 3-2).
- The probe position is in the anterior midline over the left lobe of the liver.
- The probe marker is to the patient's left.
- The probe is aimed toward the left shoulder.

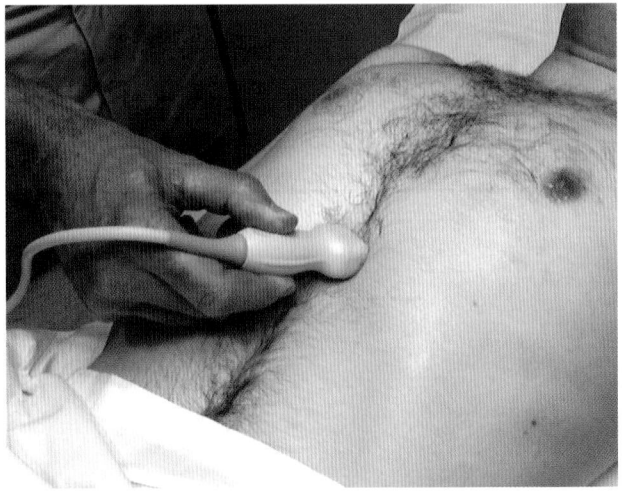

A

Figure 3-2. **A.** Transducer position for subcostal four-chamber view.

(Figures 3-2B and C continued on next page)

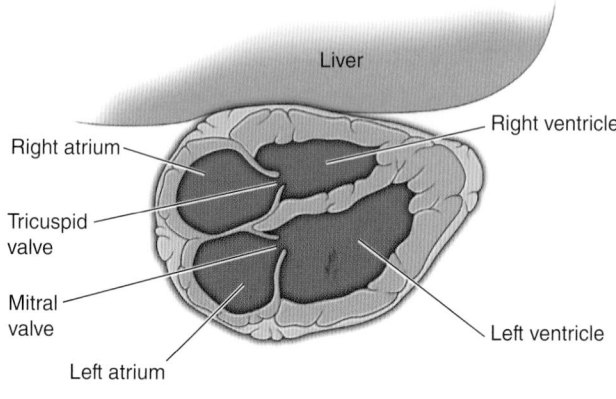

B

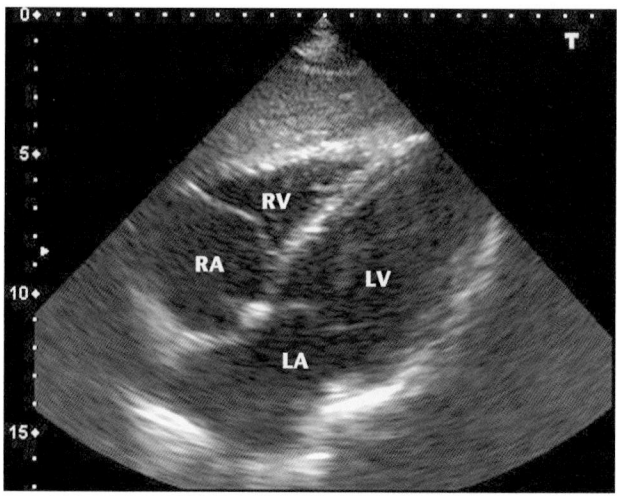

C

Figure 3-2. **B.** Relevant anatomy. **C.** Subcostal four-chamber normal ultrasound. RA = right atrium; RV = right ventricle; LA = left atrium; LV = left ventricle. (C: Courtesy of Hennepin County Medical Center.)

Subxiphoid Short-Axis View (Figure 3-3)

- The advanced view may be confusing because multiple views are obtained from one position.
- Start with a subxiphoid four-chamber view and then rotate the probe about 90 degrees counterclockwise.
- Different short-axis views can be obtained similar to parasternal short-axis views (see Figures 3-6B, 3-7, 3-8, and 3-9).
- The most useful view of the mid-ventricle at the level of the papillary muscles.

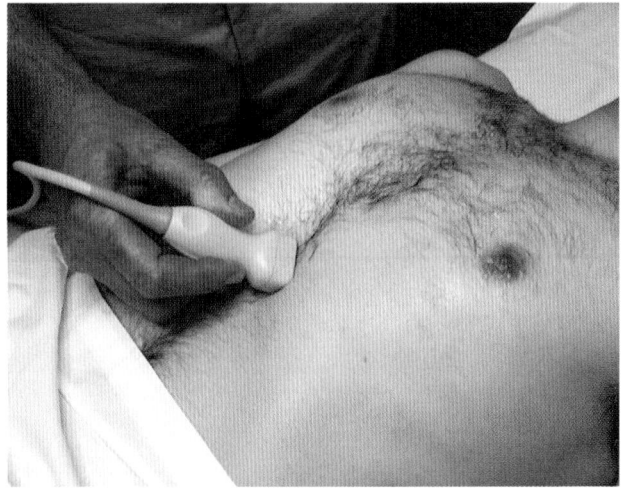

A

Figure 3-3. **A.** Transducer position for subcostal short-axis view.

(Figures 3-3B and C continued on next page)

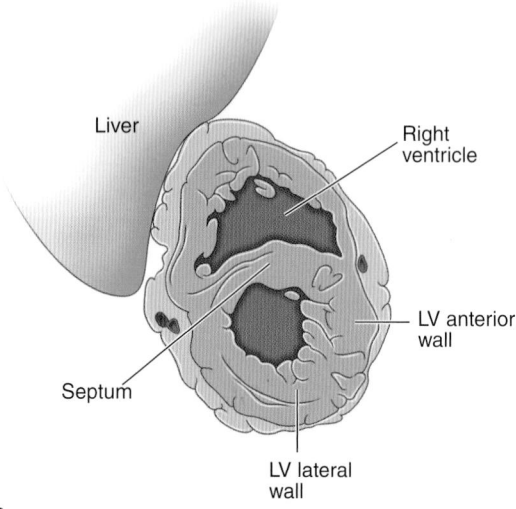

B

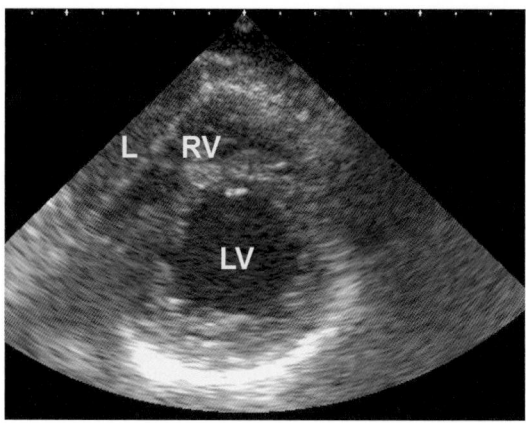

C

Figure 3-3. **B.** Relevant anatomy. **C.** Subcostal short-axis normal ultrasound. L = liver; RV = right ventricle; LV = left ventricle. (C: Courtesy of James Mateer, MD.)

Subxiphoid Long-Axis View of the Inferior Vena Cava

- The probe position is in the anterior midline over the left lobe of the liver (Figure 3-4A).

- The probe marker should be toward the feet (cardiologists point the marker toward the head).

- Sagittal view of the liver, heart, hepatic veins, and inferior vena cava (IVC) (Figure 3-4B).

- Measure the IVC diameter about 3 cm distal to the right atrium.

- IVC collapse of more than 50% with inspiration indicates normal CVP. (Figures 3-4C and 3-4D).

- IVC collapse of more than 50% with inspiration indicates elevated right-sided pressure (CVP > 10).

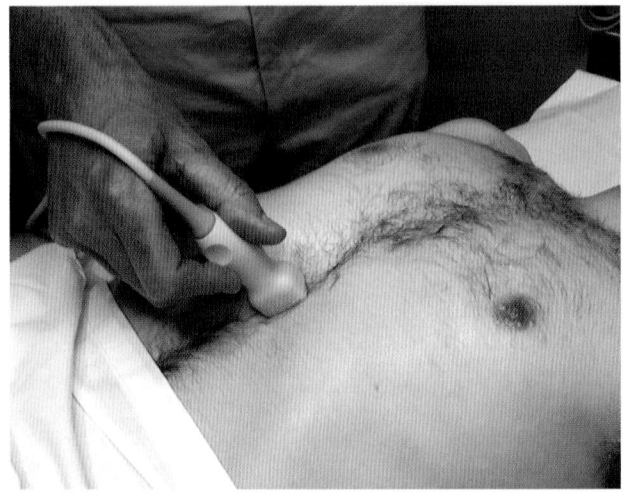

A

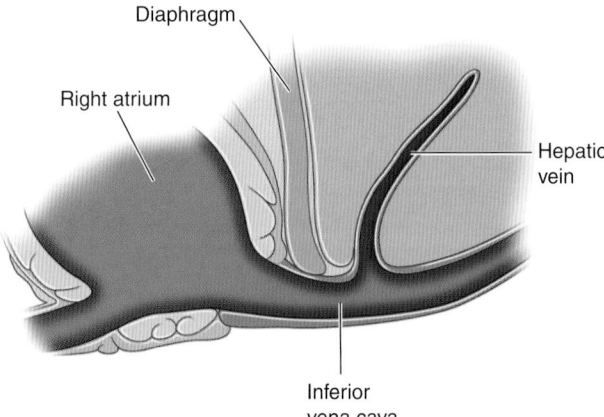

B

Figure 3-4. **A.** Transducer position for subcostal sagittal view of the IVC. **B.** Relevant anatomy.

(Figures 3-4C and D continued on next page)

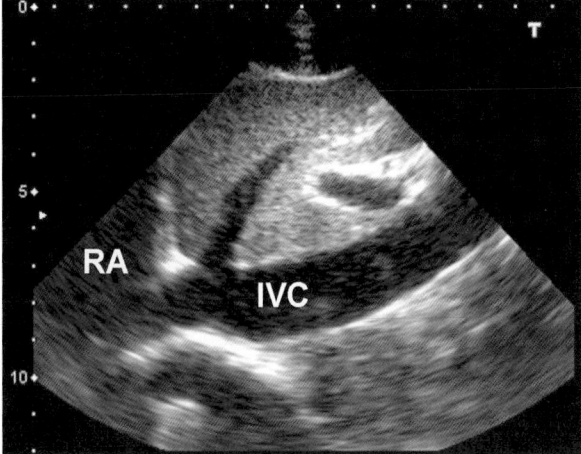

C

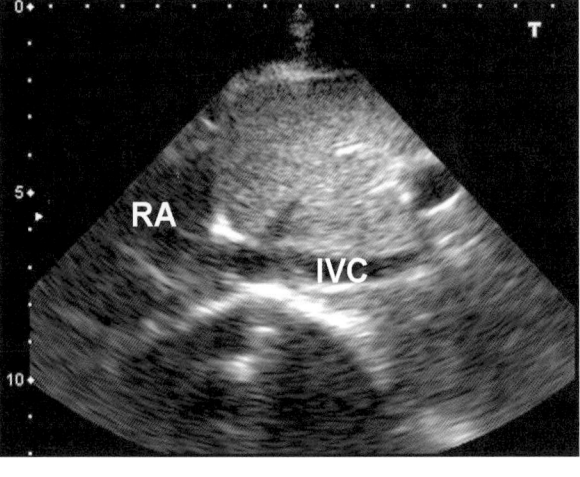

D

Figure 3-4. **C.** Proximal IVC during expiration. **D.** Proximal IVC during inspiration. IVC = inferior vena cava; RA = right atrium. (C, D: Courtesy of Hennepin County Medical Center.)

Parasternal Long-Axis View

- This is also one of the easiest cardiac views (Figure 3-5).
- The probe position is just left of the sternum in the 3rd to 4th intercostal space.
- The probe marker should be toward the patient's right shoulder (10 o'clock position).

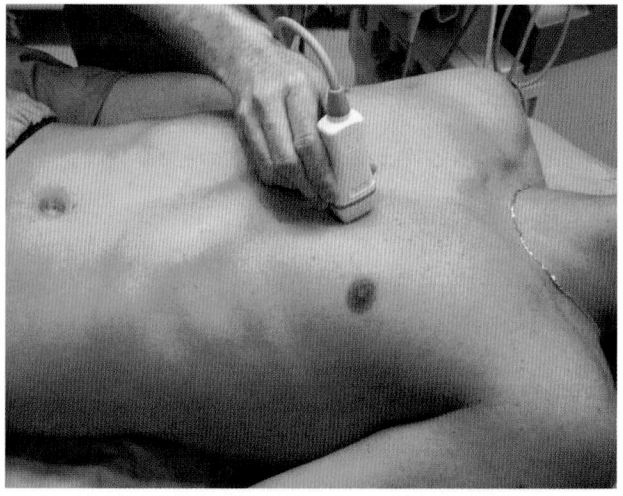

A

Figure 3-5. A. Transducer position for parasternal long-axis view. Note: May require left lateral decubitus position.

(Figures 3-5B and C continued on next page)

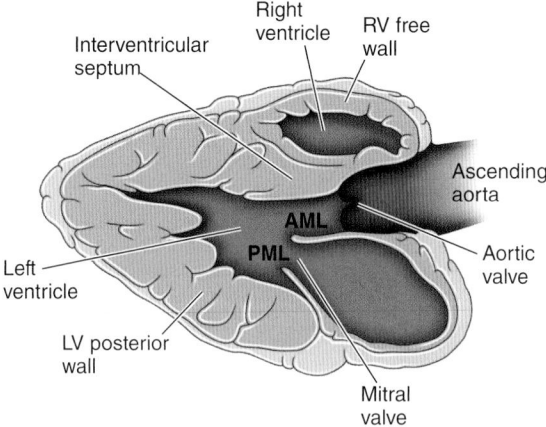

B

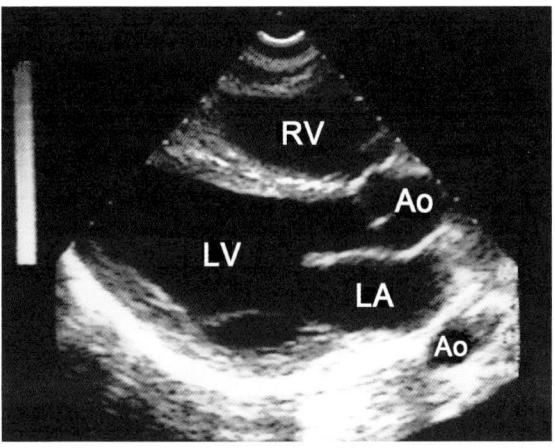

C

Figure 3-5. **B.** Parasternal long-axis diagram. **C.** Parasternal long-axis normal ultrasound. RV = right ventricle; Ao = aorta; LV = left ventricle; LA = left atrium.

Parasternal Short-Axis View

- It may be confusing because multiple views are obtained from one position (Figures 3-6 to 3-10).

- Start with a parasternal long-axis view and then rotate the probe 90 degrees clockwise.

- The best probe position is the left parasternal directly over the mitral valve.

- The probe marker should be toward the patient's left shoulder (Figure 3-6A).

- Multiple views are obtained by tilting the probe toward the apex or base (Figure 3-6B).

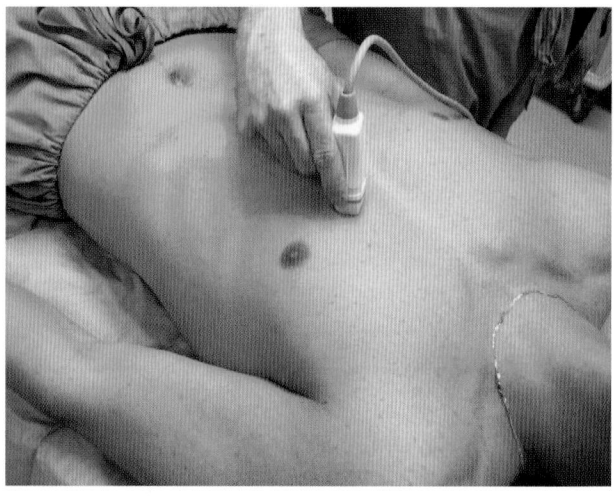

A

Figure 3-6. **A.** Transducer position for parasternal short-axis view. Note: May require left lateral decubitus position.

(Figure 3-6B continued on next page)

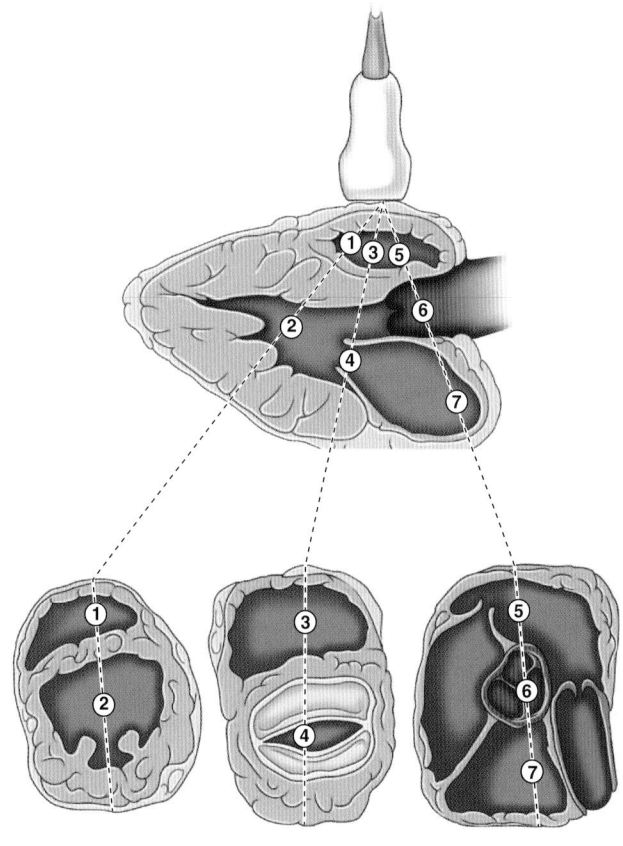

B

Figure 3-6. **B.** Diagram of short-axis views from the papillary muscle (mid-ventricle) level to the base.

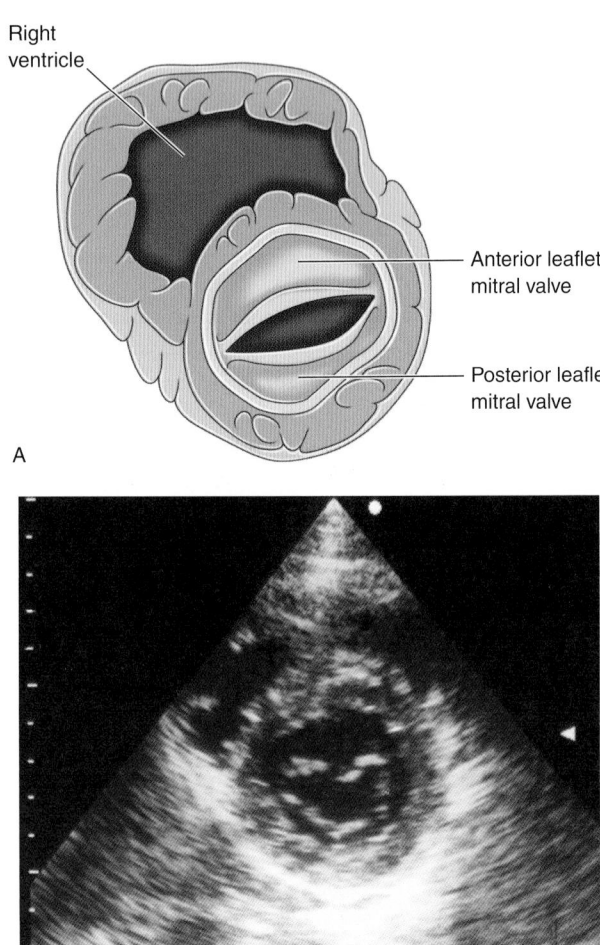

Right ventricle

Anterior leaflet mitral valve

Posterior leaflet mitral valve

A

B

Figure 3-7. **A.** Parasternal short-axis diagram at mitral valve. **B.** Parasternal short-axis normal ultrasound at mitral valve.

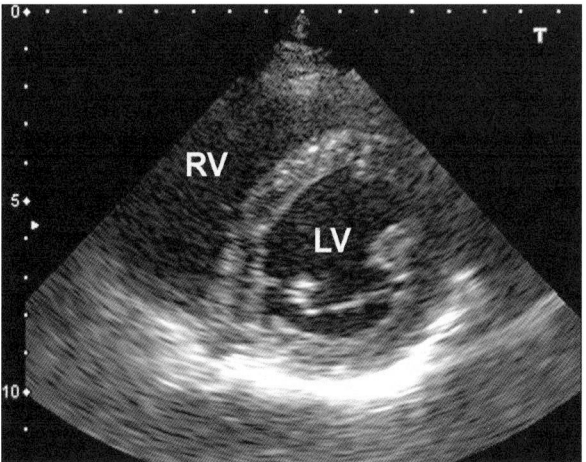

Figure 3-8. **A.** Parasternal short-axis diagram at papillary muscles (mid-ventricle). **B.** Parasternal short-axis normal ultrasound at papillary muscles (mid-ventricle). RV = right ventricle, LV = left ventricle. (B: Courtesy of Hennepin County Medical Center.)

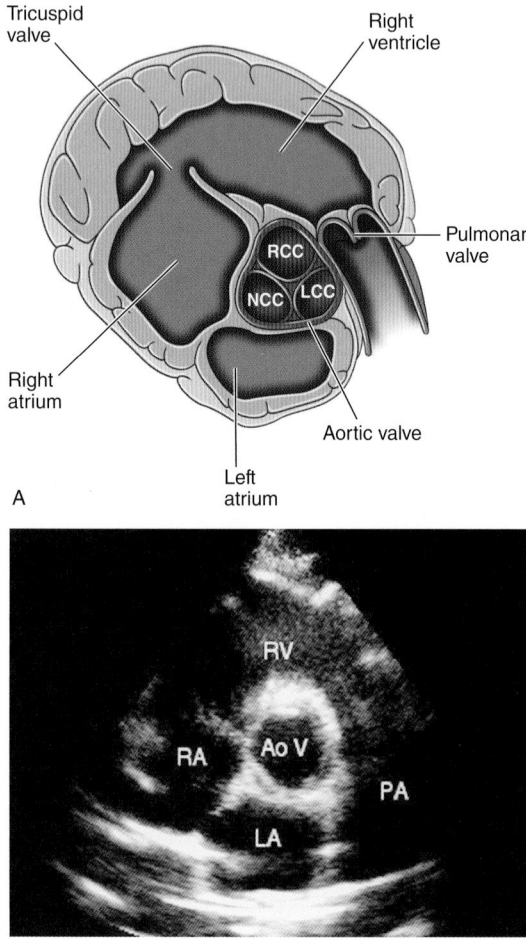

Figure 3-9. **A.** Parasternal short-axis diagram at aortic valve.
B. Parasternal short-axis normal ultrasound at aortic valve.
NCC= noncoronary cusp; RCC= right coronary cusp; LCC = left
coronary cusp; RV = right ventricle; RA = right atrium; LA = left
atrium; PA = pulmonary artery; Ao V = aortic valve.

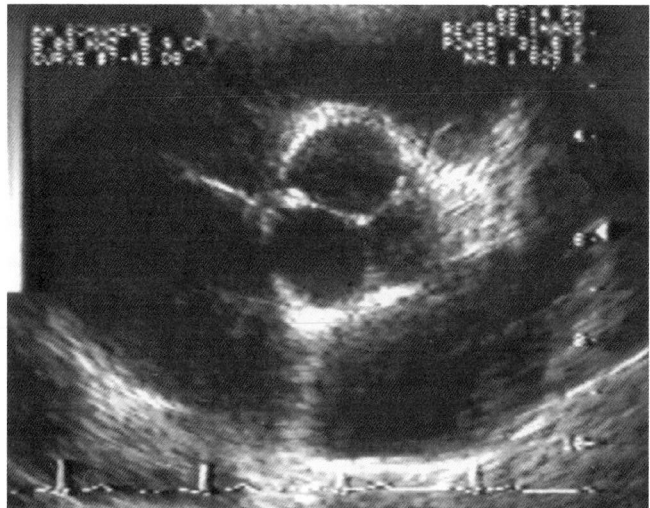

Figure 3-10. Mercedes Benz sign. Parasternal short-axis view at the aortic valve demonstrates closure of all three cusps. (Photo contributed by Lori Sens and Lori Green, Gulfcoast Ultrasound.)

Apical Four-Chamber and Five-Chamber Views

- This is one of the best views for estimating left ventricular function.
- Several views can be obtained by placing the probe at the point of maximal impulse (PMI) under the left nipple.
- May need to roll the patient to the left, especially younger patients.
- The probe marker should be to the patient's left and aimed toward the base of the heart (Figure 3-11A).
- The cardiac apex should be centered, and the left ventricle should point at the probe (Figure 3-11B and C).
- More or less of the right ventricle is visualized as the probe is rotated clockwise or counterclockwise.
- Tilting the transducer slightly anterior will bring the aortic valve into view in the center of the image (this is the five-chamber view).
- If the left ventricle is short and round, the probe position is too cephalad.

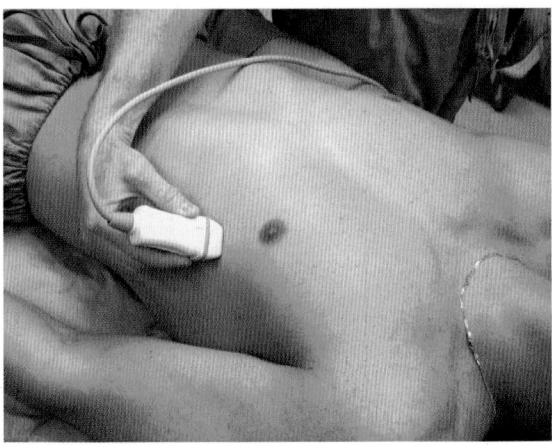

A

Figure 3-11. **A.** Transducer position for apical four-chamber view. Note: May require left lateral decubitus position with left arm elevated.

(Figures 3-11B and C continued on next page)

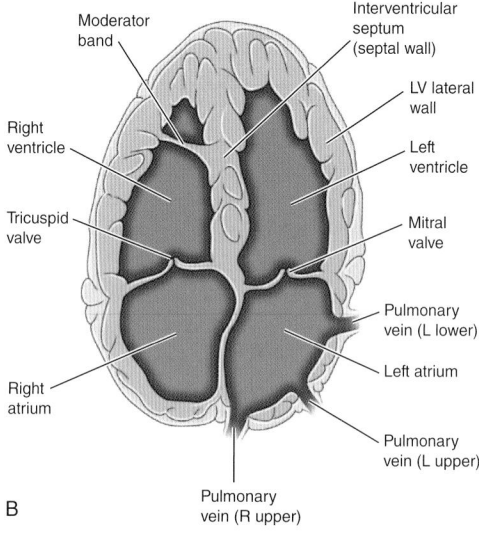

B

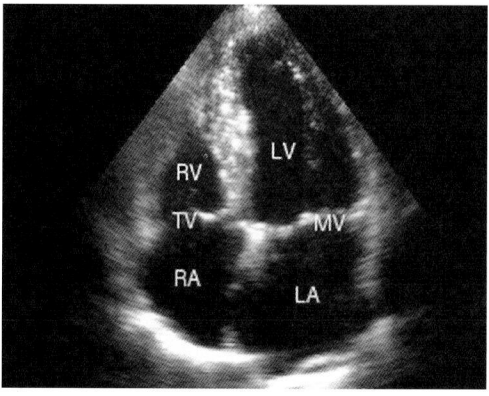

C

Figure 3-11. **B.** Apical four-chamber diagram. **C.** Apical four-chamber normal ultrasound. RV = right ventricle; LV = left ventricle; MV = mitral valve; LA = left atrium; RA = right atrium; TV = tricuspid valve. Tilting the transducer slightly anterior will bring the aortic valve into view in the center of the image, this is the five-chamber view (not shown here).

Apical Two-Chamber and Long-Axis Views

Advanced Views

- Obtain the apical four-chamber view and then rotate the probe 60 degrees counterclockwise (Figure 3-12A).

- The right side will disappear, and only the left ventricle and left atrium will be visualized (Figure 3-12B).

- The left ventricle should appear elongated and pointing at the probe (Figure 3-12C).

- Even with good technique, the anterior wall may be difficult to visualize.

- Continued counterclockwise rotation of about 30 degrees will bring the aortic valve into view on the right side of the image (this is the long-axis view).

- If the left ventricle is short and round, the probe placement is too cephalad.

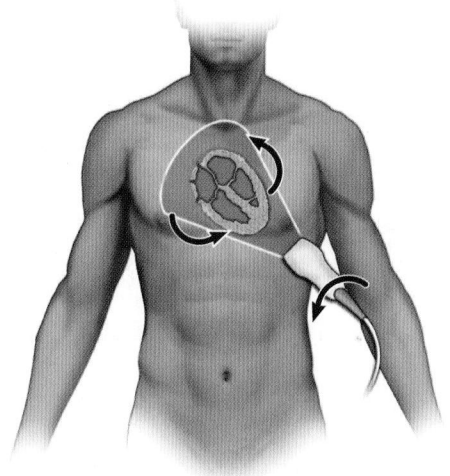

A

Figure 3-12. A. Rotation of the transducer (counterclockwise) needed to obtain the apical two-chamber and long-axis views. Beginning from the apical four-chamber view, rotate approximately 60 degrees for the two-chamber view, then another 30 degrees for the long-axis view.

(Figures 3-12B and C continued on next page)

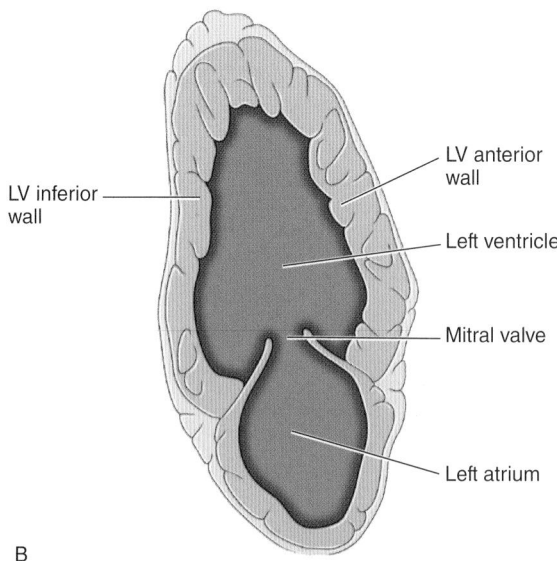

B

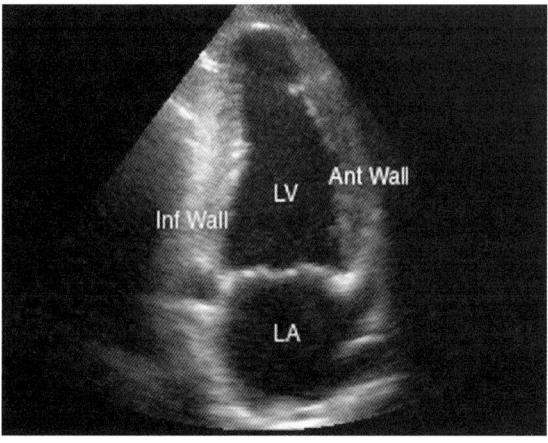

C

Figure 3-12. **B.** Apical two-chamber diagram. **C.** Apical two-chamber normal ultrasound. LV = left ventricle; LA = left atrium.

Suprasternal View

Advanced View

- The probe position is in the sternal notch (Figure 3-13A).
- The probe marker should be toward the patient's left scapula.
- The plane of the aortic arch is oblique proximally anterior and distally posterior.
- Lay the probe down and aim at the cardiac apex until the arch is visualized (Figures 3-13B and 3-13C).

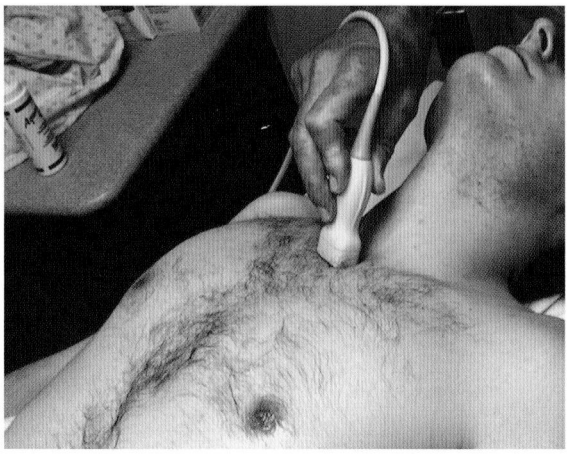

A

Figure 3-13. **A.** Transducer position for suprasternal view. From here, rotate the indicator towards the left scapula for a long axis view of the arch.

(Figures 3-13B and C continued on next page)

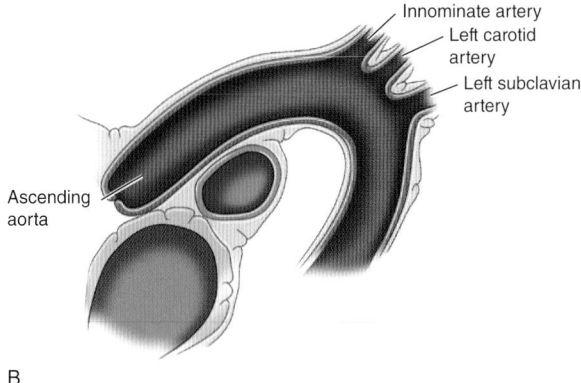

B

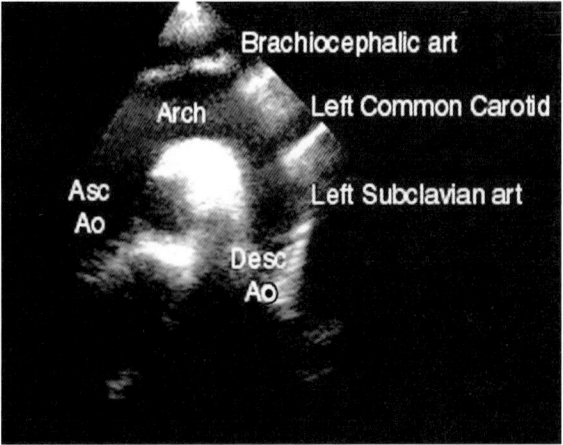

C

Figure 3-13. **B.** Suprasternal diagram. **C.** Suprasternal normal ultrasound. The branch arteries may be closely approximated as in the diagram or spread apart for some patients as in the ultrasound example. Asc Ao = ascending aorta; Desc Ao = descending aorta.

▶ TIPS TO IMPROVE IMAGE ACQUISITION

- Understand that the cardiac location and axis are different in each patient.
- Learn to acquire multiple views because some views are impossible in certain patients.
- Patient positioning: The left lateral decubitus position improves parasternal and apical images.
- Patient breathing: Inspiration improves subxiphoid views, and exhalation improves parasternal and apical views.
- Firm probe pressure improves all views.

▶ COMMON AND EMERGENT ABNORMALITIES

Pericardial Effusion

See Figures 3-14 to 3-16.

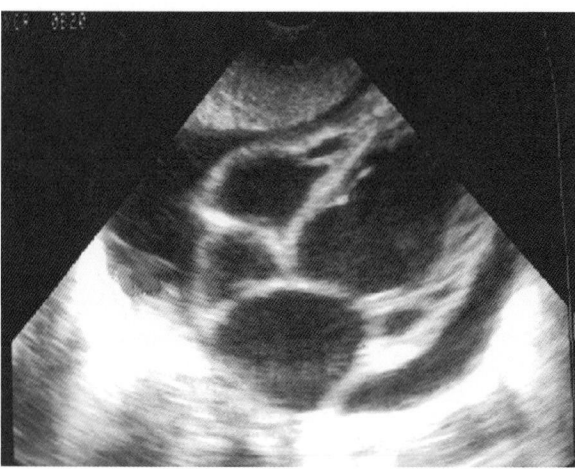

Figure 3-14. Chronic pericardial effusion (subcostal four-chamber view).

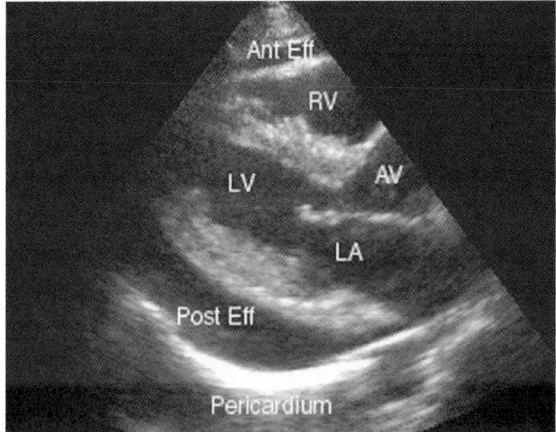

A

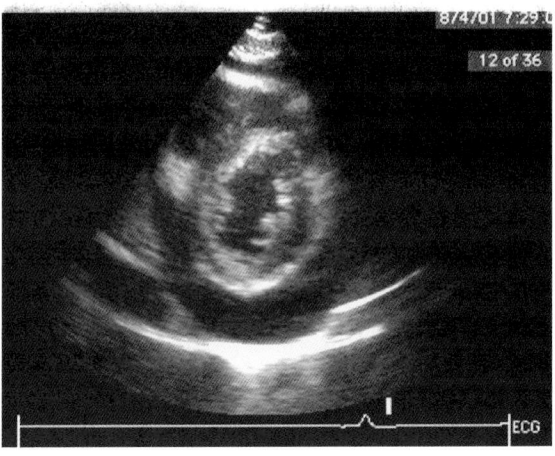

B

Figure 3-15. **A.** Pericardial effusion on the parasternal long-axis view. **B.** Parasternal short-axis view. Ant Eff = anterior effusion; AV = aortic valve; LA = left atrium; LV = left ventricle; Post Eff = posterior effusion; RV = right ventricle.

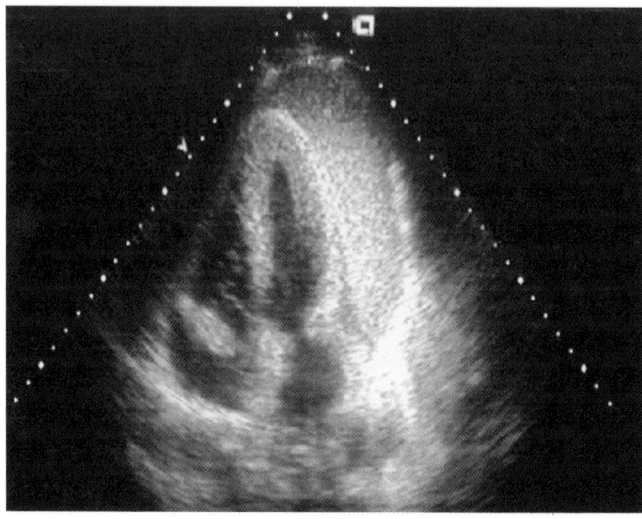

Figure 3-16. Exudative pericardial effusion (apical four-chamber view).

Cardiac Tamponade

See Figure 3-17.

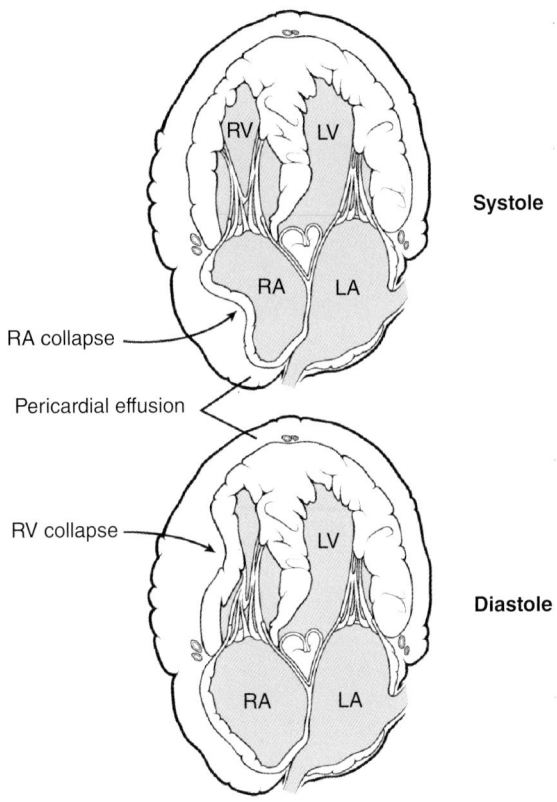

Figure 3-17. Physiology of cardiac tamponade. LA = left atrium; LV = left ventricle; RA = right atrium; RV = right ventricle.

Left Ventricular Dysfunction

Recognition of moderate or severe left ventricular dysfunction is straightforward when compared to a grossly normal exam.

vimeo.com/10341724

vimeo.com/9616959

vimeo.com/10114624

Left ventricular systolic function can be easily estimated by measuring E-point septal separation (EPSS). EPSS can be measured from the parasternal long-axis by placing M-mode through the anterior leaflet of the mitral valve. The distance is measured where the anterior leaflet comes in closest contact with the septum. A value of less than 7 mm is considered to represent normal systolic function. A value greater than 12 mm is considered to represent an ejection fraction of less than 35%. See Figure 3-18.

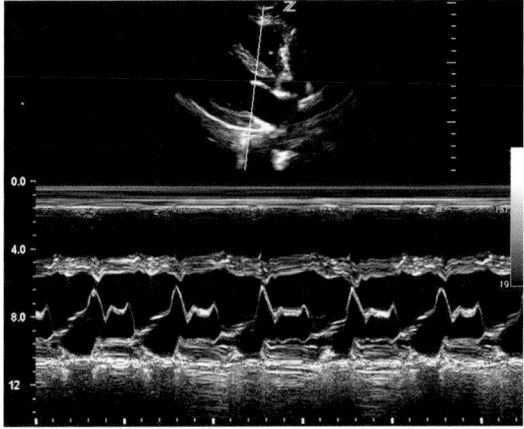

A

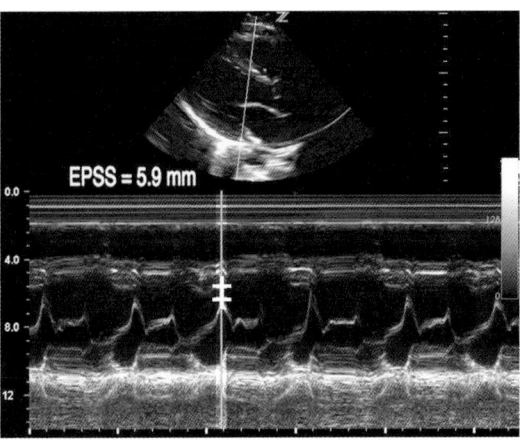

B

Figure 3-18. E-point septal separation (EPSS). M-mode at mitral leaflets, parasternal long-axis view. EPSS can be visually estimated (**A**), or it can be carefully measured (**B**). Increasing EPSS indicates worsening LV dysfunction.

Massive Pulmonary Embolism

See Figures 3-19 and 3-20.

Shock and PEA

Cardiac ultrasound can be used to help determine the etiology of shock and pulseless electrical activity (PEA).

vimeo.com/9219588

vimeo.com/9411088

vimeo.com/9610619

vimeo.com/9219736

vimeo.com/9612168

vimeo.com/10076347

vimeo.com/10086597

vimeo.com/10114530

vimeo.com/10106165

vimeo.com/10088054

vimeo.com/10087306

vimeo.com/10077971

vimeo.com/10073943

vimeo.com/10087449

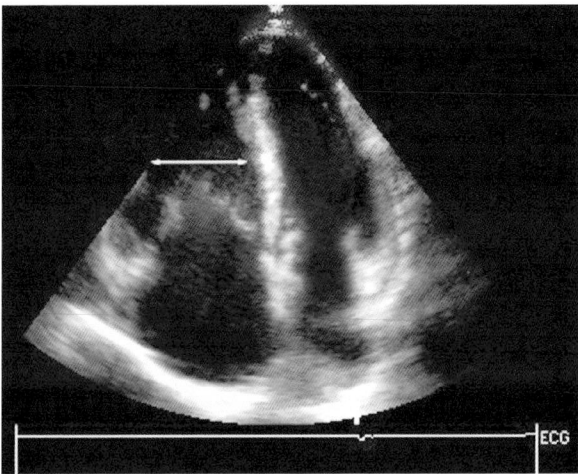

Figure 3-19. Right ventricular enlargement. The apical four-chamber diameter at the mid-right ventricle exceeds 3.5 cm.

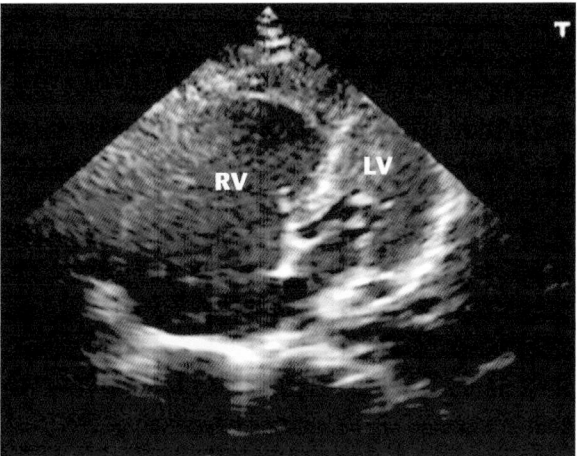

Figure 3-20. Massive pulmonary embolism. Apical view (centered over the right ventricular [RV] apex) shows severely decompensated RV that is round in shape and much larger than the left ventricle (LV).

► ADDITIONAL FINDINGS

Myocardial Ischemia

See Figures 3-21 and 3-22.

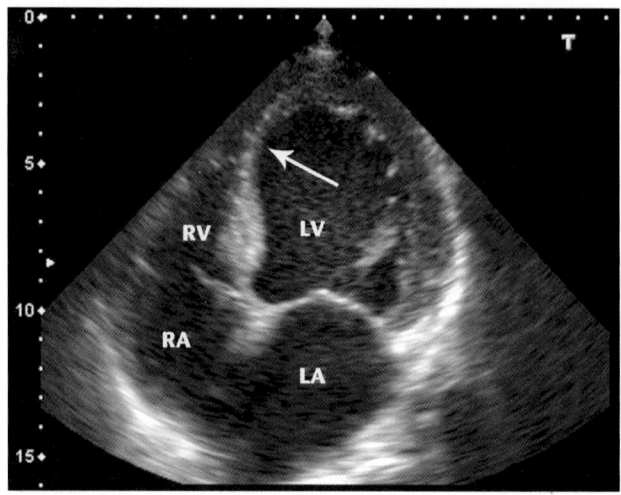

A

Figure 3-21. Chronic left ventricular (LV) infarction. **A.** Apical four-chamber view demonstrates thinning and increased echogenicity of the apical septum (*arrow*) with increased size of the LV and left atrial (LA) chambers.

(Figure 3-21B continued on next page)

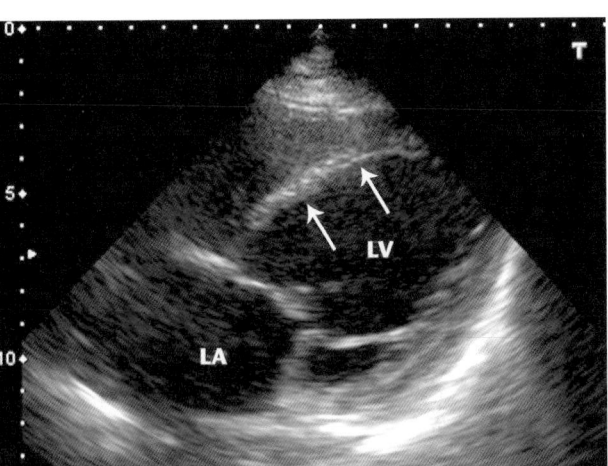

B

Figure 3-21. **B.** Subcostal four-chamber view shows chronic thinning of the entire inferior septum (*arrows*). LA = left atrium; LV = left ventricle.

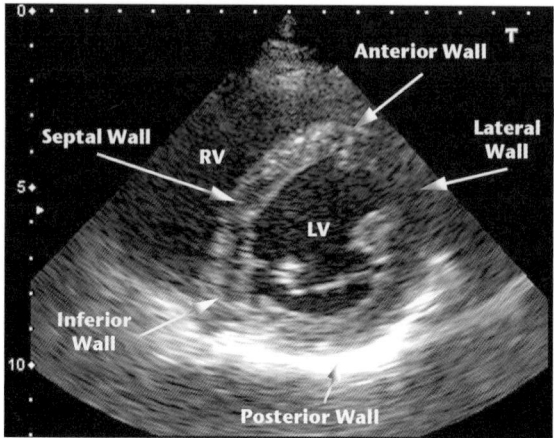

A

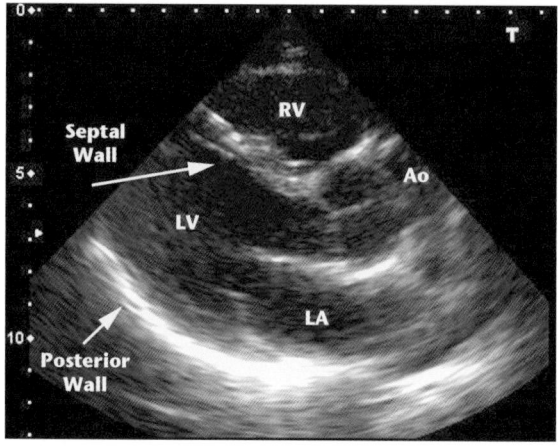

B

Figure 3-22. Left ventricular (LV) wall segments. **A.** Parasternal short-axis view. **B.** Parasternal long-axis view. RV = right ventricle; LA = left atrium; Ao = aorta.

(Figures 3-22C and D continued on next page)

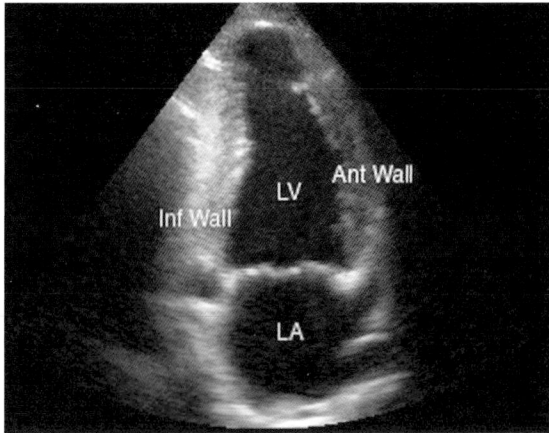

C

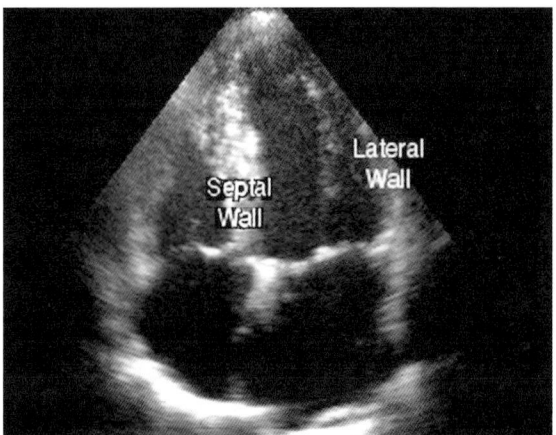

D

Figure 3-22. **C.** Apical two-chamber view. Inf = inferior; Ant = anterior. **D.** Apical four-chamber view.

(Figure 3-22E continued on next page)

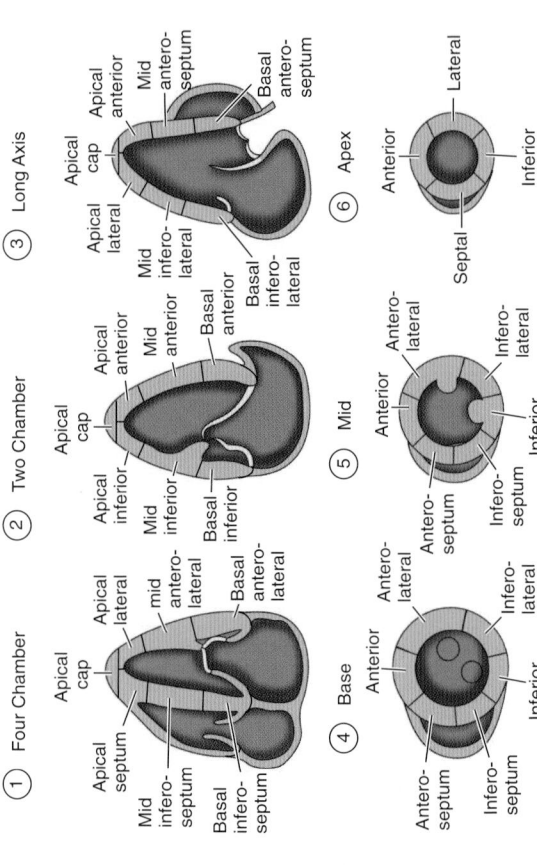

Figure 3-22. E. Left ventricular wall segments visualized on various cardiac ultrasound views.

(Figure 3-22F continued on next page)

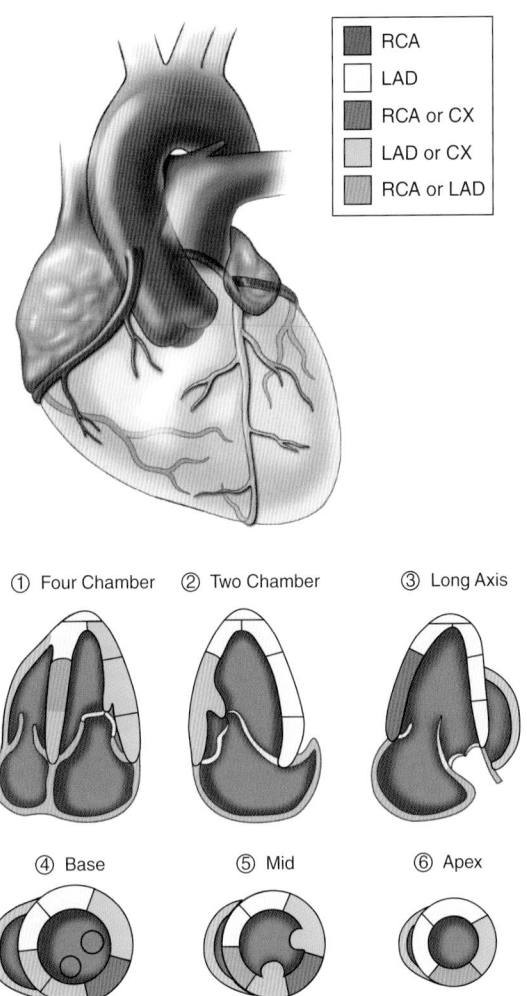

Figure 3-22. **F.** Coronary perfusion of the myocardium based on wall segments visualized in various cardiac ultrasound views. Coronary distribution varies between patients.

Valvular Abnormalities

See Figures 3-23 and 3-24.

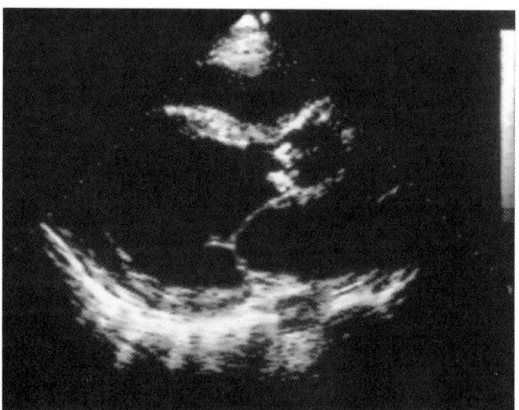

A

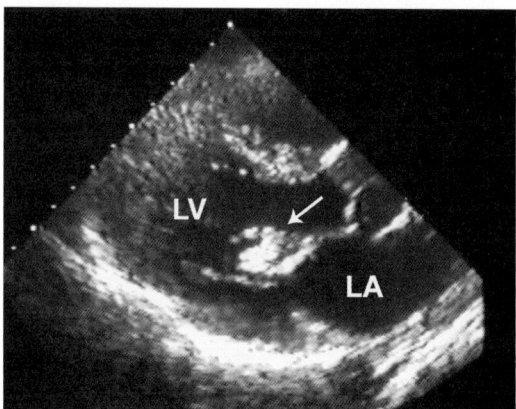

B

Figure 3-23. Endocarditis. **A.** Parasternal long-axis view reveals echogenic mobile vegetations on the aortic valve leaflets. **B.** Parasternal long-axis view with echogenic mobile vegetations on the mitral valve leaflets (*arrow*). LA = left atrium; LV = left ventricle. (Photos contributed by Lori Sens and Lori Green, Gulfcoast Ultrasound.)

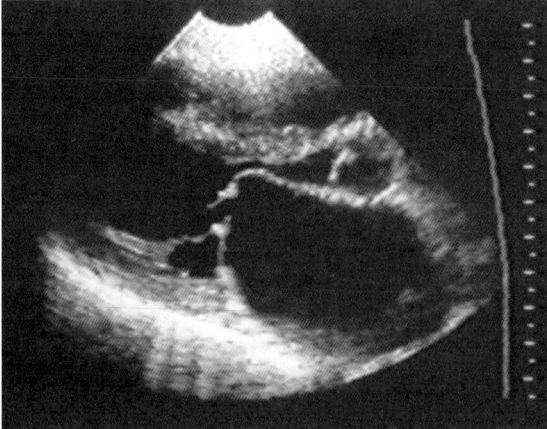

A

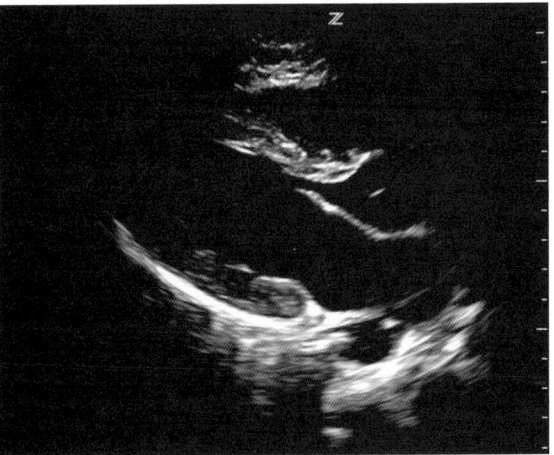

B

Figure 3-24. **A.** Mitral stenosis. Parasternal long-axis view shows the typical features: left atrial enlargement, ballooning of the valve, and a "hockey stick" appearance of the anterior leaflet. **B.** Normal (fully opened) mitral valve.

Ascending Aortic Aneurysm and Proximal Aortic Dissection

See Figures 3-25 to 3-27.

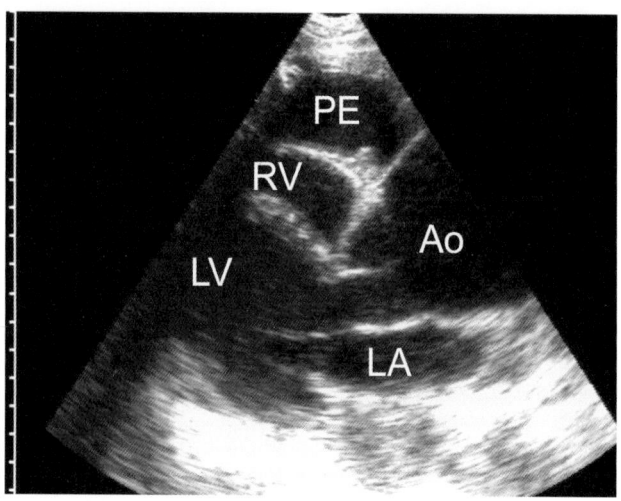

Figure 3-25. Aortic aneurysm. Parasternal long-axis view shows a 6-cm aneurysm in the ascending aorta. Pericardial fluid effusion anteriorly. Ao = aorta; LA = left atrium; PE = pericardial effusion; RV = right ventricle.

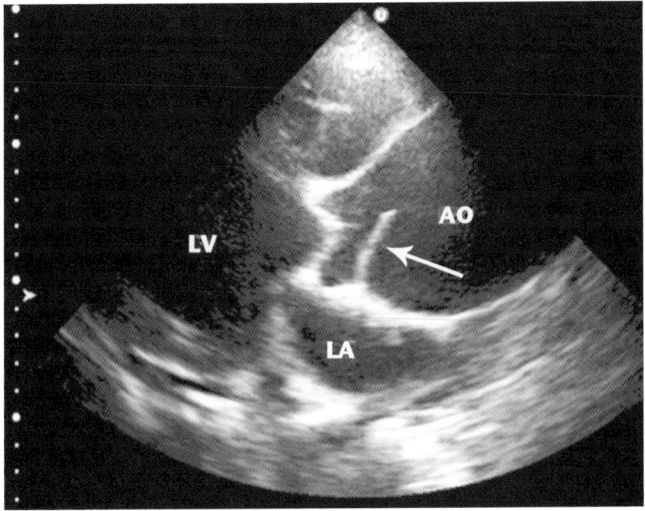

Figure 3-26. Ascending aortic aneurysm with dissection. Parasternal long-axis view shows dilated aortic root and proximal flap (*arrow*). Ao = aorta; LA = left atrium; LV = left ventricle.

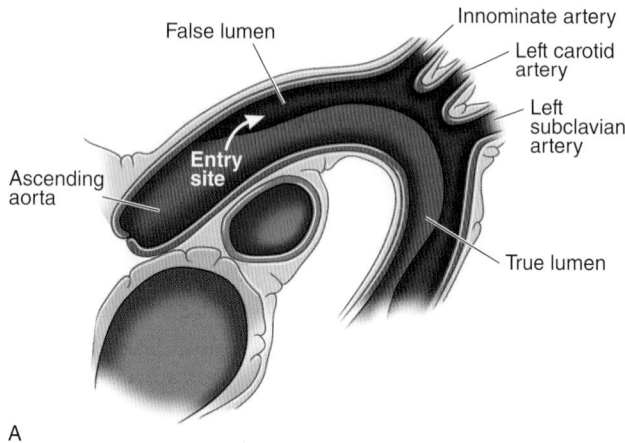

A

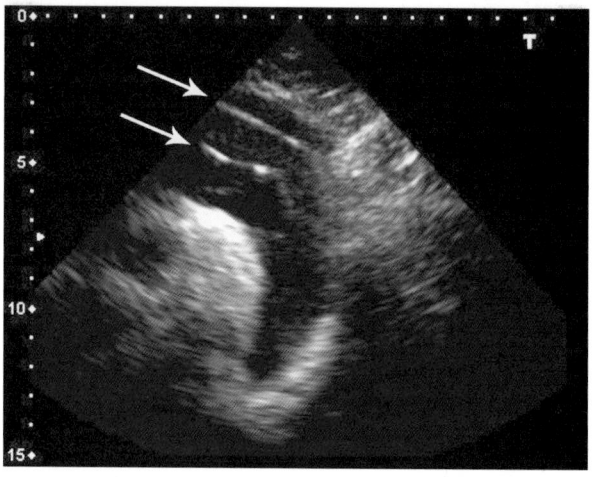

B

Figure 3-27. **A.** Type A aortic dissection diagram. **B.** Suprasternal ultrasound view of the aortic arch. The imaging plane crosses the intimal flap in two locations (*arrows*). (B: Courtesy of Hennepin County Medical Center.)

Ventricular Hypertrophy

See Figures 3-28 and 3-29.

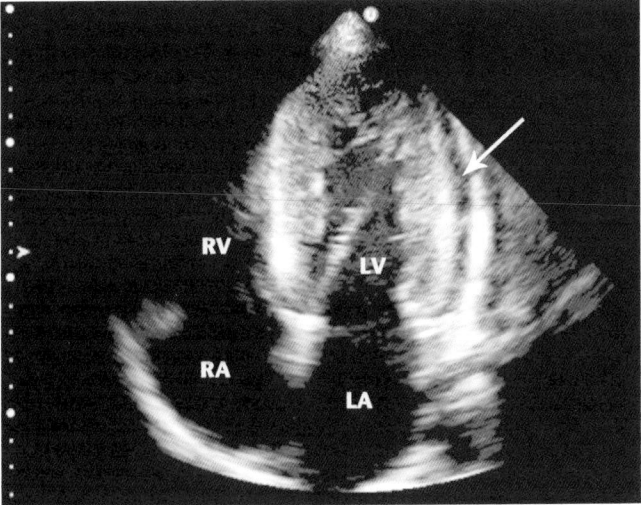

Figure 3-28. Concentric hypertrophy. Apical four-chamber view demonstrates symmetrical thickening of the left ventricular (LV) wall. A small pericardial effusion is noted adjacent to the LV (*arrow*). LA = left atrium; RA = right atrium; RV = right ventricle.

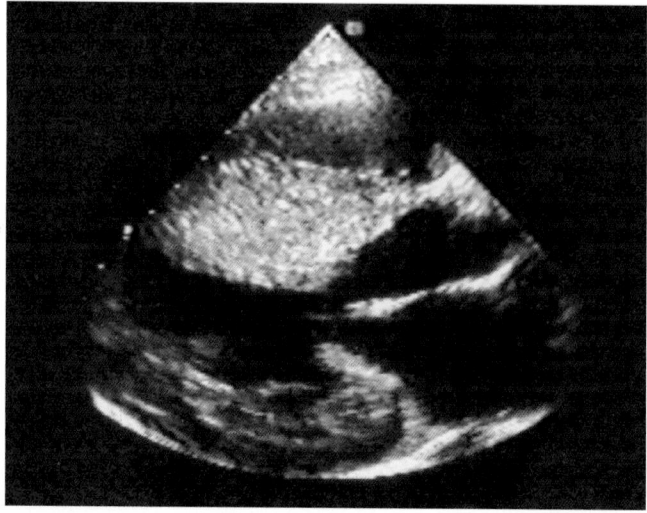

Figure 3-29. Asymmetric septal hypertrophy. A thickened, echogenic left ventricular (LV) septum is noted in the parasternal long-axis view in a patient with this condition (also known as idiopathic hypertrophic subaortic stenosis). (Photo contributed by Lori Sens and Lori Green, Gulfcoast Ultrasound.)

Thrombus

See Figure 3-30.

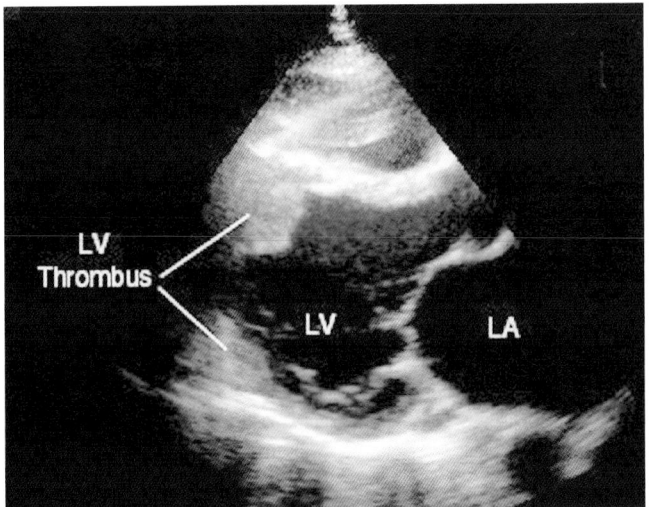

Figure 3-30. A left ventricular (LV) thrombus is located near the apex (parasternal long-axis view). LA = left atrium.

▶ PITFALLS

- Inability to obtain adequate views
- Reversed orientation
- Mistaking pericardial fat for a pericardial effusion
- Incorrect adjustment of gain
- Incorrect adjustment of depth
- Setting the dynamic range too high

For more detailed information go to the comprehensive textbook Ma and Mateer's Emergency Ultrasound, 3rd edition, Chapter 6 "Cardiac" by Robert Reardon, MD, Andrew Laudenbach, MD, and Scott Joing, MD.

CHAPTER 4
Pulmonary

▶ CLINICAL CONSIDERATIONS

- Applications of lung ultrasound are often more sensitive and specific than plain radiographs and do not expose the patient to ionizing radiation.
- In the critically ill, pathology can be diagnosed and acted on much more quickly with ultrasound than other types of imaging.

▶ CLINICAL INDICATIONS

- Evaluation of undifferentiated dyspnea
- Pneumothorax
- **Alveolar-interstitial syndromes:** cardiogenic and noncardiogenic pulmonary edema, pulmonary contusion, etc.
- **Consolidations:** pneumonia, atelectasis, etc.
- Pleural effusions
- Airway management

▶ ANATOMIC CONSIDERATIONS

- The lungs are covered by the visceral pleura, which comes into contact with the parietal pleura that lines the chest wall in normal lungs.
- The lungs have a very large surface area, and not all of the area is accessible with ultrasound; however, scanning a single spot on the bilateral upper anterior chest wall will often be diagnostic.

► TECHNIQUE AND NORMAL FINDINGS

- Most of the interpretation of lung ultrasound is based on artifacts because ultrasound does not transmit well through air.

- Lung ultrasound can be performed with a linear, curvilinear, or phased array transducer.

Pleural Interface Views

- Position the transducer in the sagittal plane with the indicator cephalad anywhere on the chest wall (Figure 4-1).

- Identify the ribs, rib shadows, and pleural interface (Figure 4-2).

- Once the pleural interface is identified, rotate the probe 90 degrees to obtain a transverse view.

- Look for respiratory motion at the pleural interface (lung sliding) and normal comet-tail and A-line artifacts.

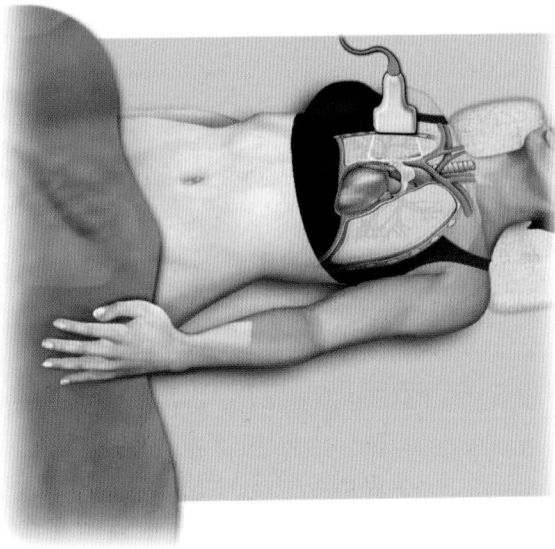

Figure 4-1. Transducer position for examination of the pleural interface.

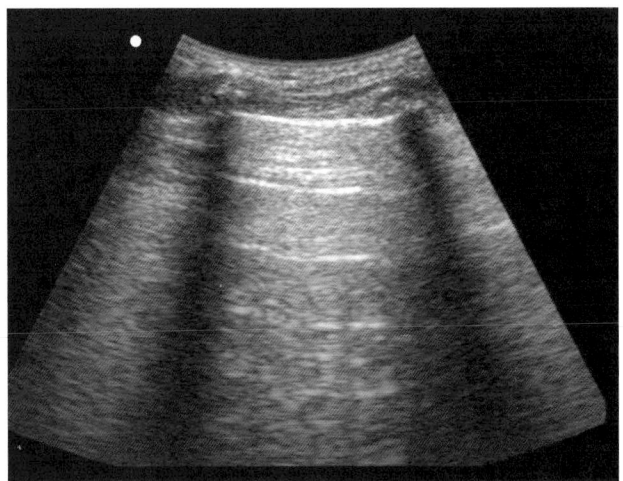

A

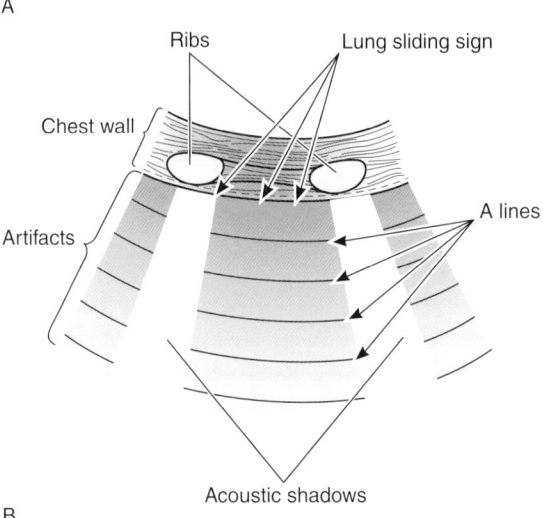

B

Figure 4-2. Normal lung. **A.** Longitudinal intercostal scan.
B. Schematic representation of the same sonographic image.

Right Lung Base View

- Position the curvilinear or phased array probe in the mid-axillary line at about the 8th to 11th rib interspace.

- Use an oblique scanning plane with the indicator pointing toward the right posterior axilla (Figure 4-3A).

- Angle the transducer cephalad to examine the right diaphragm and base of the lung with the liver at the bottom of the image (Figure 4-3B).

- This is generally a straightforward view to obtain because the liver is large and provides a good acoustic window.

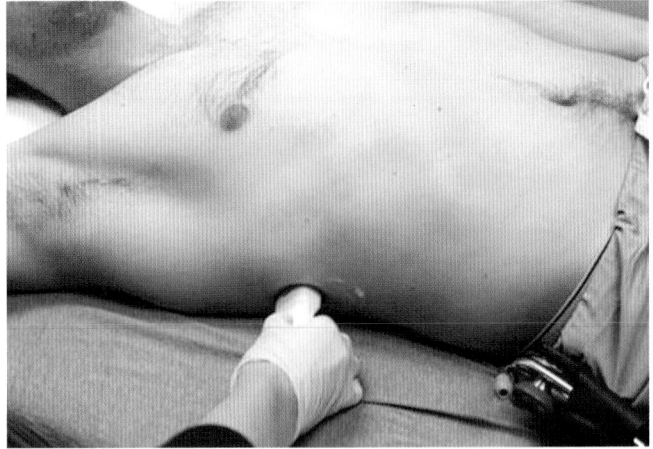

A

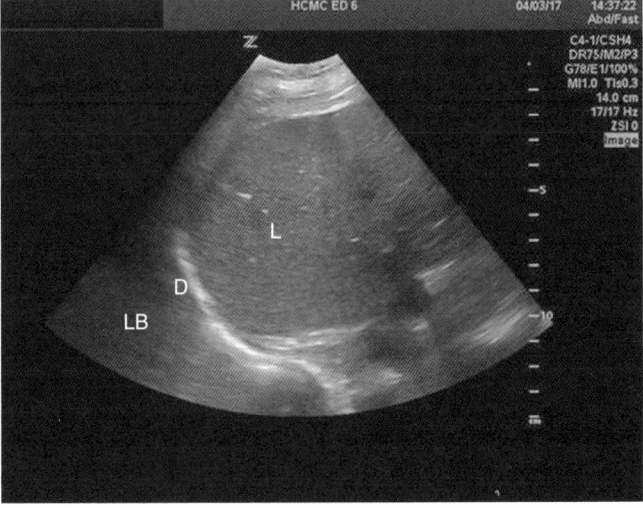

B

Figure 4-3. **A.** Transducer position for examination of right lung base. **B.** Normal right lung base. L = Liver; D = Diaphragm; LB = Lung Base.

Left Lung Base View

- Position the curvilinear or phased array probe in the posterior-axillary line at about the 7th to 9th rib interspace.

- Use an oblique scanning plane with the indicator pointing toward the left posterior axilla (Figure 4-4A).

- Angle cephalad to examine the left diaphragm and base of the lung with the spleen at the bottom of the image (Figure 4-4B).

- This is generally a more challenging view to obtain because the spleen generally does not serve as a good acoustic window.

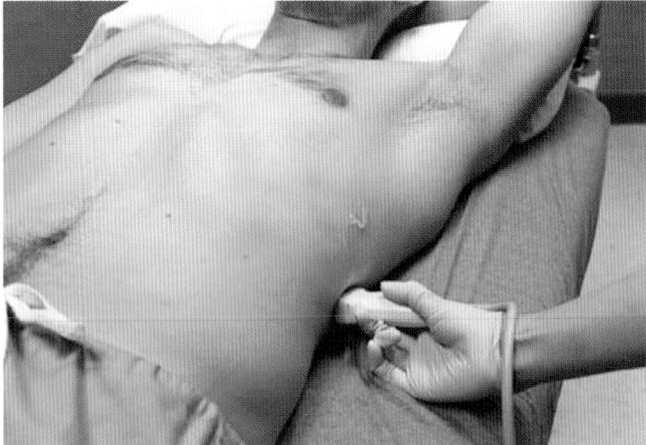

A

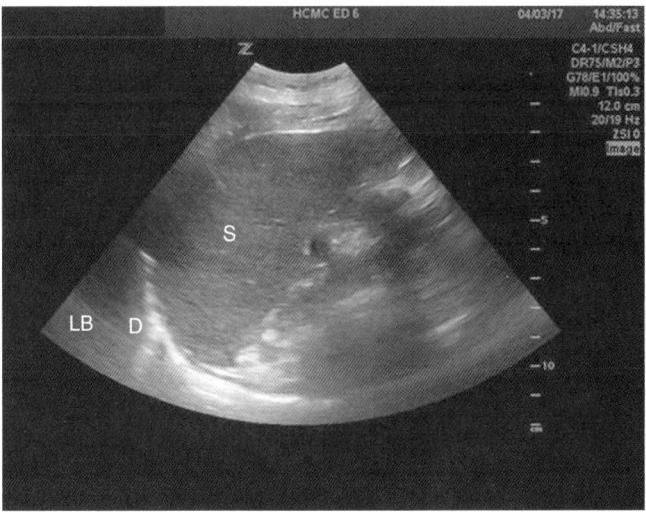

B

Figure 4-4. **A.** Transducer position for examination of the left lung base. **B.** Normal left lung base. S = Spleen; D = Diaphragm; LB = Lung Base.

▶ TIPS TO IMPROVE IMAGE ACQUISITION

- Place the transducer in the sagittal plane between two ribs to allow for more accurate identification of the pleural interface.

- Novice sonologists often better appreciate lung sliding using a linear transducer.

- Use a curvilinear or phased array transducer when evaluating the diaphragm and base of the lung.

- Decrease the depth to about 5 cm when scanning for lung sliding.

- Increase the depth to 10 to 15 cm when scanning the lung bases or for lung pathology other than pneumothorax.

- When scanning at the level of the diaphragm, changes in the respiratory cycle will result in intermittent visualization of either sliding signs or the solid organs (liver or spleen). This is referred to as the curtain sign.

▶ COMMON AND EMERGENT ABNORMALITIES

- Pneumothorax
  - A pneumothorax can be diagnosed by absence of lung sliding as demonstrated by real-time 2-D imaging, power Doppler imaging, or M-mode imaging (Figure 4-5).
  - If B-lines are detected, even in the absence of obvious lung sliding, there is no pneumothorax in that portion of the lung because the pleural interfaces have to be intact to create that artifact.

- Alveolar-interstitial syndromes (Figures 4-6 to 4-8)
  - Pathologic B-lines are defined as more than 3 comet-tail artifacts per rib space.
  - A focal area of B-lines could be consistent with either pneumonia or pulmonary contusion.

- Consolidations (Figures 4-9 and 4-10)

- Effusions (Figure 4-11)

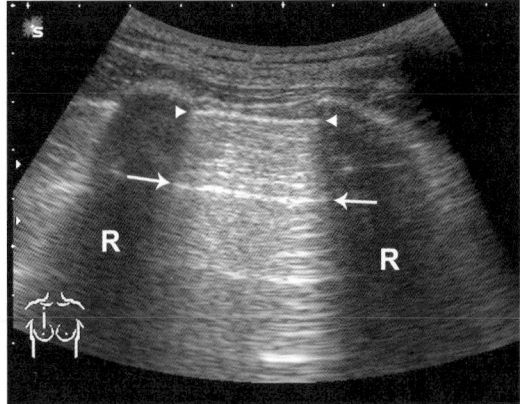

A

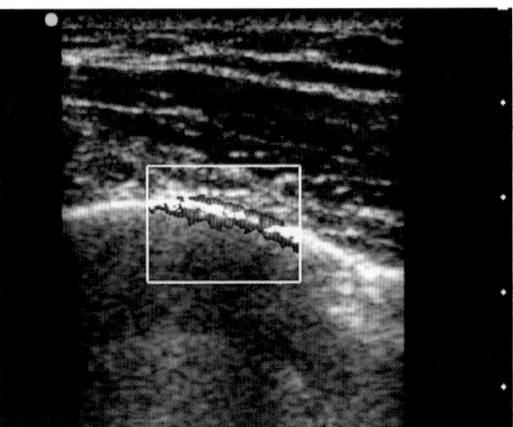

B

Figure 4-5. **A.** 2-D ultrasound image of the pleural interface. Absence of lung sliding at the pleural interface (*arrowheads*) in real-time is indicative of a pneumothorax. A-lines (*arrows*) may be present with normal lung sliding or with a pneumothorax. **B.** Power Doppler of the pleural interface demonstrates lung sliding with color.

(Figure 4-5C continued on next page)

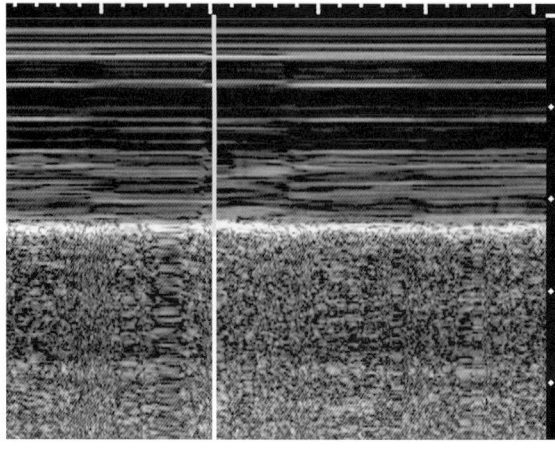

C

Figure 4-5. **C.** M-mode ultrasound of normal lung at 7.5 to 10 MHz ("seashore sign"). Granular artifacts below the bright pleural line represent normal lung sliding on M-mode.

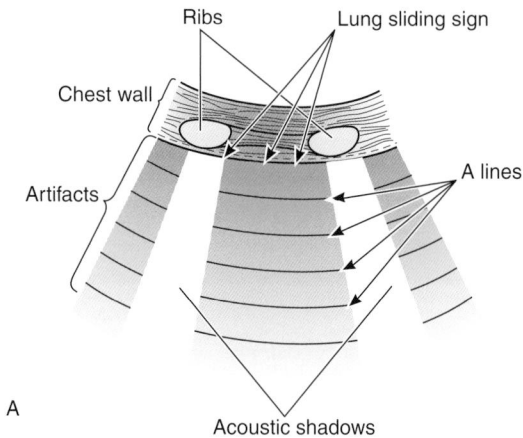

A

Figure 4-6. Pulmonary ultrasound to evaluate for extravascular lung water. **A.** Normal "dry lung" has a prominent A-line pattern.

(Figures 4-6B and C continued on next page)

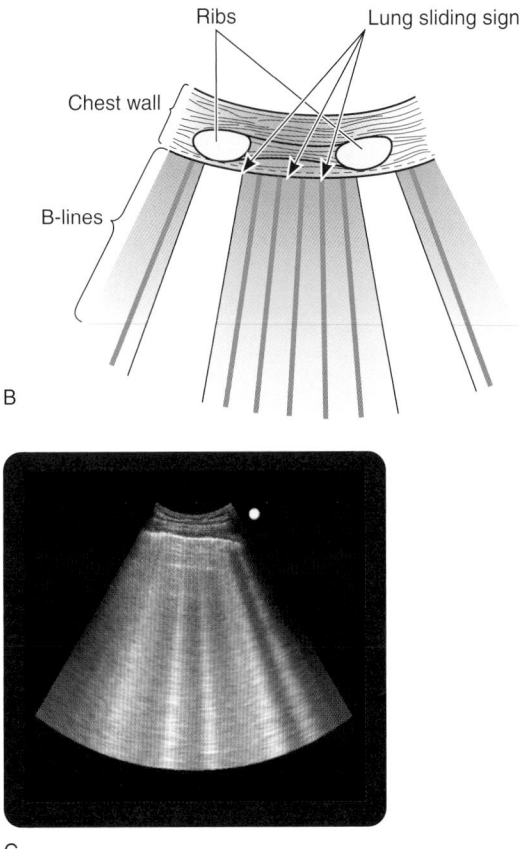

Figure 4-6. **B.** Prominent B-line pattern is consistent with "wet lung." **C.** Corresponding ultrasound image demonstrating B-lines.

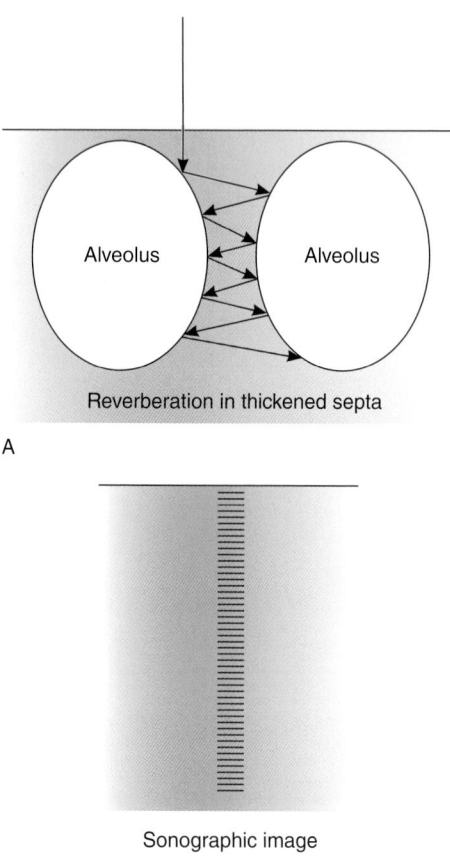

Figure 4-7. Why B-lines are present in alveolar-interstitial syndromes. **A.** The ultrasound wave reverberates in the soft tissue or thickened interalveolar/interlobular septa. **B.** The ultrasound machine generates a vertical line formed by innumerable tiny horizontal lines that represent each reflection.

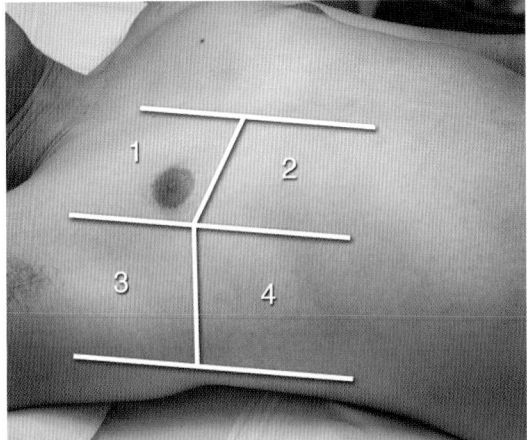

Figure 4-8. Eight-region exam for assessment of cardiogenic pulmonary edema. Two or more positive regions bilaterally define a positive exam.

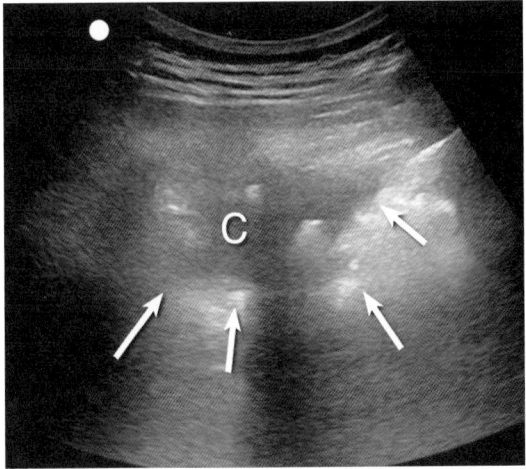

Figure 4-9. Pneumonia. Note the irregular limits (*arrows*) of the consolidation (C). The pleural line is not visible because there is no alveolar air to generate the lung sliding sign.

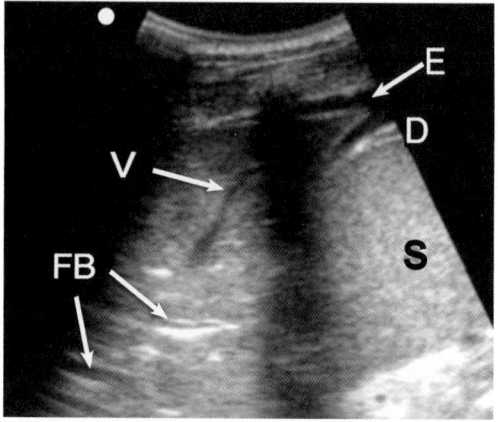

A

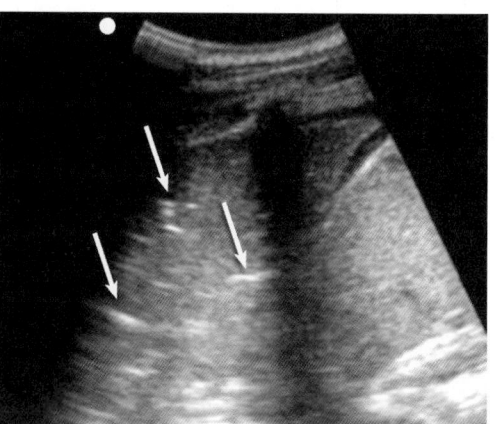

B

Figure 4-10. A. Left lower lobe pneumonia at the lateral costophrenic recess. Fluid bronchograms (FB) can be seen. They have much more echogenic walls than vessels (V) and do not demonstrate flow with Doppler exam. A tiny pleural effusion (E) is seen above the diaphragm (D) overlying the spleen (S). **B.** Dynamic air bronchograms. Movement of secretions could be seen within the air bronchograms (*arrows*) in real time.

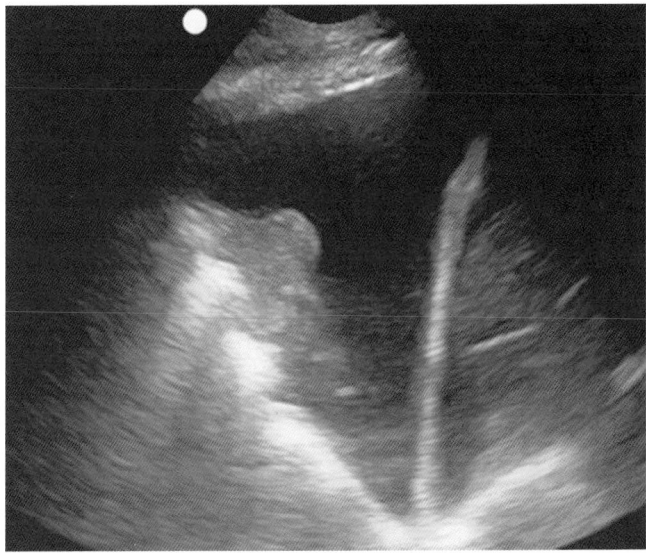

Figure 4-11. Pleural effusion. Corresponding ultrasound image. Also note the compressive atelectasis at the base of the lung.

▶ ADDITIONAL FINDINGS

- Mirror artifact (Figure 4-12)

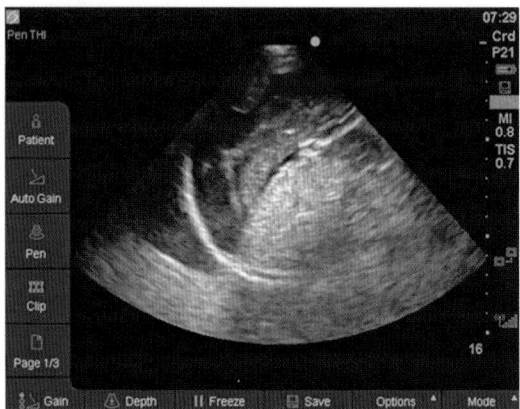

Figure 4-12. Mirror artifact. The diaphragm is a reflective surface that produces a mirror image reflecting subdiaphragmatic contents above the diaphragm. In this image, subdiaphragmatic free fluid is reflected above the diaphragm, making it appear as if there is a pleural effusion.

▶ PITFALLS

- Not appreciating other conditions that result in absence of lung sliding, such as apnea, pulmonary blebs, main-stem intubation, status-post pleurodesis, adhesions, and subcutaneous air.

- Misidentifying fascia or muscle planes of the chest wall as the pleural line.

- Mistaking movement of the muscles in the chest wall as lung sliding.

- Mistaking a mirror artifact from free fluid under the diaphragm for a pleural effusion or hemothorax.

- Misidentifying abdominal and cardiac structures for pulmonary pathology when scanning the lower chest.

- Only scanning one spot on the chest wall when any place the lung comes into contact with the chest wall can be imaged.

For more detailed information go to the comprehensive textbook Ma and Mateer's Emergency Ultrasound, 3rd edition, Chapter 7, by Fernando Silva, MD and Lisa Mills, MD.

CHAPTER 5
Critical Care

► CLINICAL CONSIDERATIONS

- In the critically ill patient, a wide variety of ultrasound applications can be used to make rapid diagnoses and optimize resuscitation efforts.
- In undifferentiated shock, "whole body" ultrasound can be used to evaluate for the cause of shock in order to rapidly focus treatment.

► CLINICAL INDICATIONS

- Cardiac arrest and near-arrest states
- Evaluation of undifferentiated hypotension
- Assessment of volume status and fluid requirements
- Assessment of shortness of breath or respiratory distress
- Evaluation of deep vein thrombosis (DVT)
- Evaluation of abdominal sources of shock or sepsis
- Critical ultrasound-guided procedures

► TECHNIQUE AND NORMAL FINDINGS

- Ultrasound applications include assessment of cardiac function, lungs, inferior vena cava (IVC), abdomen, and lower extremity vasculature. Details of these exams are outlined in Chapters 2, 3, 4, 6, 7, 8, and 11 of this book.

▶ PRACTICAL TIPS FOR ULTRASOUND IN THE CRITICALLY ILL

- Combining examination of the lungs, heart, and IVC can more accurately determine the cause of undifferentiated shock and a patient's volume status.

- The cardiac exam in those with undifferentiated hypotension or acute dyspnea is used to evaluate for left ventricular systolic function, right ventricular size, pericardial effusion, large wall motion abnormalities, and valvular abnormalities (Figure 5-1).

- The thoracic exam in those with undifferentiated hypotension or acute dyspnea is used to evaluate for presence or absence of B-lines and lung sliding.

- The IVC exam in those with undifferentiated hypotension or acute dyspnea is used to evaluate for size and collapsibility of the IVC (Figures 5-2 and 5-3).

- The combination of a flat, collapsing IVC, hyperdynamic cardiac contractility, and dry lungs can represent hypovolemic or distributive (septic) shock (Figure 5-4).

- The combination of a large, noncollapsing IVC, poor cardiac contractility, and wet lungs is consistent with cardiogenic shock (Figures 5-5 and 5-6).

- The combination of a large, noncollapsing IVC, hyperdynamic or normal cardiac contractility, and dry lungs is consistent with obstructive shock (eg, pulmonary embolism [PE], tamponade) (Figure 5-7).

- The majority of patients with a massive PE will have a lower extremity DVT that is straightforward to diagnose on a simple two-point compression exam (Figure 5-8).

- Palpation of pulses in patients with cardiac arrest has been shown to be inaccurate. Using ultrasound to determine if cardiac activity is present in combination with palpating pulses is more reliable than pulse checks alone.

- Critically ill patients are often volume depleted and this can make imaging both the heart and IVC more challenging. Scanning the heart and IVC from multiple windows will improve views (Figure 5-9).

- Subcutaneous air of the chest wall can make cardiac imaging difficult or impossible. In these patients, sometimes the only cardiac view that can be obtained is the subcostal view.

- Abdominal sources of shock are often missed or overlooked. Use the FAST exam to evaluate for causes of atraumatic intra-abdominal hemorrhage. Scan the abdominal aorta to evaluate for an abdominal aortic aneurysm (AAA), and scan the kidneys and gallbladder to evaluate for abdominal causes of sepsis (eg, cholecystitis, infected obstructing renal calculus, renal abscess).

- The critically ill often require central venous access. Ultrasound can be used to rapidly and safely guide line insertion (Figures 5-10 and 5-11).

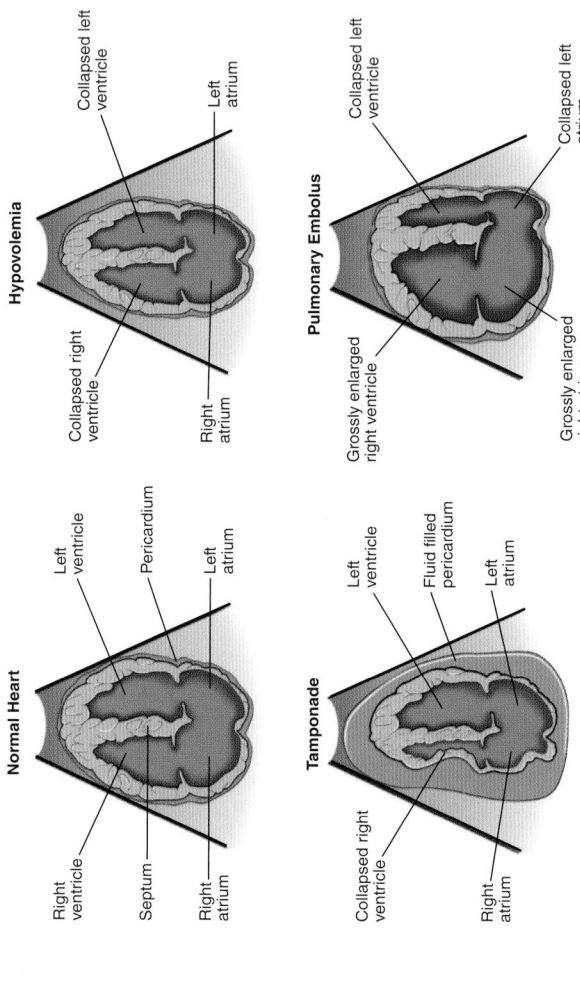

Figure 5-1. Relative cardiac chamber size in different shock states.

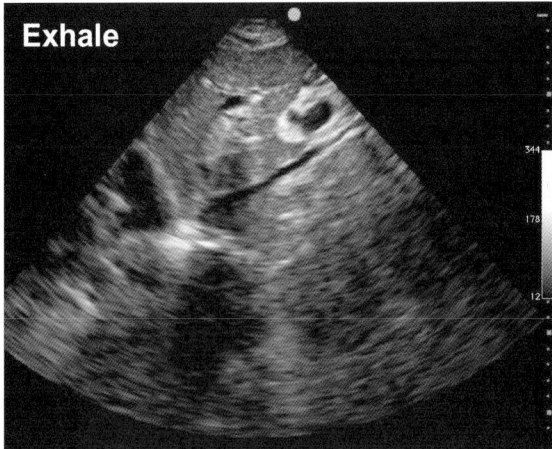

A

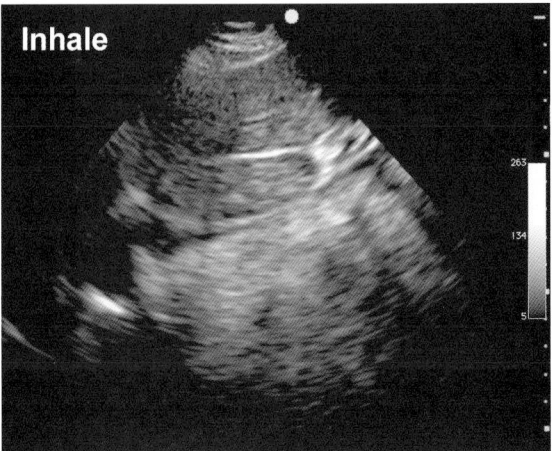

B

Figure 5-2. IVC findings consistent with low central venous pressure. Longitudinal view of the IVC during exhalation (**A**) and inhalation (**B**). Note narrow initial diameter (<1 cm) and complete collapse with inhalation.

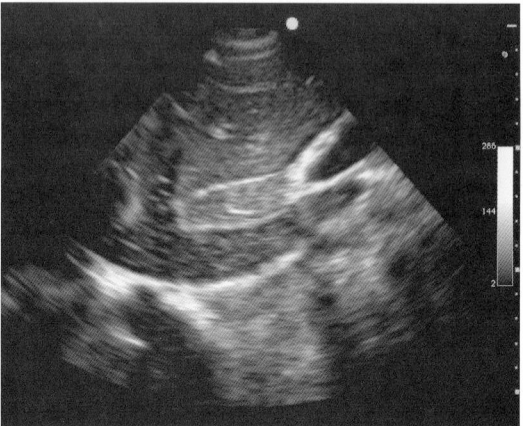

A

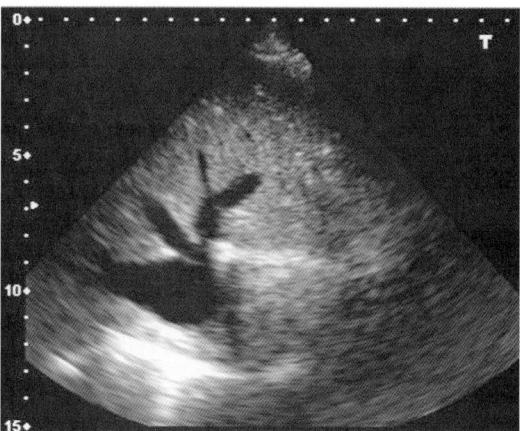

B

Figure 5-3. IVC findings consistent with high central venous pressure. **A.** Longitudinal view of the IVC shows a large diameter (≥2 cm) and spontaneous contrast. There was no change with respirations on real-time views. Also note dilated hepatic veins branching anteriorly. **B.** Corresponding transverse view of the IVC.

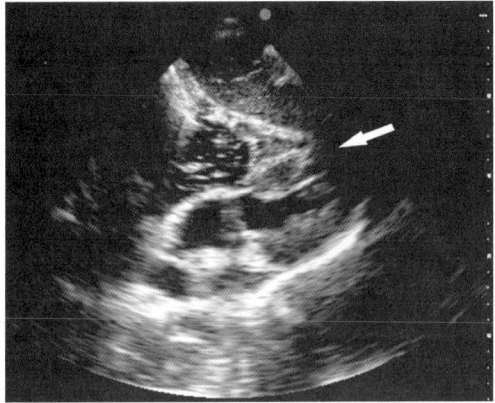

A

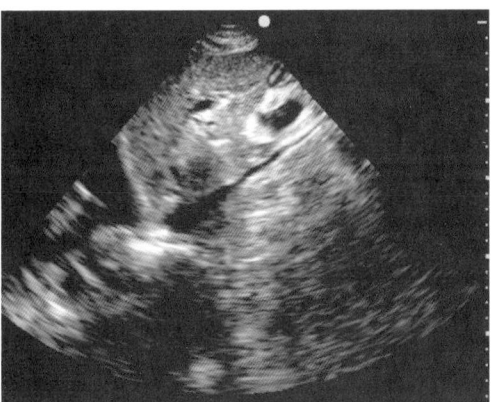

B

Figure 5-4. Hypovolemic or distributive shock. **A.** Subcostal four-chamber cardiac view with position of interventricular septum indicated (*arrow*). Left ventricular and right ventricular chambers are ≤2 cm in diameter. **B.** Long-axis view of the IVC. The findings of a small hyperdynamic heart and completely collapsed IVC are consistent with hypovolemic or distributive shock. The provider should consider looking for an abdominal aortic aneurysm or abdominal sources of hemorrhage or sepsis. This patient had urosepsis and acute renal failure.

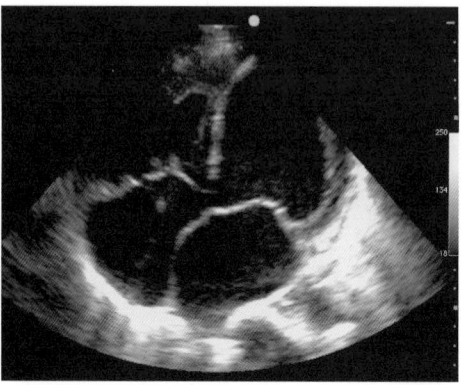

A

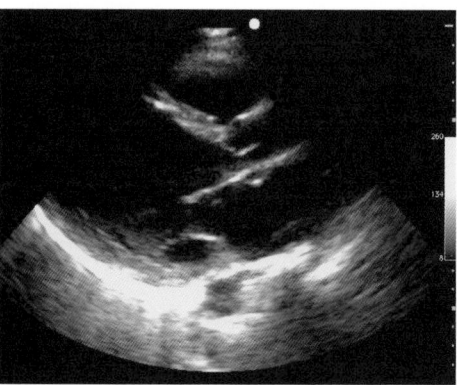

B

Figure 5-5. Acutely decompensated heart failure and cardiogenic shock. **A.** Apical four-chamber view. **B.** Parasternal long-axis view. Obvious changes associated with chronic heart disease, including biatrial and biventricular enlargement. These findings suggest that shock could be cardiogenic in etiology. Supporting evidence can be obtained by assessing the lungs and other body regions looking for other possible causes of shock. This patient was found to have a normal abdominal aorta and diffuse bilateral B-lines on pulmonary ultrasound, consistent with pulmonary edema from heart failure.

(Figure 5-5C continued on next page)

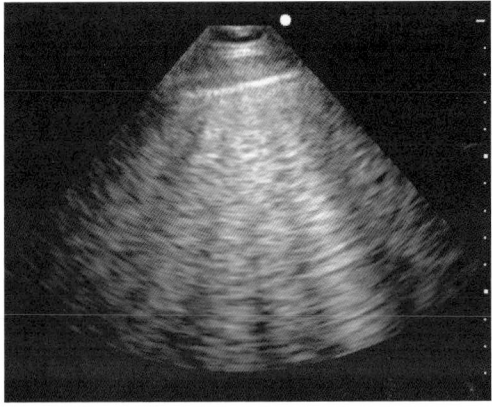

C

Figure 5-5. **C.** The static lung image demonstrates multiple diffuse B-lines emanating from the entire pleural surface (more obvious during real-time exam). Using a curved or phased array transducer, these lines can be seen to radiate to the full depth of the image. (Image C courtesy of James Mateer, MD.)

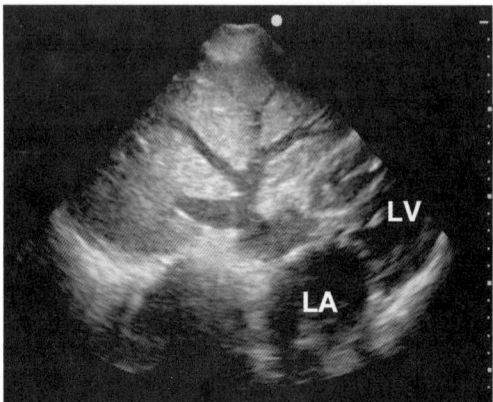

A

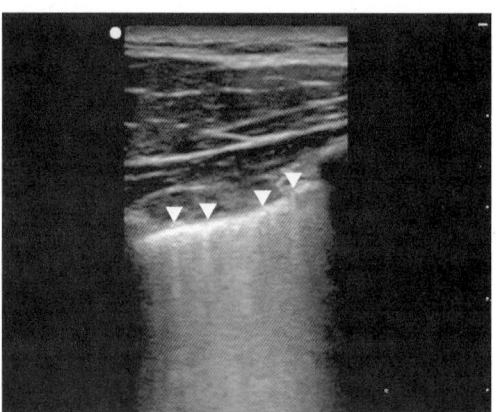

B

Figure 5-6. Cardiogenic shock. **A.** Subcostal four-chamber view angled toward the midline. LA enlargement is noted, and dilated hepatic veins are seen with spontaneous echo contrast noted on real-time exam. These are all signs of poor forward flow and cardiogenic shock. **B.** High-frequency linear array image of the pleura. The finding of a diffuse bilateral B-line pattern on lung ultrasound is diagnostic for pulmonary edema. The origins of the B-lines are indicated (*arrowheads*) and were obvious on real-time exam. LA = left atrial; LV = left ventricle.

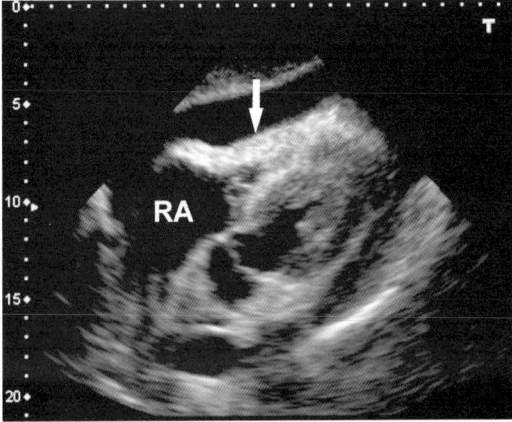

A

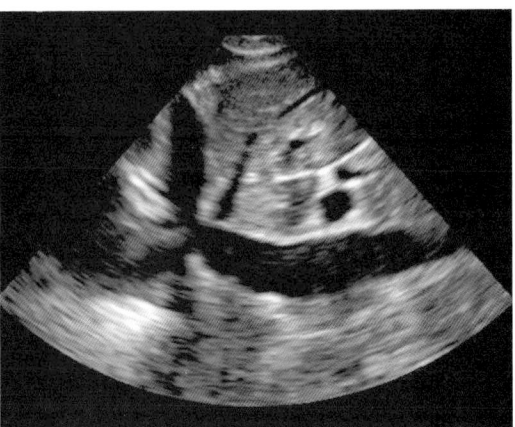

B

Figure 5-7. Cardiac tamponade. The classic ultrasound finding of tamponade is early-diastolic collapse of the right ventricle. **A.** Subcostal four-chamber view with right atrium visible, but right ventricular chamber is completely collapsed (*arrow*). A moderate-to-large pericardial effusion is surrounding the heart. **B.** A dilated fixed IVC is supportive evidence of the hemodynamic significance of the pericardial effusion. RA = right atrium.

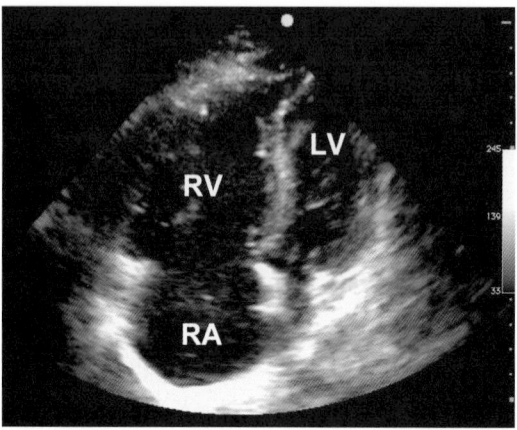

A

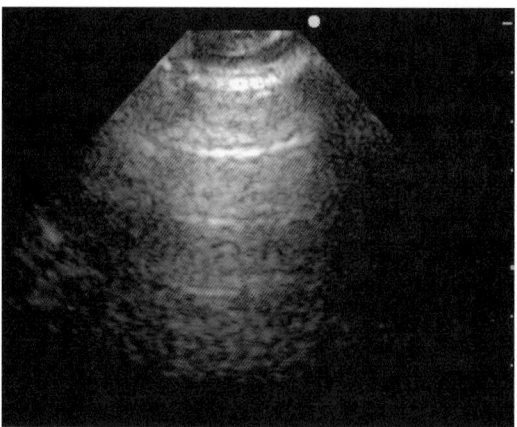

B

Figure 5-8. Massive PE. This patient presented with hypotension and severe dyspnea. **A.** Apical view of RV and RA. Dilated and poorly functioning RV noted on real-time views. RV = right ventricle, RA = right atrium, LV = left ventricle. **B.** Intact lung sliding and A-line pattern on lung ultrasound (phased array transducer) rule out pneumothorax and pulmonary edema.

(Figure 5-8C continued on next page)

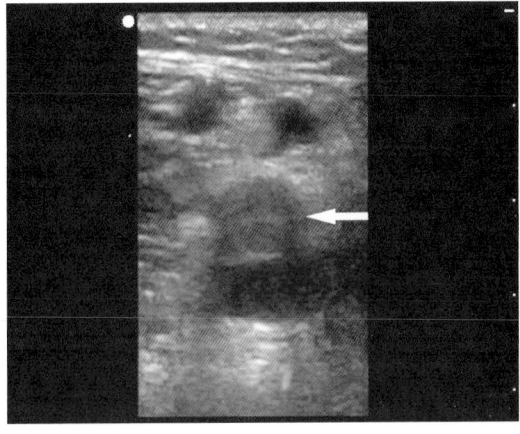

C

Figure 5-8. **C.** Right popliteal vein is noncompressible and contains echogenic clot (*arrow*).

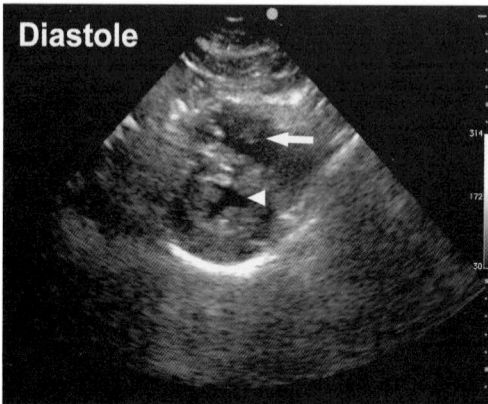

A

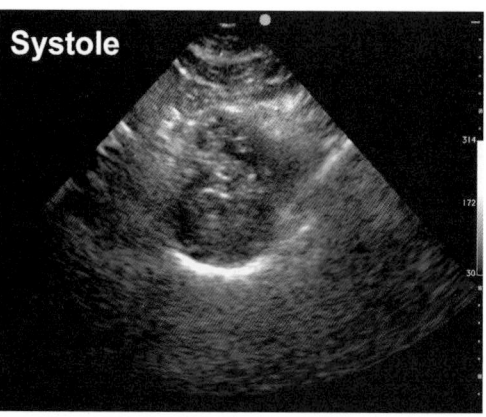

B

Figure 5-9. Underfilled hyperdynamic heart, parasternal short-axis views. **A.** The left ventricular chamber is very small at the end of diastole (*arrowhead*) and the right ventricular chamber is barely visible (*arrow*). **B.** The left ventricle and right ventricle are completely obliterated during systole, an accurate indicator of severe volume depletion. This patient presented in PEA from a ruptured abdominal aortic aneurysm.

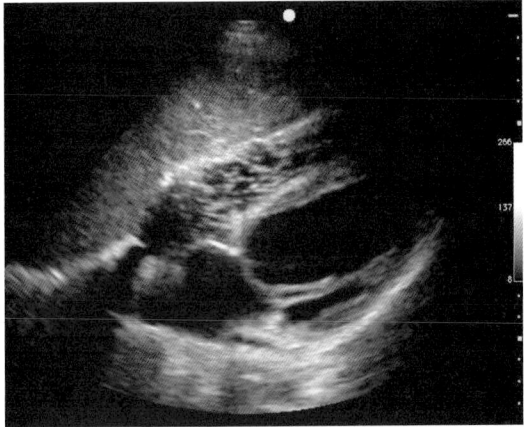

A

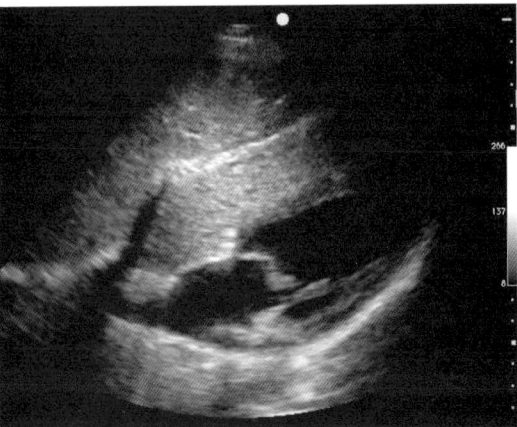

B

Figure 5-10. Cardiac bubble test to confirm IV location of central venous catheters—subcostal four-chamber view. Ten mL of sterile saline is rapidly injected into the catheter. **A.** Bubbles immediately begin to appear in the right ventricle. **B.** Then the right side of the heart becomes completely opacified.

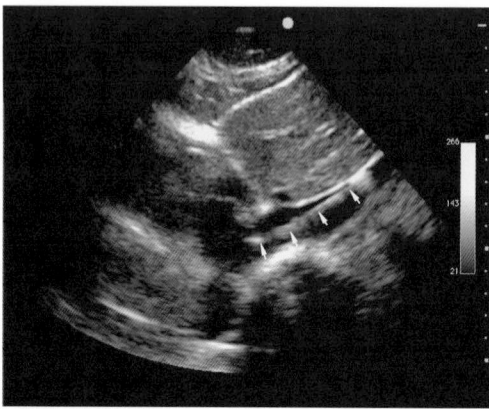

A

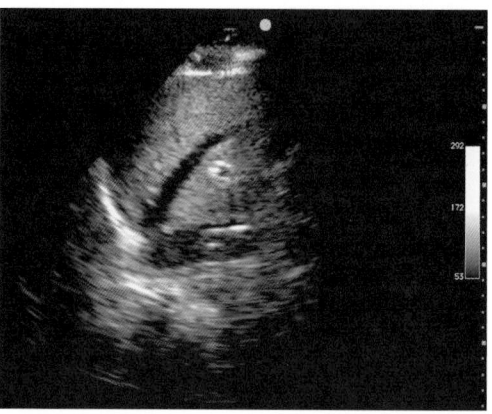

B

Figure 5-11. Visualization of guidewire in the IVC to predict proper placement of central venous catheters—longitudinal view of IVC in upper abdomen. This technique helps assure that the guidewire is in a vein and that the tip of the catheter will ultimately reside within the central venous circulation. **A.** The guidewire is clearly visualized (*arrows*) inside the IVC after insertion from the right internal jugular vein. **B.** In a separate case, the J-shaped tip of the guidewire is clearly visualized inside the IVC after insertion from the left femoral vein.

▶ PITFALLS

- Anchoring on one diagnosis too early and not completing a "whole body" ultrasound assessment in the critically ill patient.

- Failing to combine lung, cardiac, and IVC ultrasound exams to more thoroughly assess volume status.

- Relying on IVC imaging alone to assess volume status, as this can be misleading.

- Over-reliance of pulse checks in cardiac arrest cases.

For more detailed information go to the comprehensive textbook Ma and Mateer's Emergency Ultrasound, 3rd edition, Chapter 8, by Gavin Budhram, MD, Robert Reardon, MD, and David Plummer, MD.

CHAPTER 6
Abdominal Aortic Aneurysm

▶ CLINICAL CONSIDERATIONS

- Ruptured abdominal aortic aneurysms (AAAs) cause 30,000 deaths per year in the United States.
- A total of 30% to 60% are initially misdiagnosed.
- Patients often present with vague symptoms and normal vital signs.
- Rapid diagnosis after rupture decreases mortality.
- Diagnosis before rupture carries a much lower mortality.
- Bedside ultrasound is nearly 100% accurate for diagnosing AAA.

▶ CLINICAL INDICATIONS

- Patients older than age 50 years with abdominal, back, flank, or groin pain
- Unexplained hypotension, dizziness, or syncope
- Cardiac arrest
- Screening for AAA in patients at risk

▶ ANATOMIC CONSIDERATIONS

- The upper abdominal aorta is easier to visualize.
- The most common site of an AAA is the distal abdominal aorta.
- The proximal abdominal aorta contains anterior branches (Figure 6-1).
- The distal abdominal aorta bifurcates at the level of the umbilicus.
- Ultrasound windows must consider common bowel gas patterns (Figure 6-2).

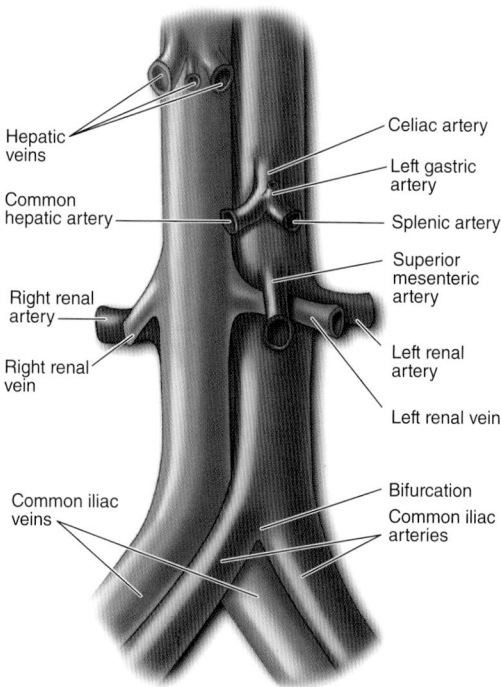

Figure 6-1. Branches of the abdominal aorta and inferior vena cava.

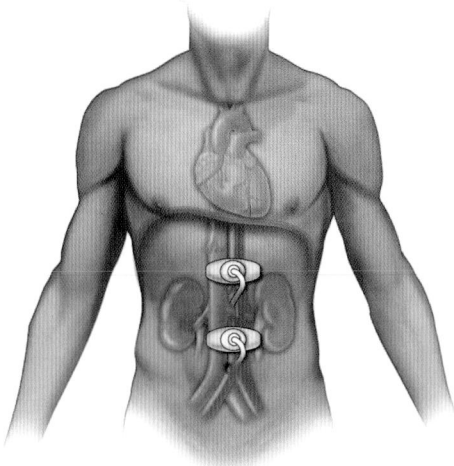

Figure 6-2. Ultrasound transducer positions for imaging the abdominal aorta. The length of the aorta can be imaged using sweeping views from these transducer positions. This can avoid potential interference from gas in the transverse colon.

▶ TECHNIQUE AND NORMAL FINDINGS

Transverse Views

- Start with the transverse plane in the upper abdominal aorta and the indicator aimed toward the patient's right (Figures 6-3 and 6-4).
- Move distally to visualize the entire abdominal aorta (Figure 6-5).
- Follow the aorta distally until it bifurcates (Figure 6-6).

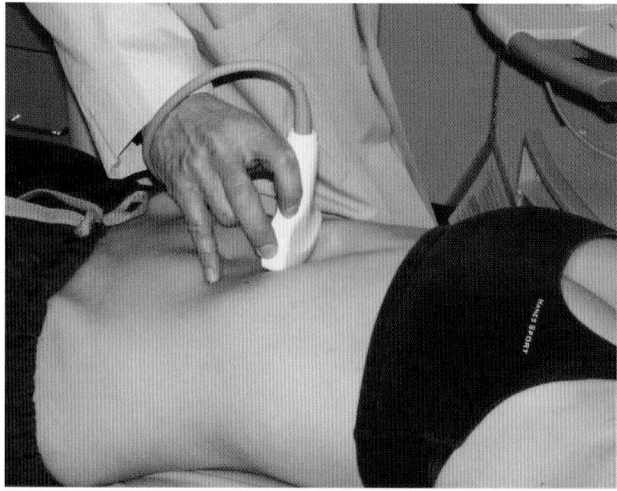

Figure 6-3. Initial transducer position for complete imaging of the abdominal aorta—transverse with indicator to the patient's right.

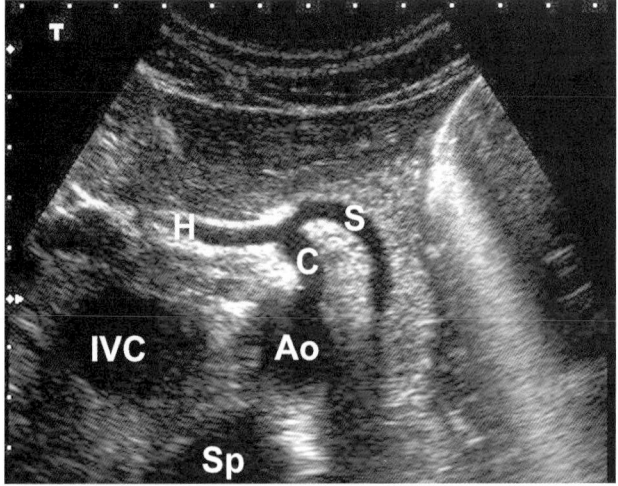

Figure 6-4. Transverse view of the upper aorta (at the level of the celiac trunk). By using a large convex probe in a thin patient, the relative positions of the anatomical landmarks can be visualized. The liver serves as an acoustic window to the structures below. The aorta and inferior vena cava (IVC) are immediately above the spine. Ao = aorta; C = celiac artery; H = hepatic artery; S = splenic artery; Sp = spine.

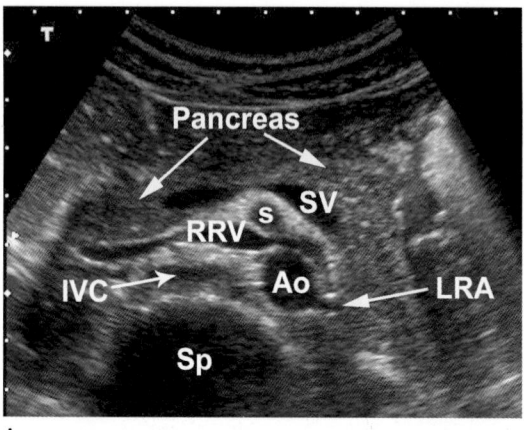

A

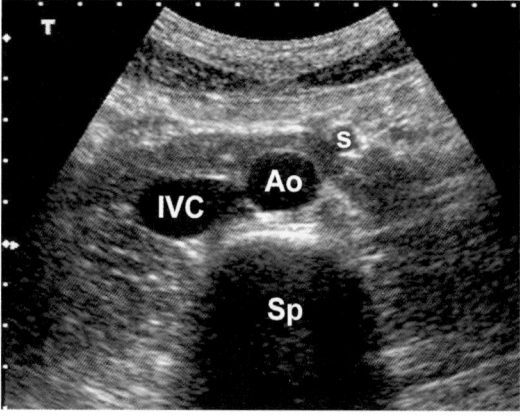

B

Figure 6-5. A. Transverse view of the middle portion of the abdominal aorta (at a level just below the branching point for the superior mesenteric artery [SMA]). **B.** Transverse view of the distal abdominal aorta (at a level above the bifurcation). Ao = aorta; IVC = inferior vena cava; LRA = left renal artery; RRV = right renal vein; s = superior mesenteric vein (or artery); Sp = spine; SV = splenic vein.

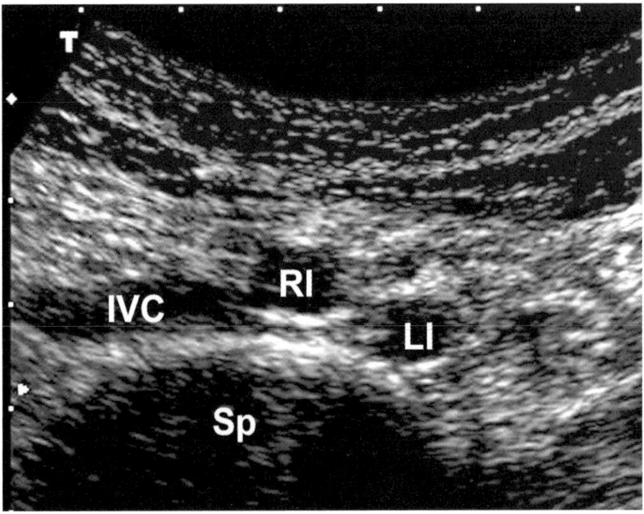

Figure 6-6. Transverse view of the bifurcation of the abdominal aorta. IVC = inferior vena cava; Ll = left iliac artery; Rl = right iliac artery; Sp = spine.

Longitudinal Views

- Start with the longitudinal plane in the upper aorta and the indicator aimed toward the patient's head (Figure 6-7).

- Tilt the probe from midline slightly toward the patient's left to visualize the aorta (Figure 6-8).

- Tilt the probe slightly toward the patient's right to visualize the inferior vena cava (IVC) (Figure 6-9).

- Move distally to visualize the entire abdominal aorta.

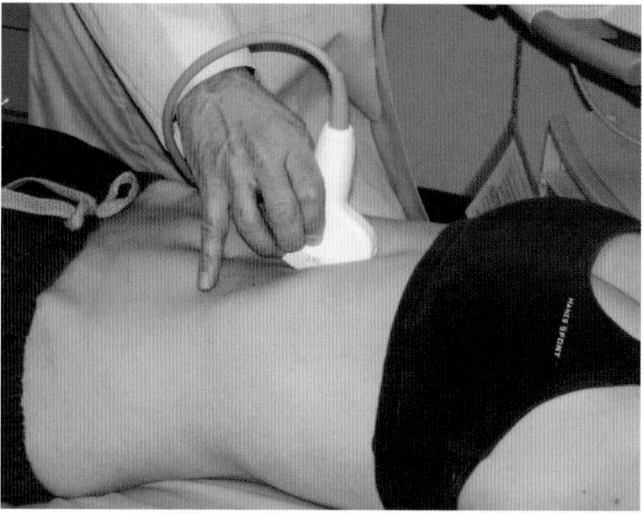

Figure 6-7. Transducer position for longitudinal views of the aorta. The indicator is cephalad.

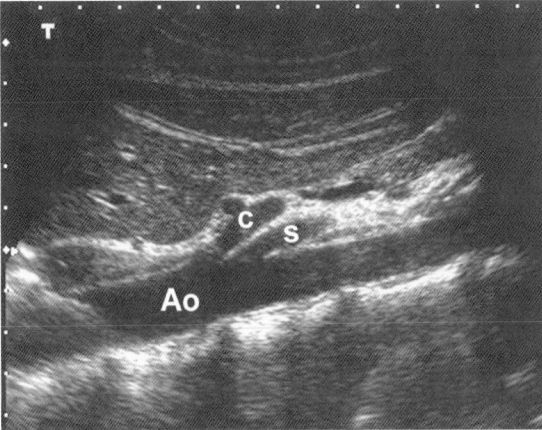

Figure 6-8. Longitudinal view of the abdominal aorta. The celiac artery (c) is the first vessel to branch off the aorta. The superior mesenteric artery (s) is immediately below the celiac artery and courses parallel to the aorta (Ao).

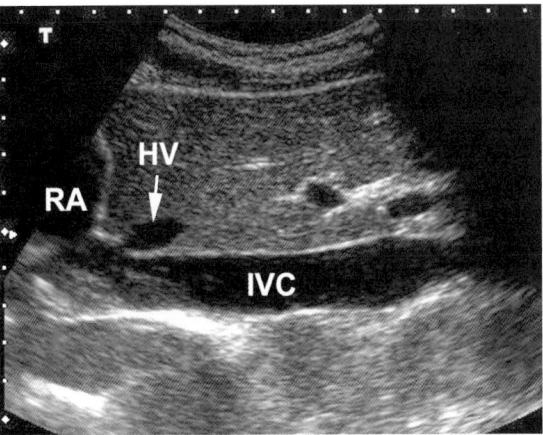

Figure 6-9. Longitudinal view of the inferior vena cava (IVC). HV = hepatic vein; RA = right atrium.

Coronal Views

- Use if the abdominal aorta cannot be visualized with midline anterior views.

- Start in the midaxillary line using the liver as an acoustic window (Figure 6-10).

- The aorta is visualized deep to the IVC (Figure 6-11).

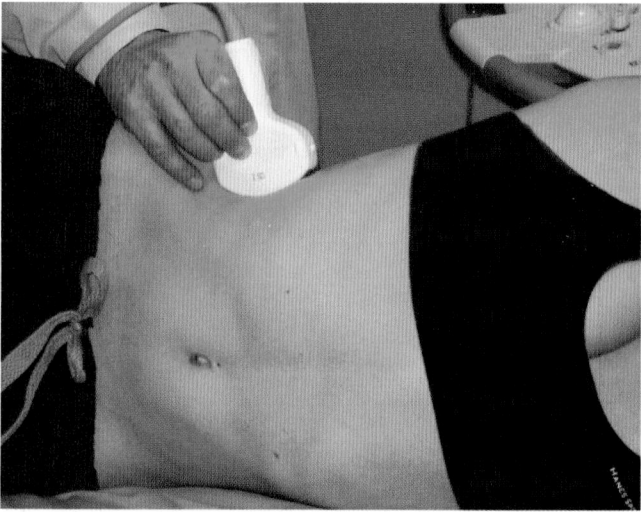

Figure 6-10. Transducer position for coronal views of the aorta. The indicator is cephalad.

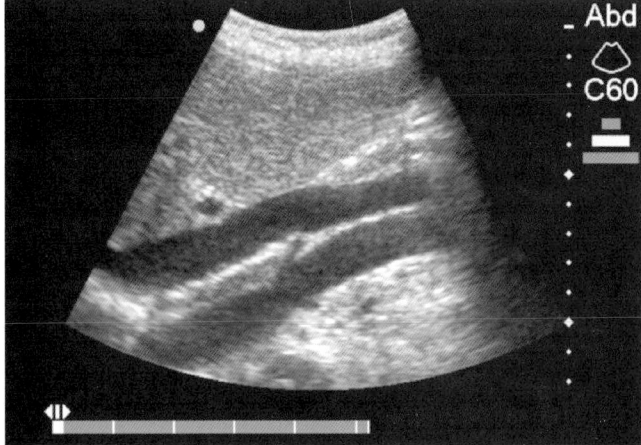

Figure 6-11. Coronal view of the aorta. The inferior vena cava is above the aorta in this right coronal view. Both renal arteries are seen branching off the aorta at a 45-degree angle (forming an arrowhead appearance in the mid aorta). The renal arteries are not routinely visualized in this view.

▶ TIPS TO IMPROVE IMAGE ACQUISITION

- Push firmly to move bowel and get the transducer closer to the aorta.
- Look for the spine as a landmark.
- Change probes or presets.
- Increase depth.
- Reposition the patient in the left lateral decubitus position.

▶ COMMON AND EMERGENT ABNORMALITIES

- Aneurysm of distal abdominal aorta (Figures 6-12 to 6-15)
- Iliac artery aneurysm and isolated proximal AAA (Figure 6-16)

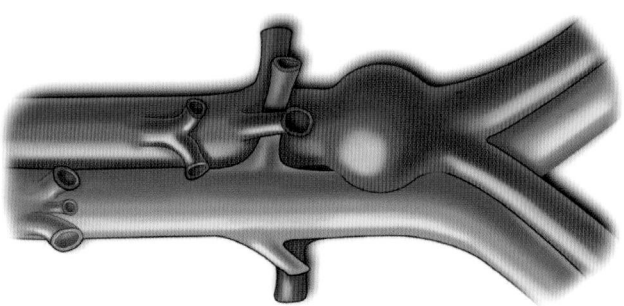

Figure 6-12. Fusiform aneurysm.

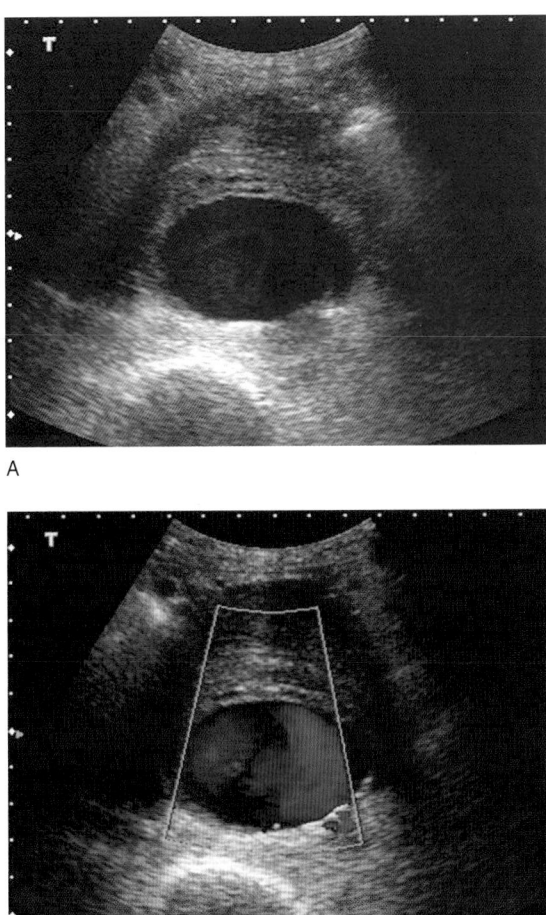

A

B

Figure 6-13. A 7-cm abdominal aortic aneurysm (AAA) with anterior mural thrombus. **A.** Transverse view. **B.** Color Doppler confirms that this is a vascular structure and that only the posterior portion of the dilated aorta is patent.

(Figure 6-13C continued on next page)

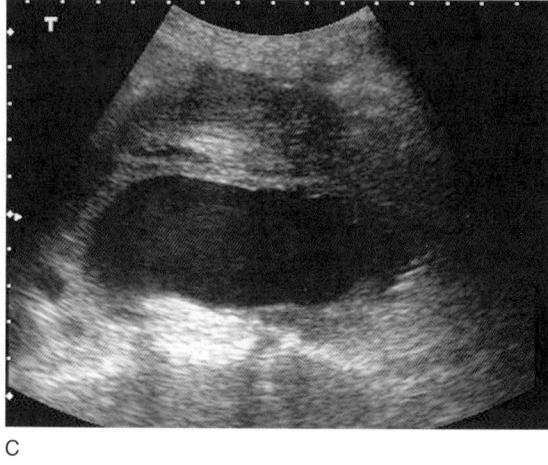

C

Figure 6-13. C. Longitudinal view of the same 7-cm AAA with anterior mural thrombus.

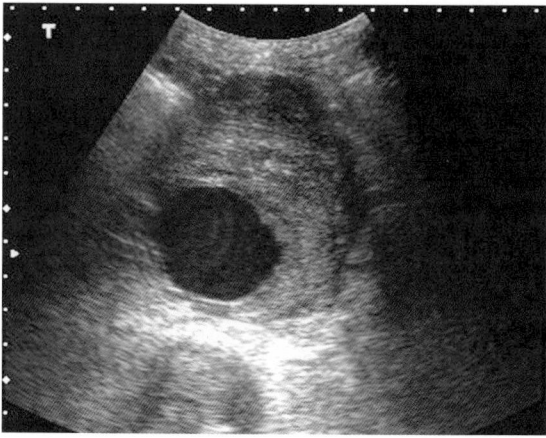

Figure 6-14. A 7-cm abdominal aortic aneurysm with anterior and lateral mural thrombus. Transverse view.

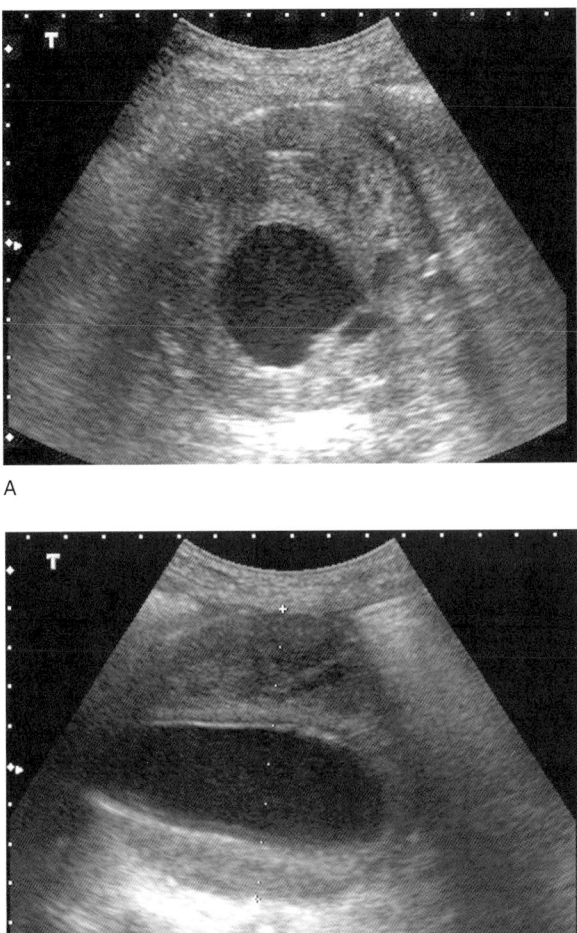

A

B

Figure 6-15. An 8-cm abdominal aortic aneurysm with circum-ferential mural thrombus. **A.** Transverse view. **B.** Longitudinal view.

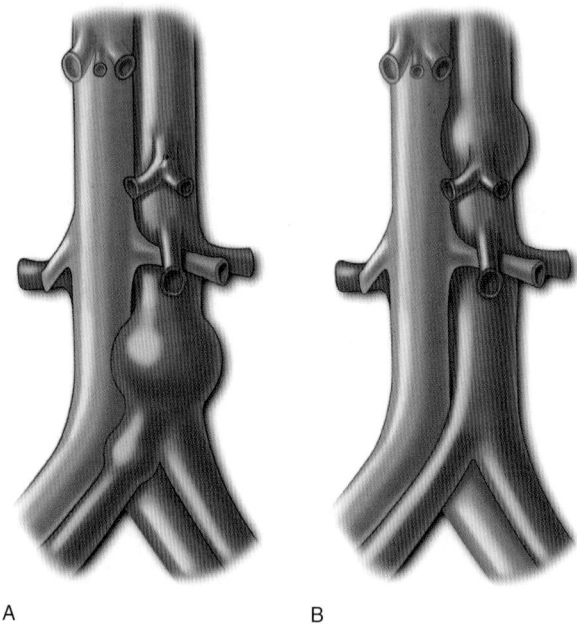

A   B

Figure 6-16. (**A**) Iliac artery aneurysm. A fusiform AAA with extension into the right common iliac artery is illustrated. (**B**) Isolated proximal AAA (uncommon).

▶ ADDITIONAL FINDINGS

- Blood in Morison's pouch from free rupture (Figure 6-17)
- Aortic dissection (Figure 6-18)

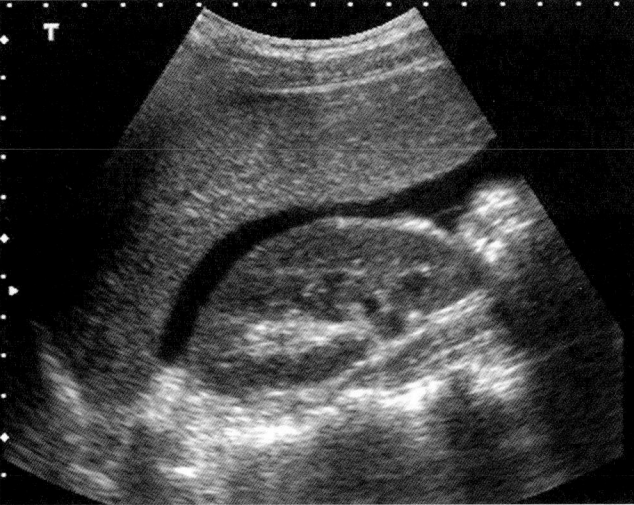

Figure 6-17. Hemoperitoneum—blood in Morison's pouch. This is unusual and is a bad sign. Bleeding is usually contained in the retroperitoneal space in patients who live after a ruptured abdominal aortic aneurysm.

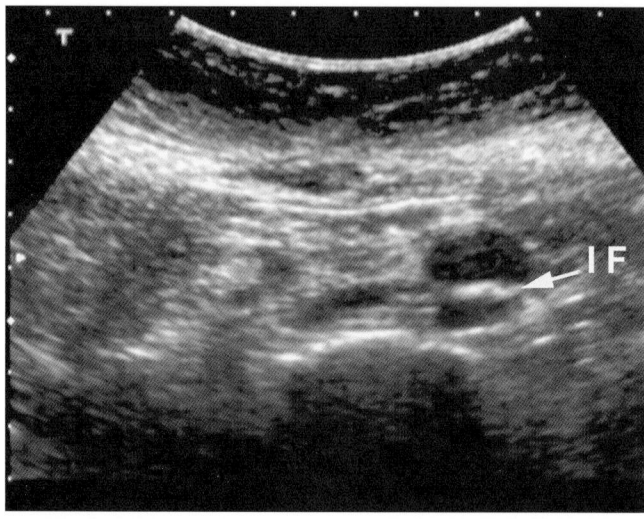

A

Figure 6-18. Acute abdominal aortic dissection. **A.** Transverse view showing intimal flap (IF).

(Figure 6-18B continued on next page)

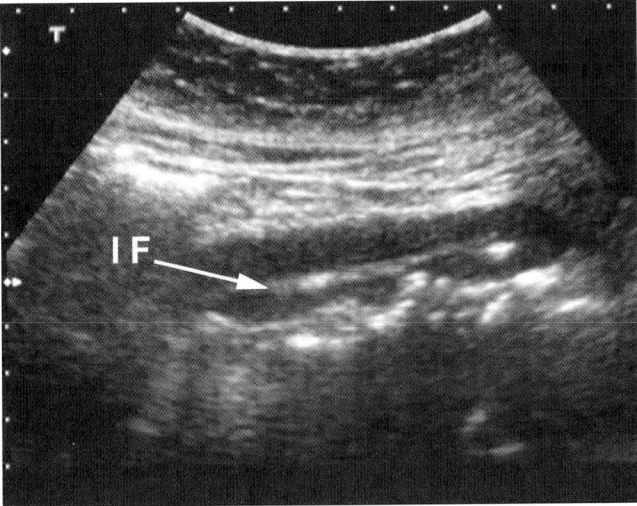

B

Figure 6-18. Abdominal aortic dissection. **B.** Longitudinal view showing intimate flap (IF).

▶ PITFALLS

- Poor quality images because of excess bowel gas or obesity.
- Confusing the aorta and IVC.
- Confusing the spine shadow with an AAA.
- AAAs usually rupture into the retroperitoneal space (not the intraperitoneal space), so the actual hemorrhage is not detected with ultrasound.
- Not imaging the aorta because another diagnosis is thought to be more likely (i.e., renal colic, inguinal hernia, or musculoskeletal back pain).
- Not pushing firmly enough or allowing time for bowel gas to dissipate.

For more detailed information go to the comprehensive textbook Ma and Mateer's Emergency Ultrasound, 3rd edition, Chapter 9 "Abdominal Aortic Aneurysm" by Robert Reardon, MD, Michelle Clinton, MD, Frank Madore, MD and Thomas Cook, MD.

CHAPTER 7
Hepatobiliary

▶ CLINICAL CONSIDERATIONS

- Hepatobiliary disease is very common in emergency and acute care settings.
- Ultrasound is the best initial diagnostic test for cholelithiasis, cholecystitis, and biliary obstruction.
- Several studies demonstrate that emergency physicians can acquire and interpret biliary ultrasound images with skill similar to traditional imaging providers.

▶ CLINICAL INDICATIONS

- Gallstones and biliary colic
- Acute cholecystitis
- Jaundice and biliary duct dilatation
- Abdominal sepsis
- Ascites
- Hepatic abnormalities

▶ ANATOMIC CONSIDERATIONS

- The gallbladder is divided into the fundus, body, and neck.
- The gallbladder body is contiguous with the inferior surface of the liver and narrows at the neck.
- The portal vein (PV) enters the hepatic hilum adjacent to the gallbladder neck.
- The common hepatic duct exits the hepatic hilum and is joined by the cystic duct to form the common bile duct (CBD) (Figure 7-1).

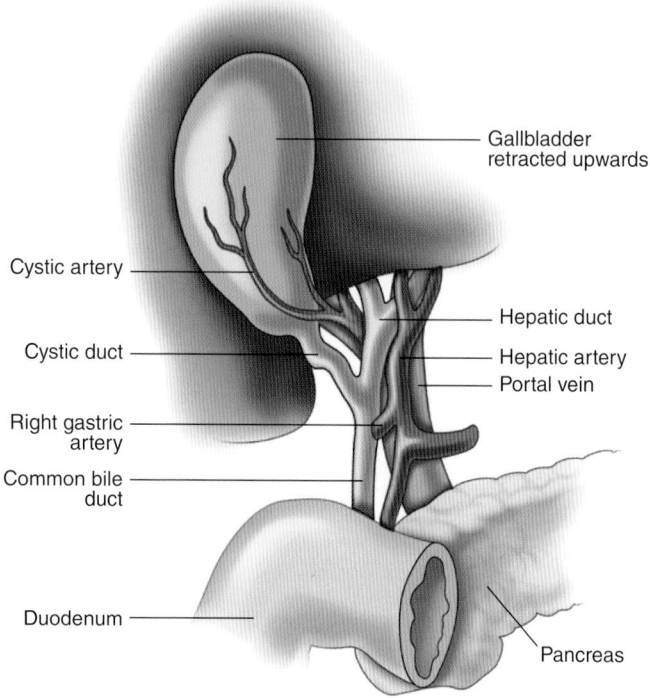

Figure 7-1. Normal anatomy. The diagram depicts the relationships in the porta hepatis. The triangle of Calot is bordered by the edge of the liver, the cystic duct, and the hepatic duct. (Redrawn from Schwartz et al. *Principles of Surgery,* 6th ed. New York, NY: McGraw-Hill, 1994:1368.)

▶ TECHNIQUE AND NORMAL FINDINGS

- The gallbladder can be scanned from the subcostal or intercostal approach.
- Proper patient positioning and breath-holding are important.
- Scan the gallbladder in two planes from the fundus to the neck and measure the anterior gallbladder wall (>3 mm is abnormal) and the CBD. A CBD internal diameter smaller than 7 mm is normal depending on the patient's age and cholecystectomy status.

Longitudinal Views of the Gallbladder

- Place the probe under the right costal margin in the midclavicular line with the indicator toward the patient's head. This usually provides a longitudinal or oblique image of the gallbladder (Figure 7-2).
- Rotate the probe as needed to obtain a true longitudinal image of the gallbladder.

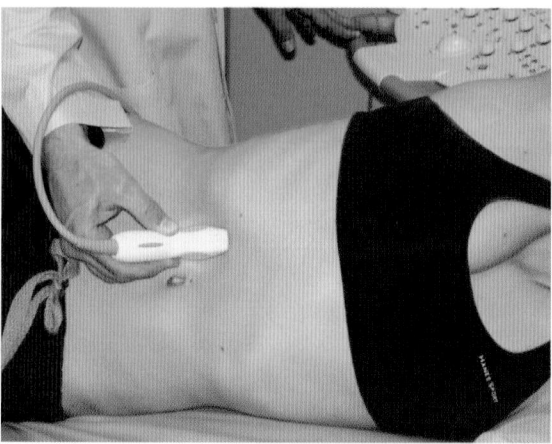

A

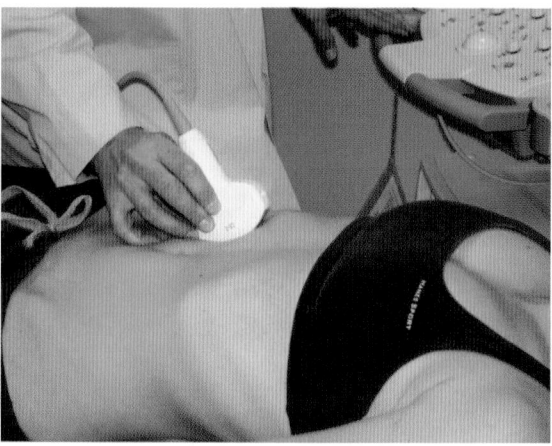

B

Figure 7-2. Longitudinal views of the gallbladder. **A.** Initial probe position with the patient in the lateral decubitus position. **B.** Initial probe position with the patient in the supine position. Gallbladder imaging is often facilitated with a deep inspiratory hold. The probe is angled cephalad under the rib margins.

(Figures 7-2C and D continued on next page)

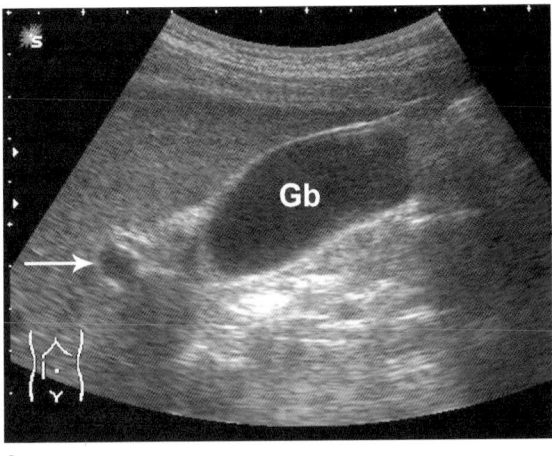

C

D

Figure 7-2. Longitudinal views of the gallbladder (Gb).
C. Corresponding ultrasound image with the portal vein indicated
(*arrow*). **D.** Color Doppler may assist in differentiating vascular
structures from the common bile duct and gallbladder.

Transverse Views of the Gallbladder

- From the longitudinal view, rotate the probe 90 degrees counterclockwise to obtain transverse images of the gallbladder (Figure 7-3).

- Scan through the entire gallbladder from the fundus to the neck in the transverse plane.

- Measure the anterior wall of the gallbladder and CBD.

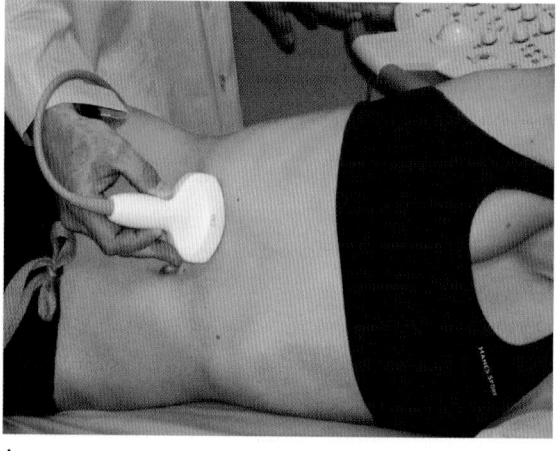

A

Figure 7-3. Transverse views of the gallbladder. **A.** Initial probe position with patient in the lateral decubitus position.

(Figures 7-3B and C continued on next page)

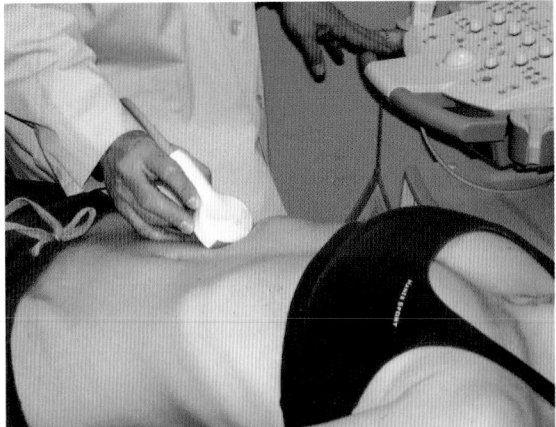

B

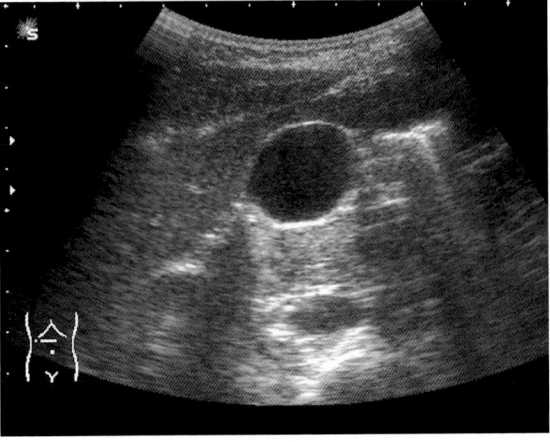

C

Figure 7-3. **B.** Initial probe position with patient in the supine position. Note the deep inspiration used and cephalad angulation of the probe to view under rib margins. **C.** Corresponding ultrasound image. Shadowing is from adjacent bowel gas outside the gallbladder.

Intercostal Views of the Gallbladder

- If subcostal imaging is difficult, consider intercostal views (Figure 7-4), which are helpful when the gallbladder is positioned under the ribs or the patient is unable to take or hold a deep breath.

- Position the transducer in the anterior axillary line in the lower rib interspaces.

- Start in the sagittal orientation with the indicator toward the patient's head.

- Rotate the transducer as needed to obtain longitudinal and transverse images of the entire gallbladder as above.

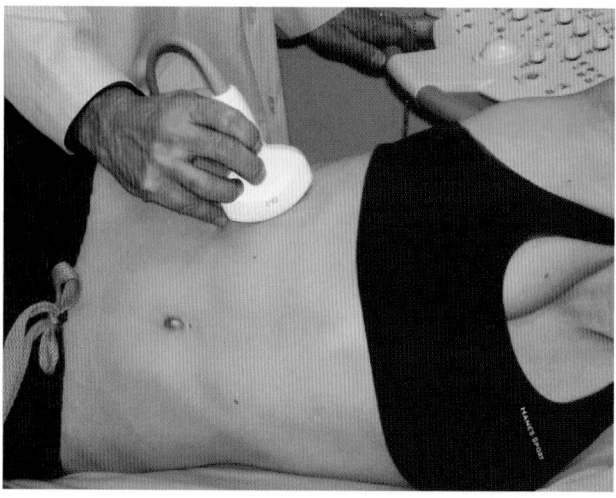

A

Figure 7-4. Intercostal views of the gallbladder. **A.** Initial probe position with the patient in the lateral decubitus position. The initial imaging plane is aligned parallel to the ribs.

(Figure 7-4B continued on next page)

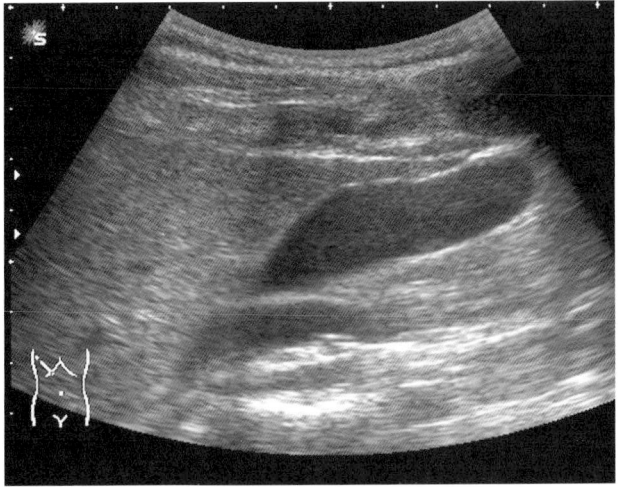

B

Figure 7-4. Intercostal view of the gallbladder. **B.** Corresponding ultrasound image. A small segment of the portal vein is seen below the neck of the gallbladder.

Imaging of the Main Portal Triad

- The main portal triad consists of the main PV, hepatic artery, and CBD.

- Identify the longitudinal axis of the PV. This varies in each patient and lies somewhere between the sagittal and transverse planes (Figure 7-5A).

- Rotate the probe 90 degrees counterclockwise from the longitudinal axis to obtain a transverse image of the PV, CBD (anterior/lateral to the PV on the image), and the hepatic artery (anterior/medial to the PV on the image) (Figures 7-5B and 7-6).

- Differentiate the duct from the artery and vein using color Doppler if needed (Figure 7-7).

- Measurement of the CBD is made from inner wall to inner wall. A normal CBD is smaller than 7 mm.

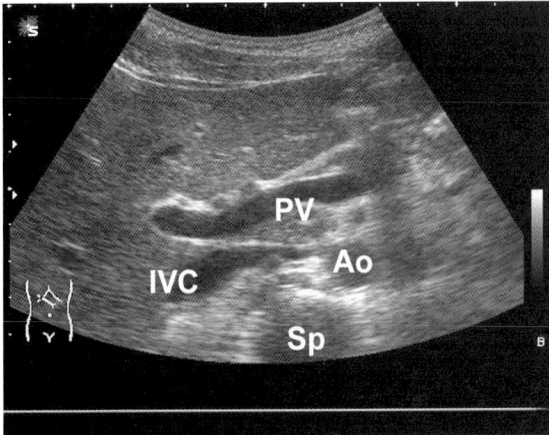

Figure 7-5. Portal vein and normal common bile duct.
A. Longitudinal view of the portal vein (PV). Ao = aorta; IVC = inferior vena cava; Sp = spine. **B.** Transverse view of the portal vein (PV). Gb = gallbladder; CBD = common bile duct; IVC = inferior vena cava.

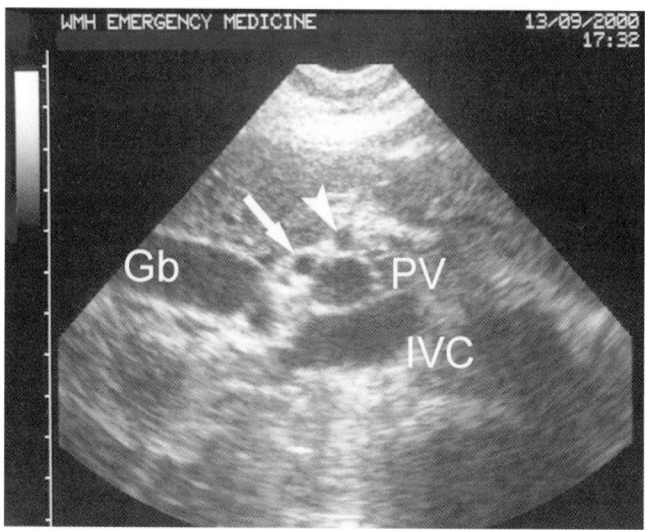

Figure 7-6. Short-axis view of the portal vein (PV) with the associated common bile duct (anterior/lateral; *arrow*) and hepatic artery (anterior/medial; *arrowhead*). The relative positions of the gallbladder (Gb) and inferior vena cava (IVC) are noted.

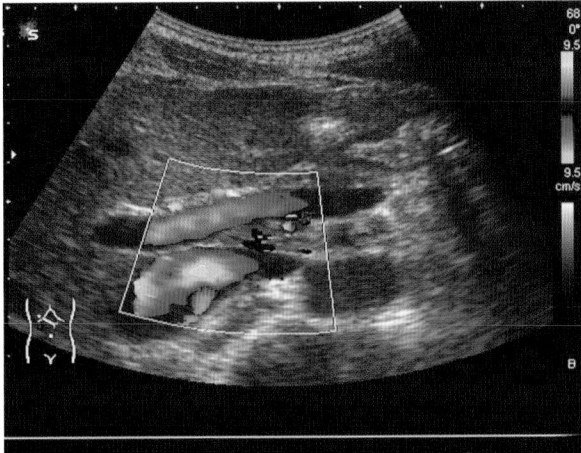

A

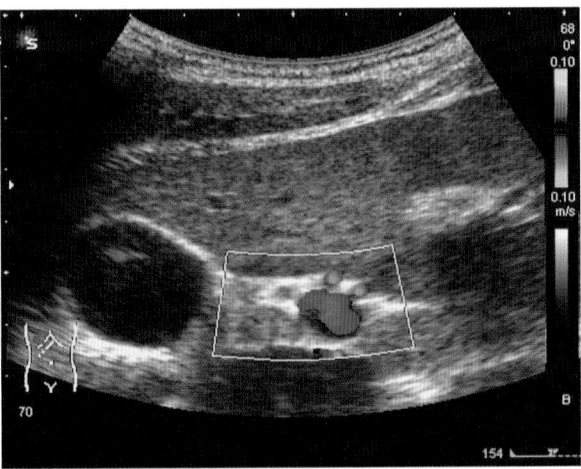

B

Figure 7-7. **A.** Longitudinal color Doppler image of the portal triad above the IVC. **B.** Transverse image showing color flow in the portal vein and duplicated hepatic artery. The CBD is identified by the lack of color flow.

► TIPS TO IMPROVE IMAGE ACQUISITION

- Patient positioning: The left lateral decubitus position is usually best.
- Patient breathing: A deep inspiration will move the gallbladder down closer to the transducer in the subcostal position.
- To help visualize a contracted gallbladder, find the longitudinal axis of the main PV and follow it to the hepatic hilum, where it exits the liver adjacent to the neck of the gallbladder (Figure 7-8).
- If there is difficulty imaging a contracted gallbladder, consider waiting a few hours to allow bile to reaccumulate and then repeating the ultrasound.
- To avoid missing mobile stones hiding in the gallbladder neck, move the patient into different positions during the exam so that gallstones will roll into the fundus.
- Understand that the gallbladder often varies in shape, size, and position of the fundus (Figures 7-9 to 7-11).

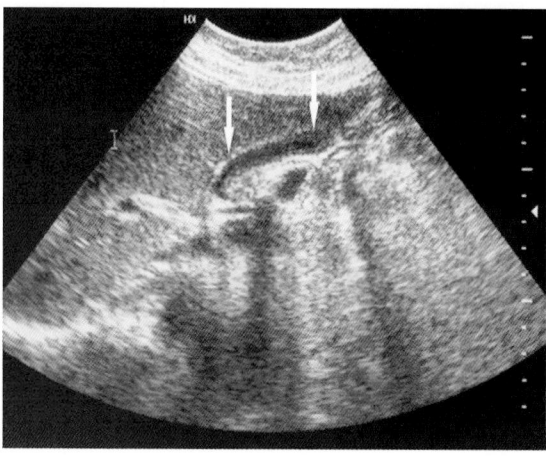

Figure 7-8. Contracted gallbladder. This can be difficult to detect (*arrows*) and may demonstrate a nonpathologically thickened wall. (Photo contributed by Lori Sens, Gulfcoast Ultrasound.)

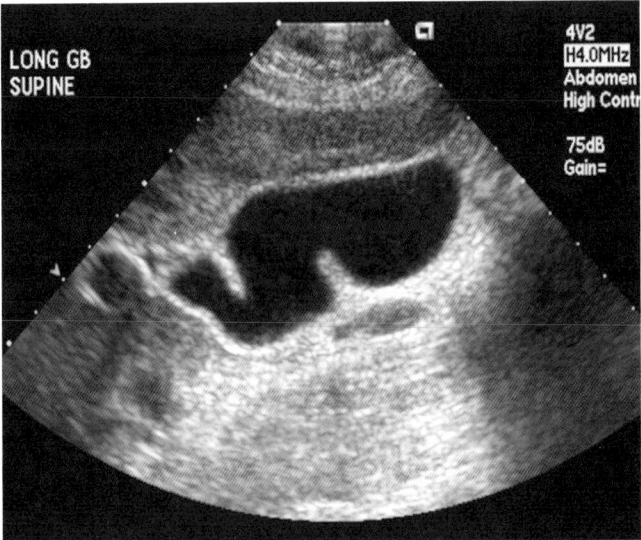

Figure 7-9. Longitudinal view of the gallbladder demonstrates nonshadowing mucosal folds on the midposterior wall and the anterior neck areas.

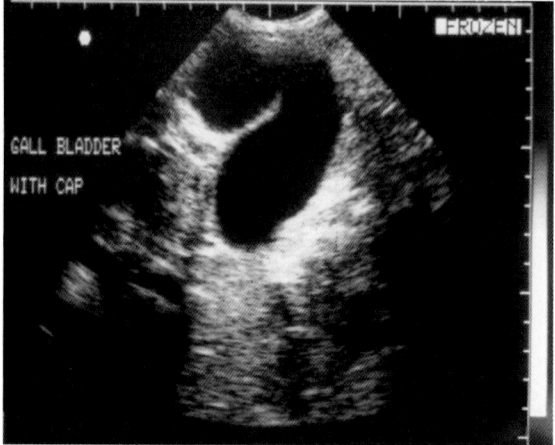

A

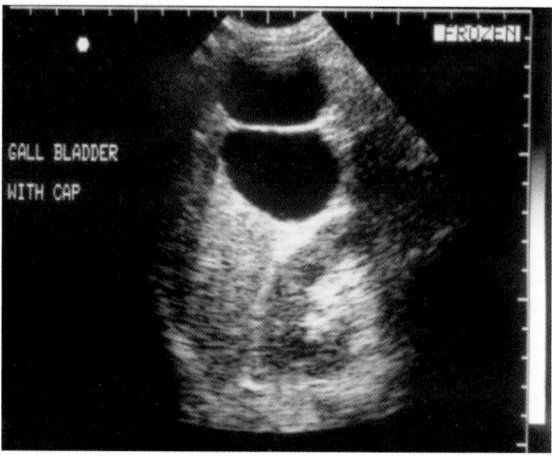

B

Figure 7-10. Phrygian cap. **A.** Longitudinal view demonstrates a folded gallbladder at the fundus. **B.** Transverse view of the same patient creates the illusion of a double gallbladder in this plane.

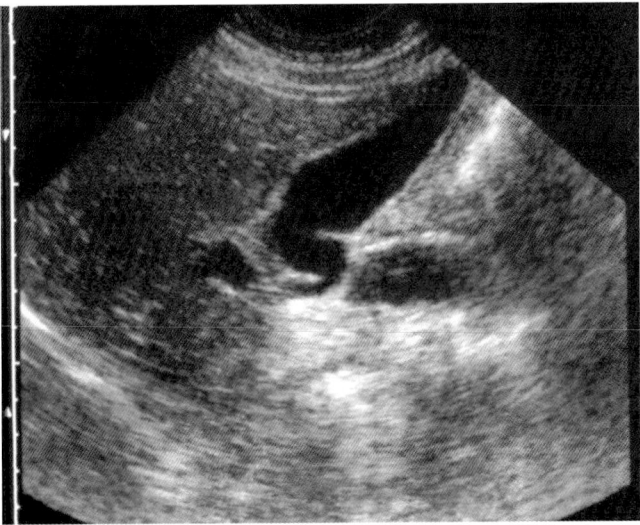

Figure 7-11. Hartman's pouch. Long-axis view of the gallbladder neck (Hartman's pouch) demonstrates the spiral valves of Heister. (Photo contributed by Lori Sens and Lori Green, Gulfcoast Ultrasound.)

► COMMON AND EMERGENT ABNORMALITIES

Cholelithiasis

See Figures 7-12 to 7-17.

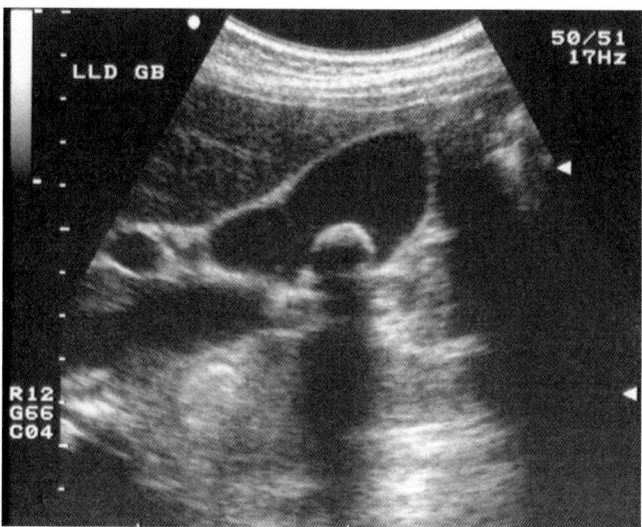

Figure 7-12. Longitudinal view of the gallbladder demonstrating a large solitary stone with prominent posterior acoustic shadowing. (Photo contributed by Lori Sens, Gulfcoast Ultrasound.)

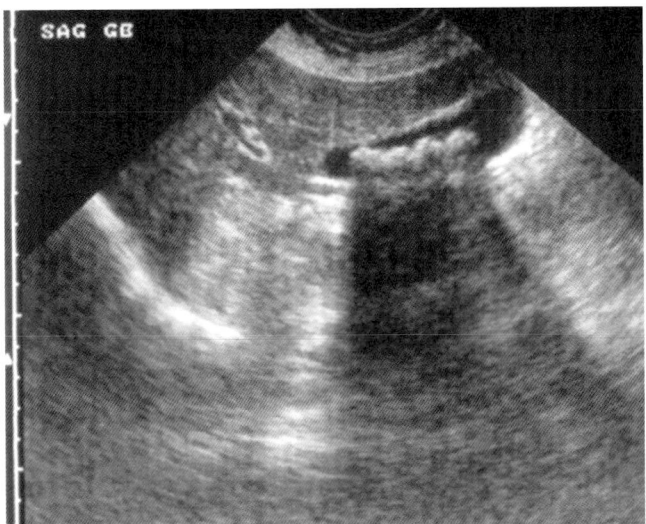

Figure 7-13. Longitudinal view of the gallbladder demonstrating multiple moderate-sized stones resembling "peas in a pod" also with prominent posterior acoustic shadowing. (Photo contributed by Lori Sens and Lori Green, Gulfcoast Ultrasound.)

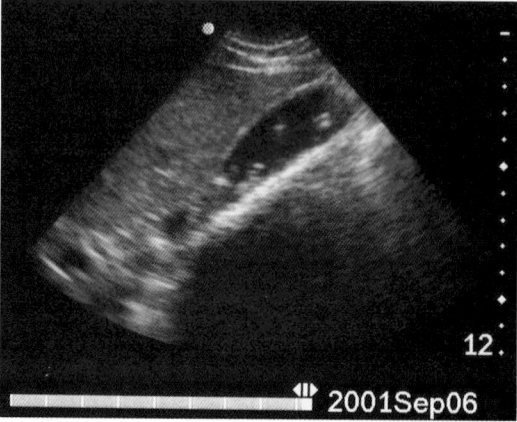

A

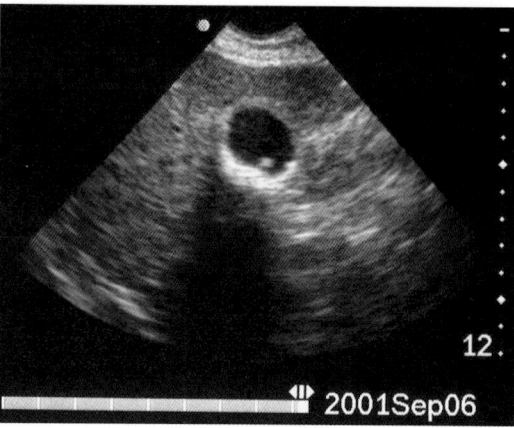

B

Figure 7-14. **A.** Longitudinal view of the gallbladder shows multiple polyps suspended inside the wall. The dense posterior shadowing is from multiple tiny stones (sand-like) layering along the posterior wall of the gallbladder. **B.** Transverse view. The posterior layering of the sand-like stones and the source of the shadowing are best appreciated in this view.

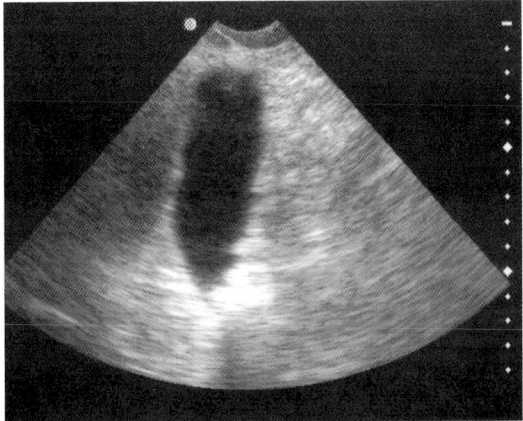

A

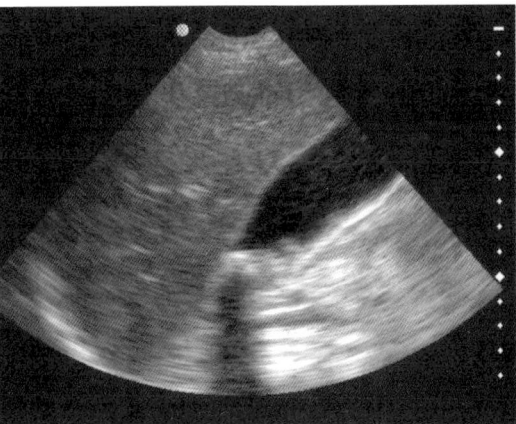

B

Figure 7-15. **A.** Longitudinal view with the probe positioned at the tip of the gallbladder. Cholelithiasis is not obvious. **B.** Intercostal oblique view of the same patient. The impacted stone in the gallbladder neck and prominent shadowing are more obvious in this view.

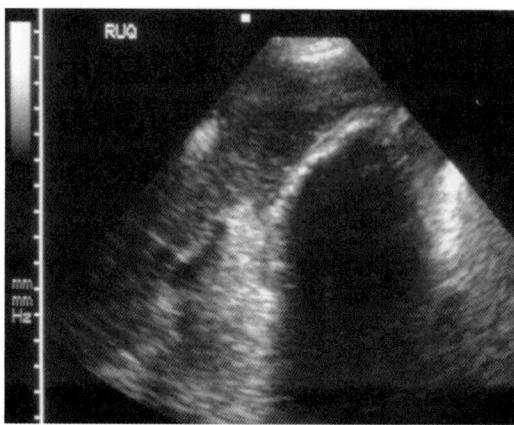

Figure 7-16. The wall echo shadow sign. Note the superficial echogenic line arising from the near wall of the gallbladder, an intervening anechoic stripe generated from bile when present, and a posterior brightly echogenic line representing stone material followed by a prominent posterior acoustic shadow.

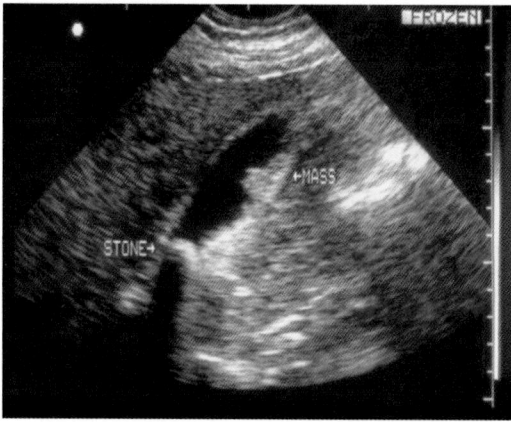

Figure 7-17. Tumefactive sludge. Dense polypoid sludge can be mistaken for a gallbladder wall tumor (*MASS*). The patient also has a stone impacted in the gallbladder neck (*STONE*).

Cholecystitis

See Figures 7-18 and 7-19.

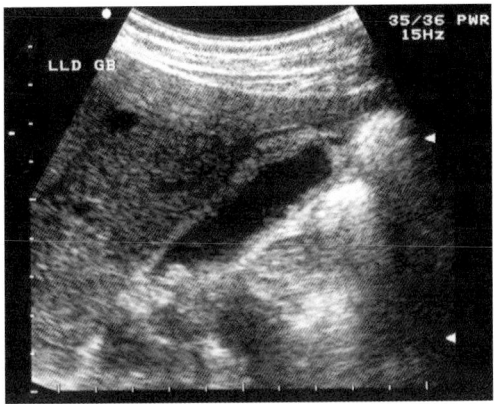

A

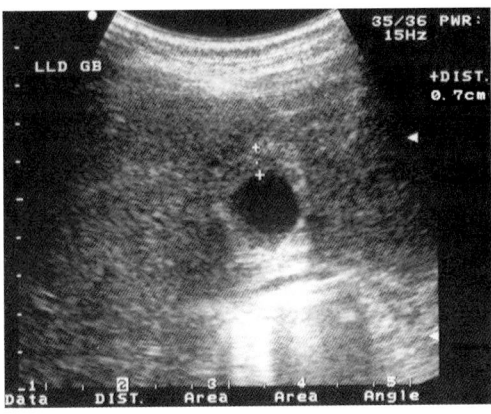

B

Figure 7-18. Cholecystitis. **A.** Longitudinal view of a gallbladder (Gb) with abnormal thickening of the wall. The bright echoes and shadowing below the Gb are from gas within the colon. **B.** Transverse view. Wall thickness measures 7 mm. (Photos contributed by Lori Sens, Gulfcoast Ultrasound.)

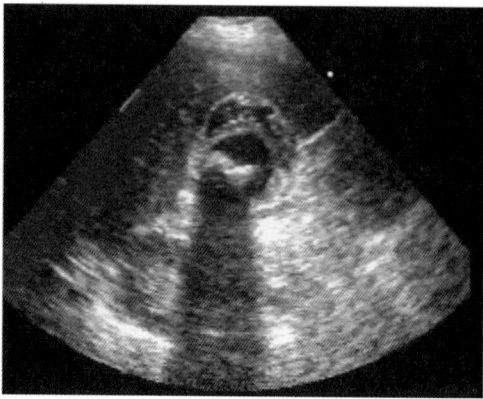

A

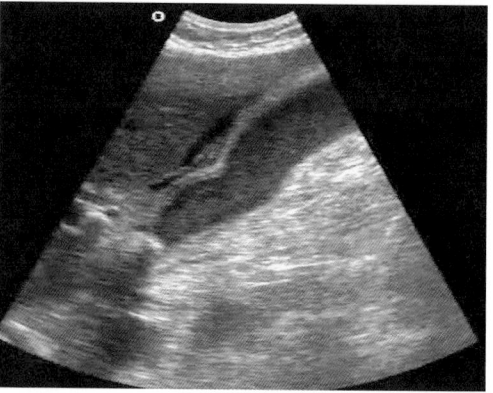

B

Figure 7-19. Cholecystitis. **A.** Transverse view of the gallbladder shows marked thickening of the anterior wall and associated edema separating the layers of the wall. Cholelithiasis with shadowing is obvious. **B.** Hemorrhagic cholecystitis. Internal echoes caused by bleeding from sloughing of the gallbladder mucosa. The wall of the gallbladder is thickened and may have a striated appearance. Note the shadowing stone lodged in the gallbladder neck.

Biliary Obstruction

See Figures 7-20 to 7-21.

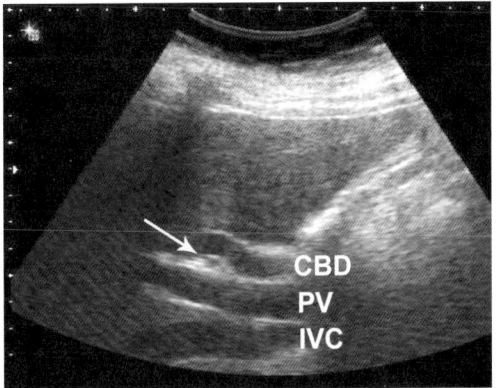

A

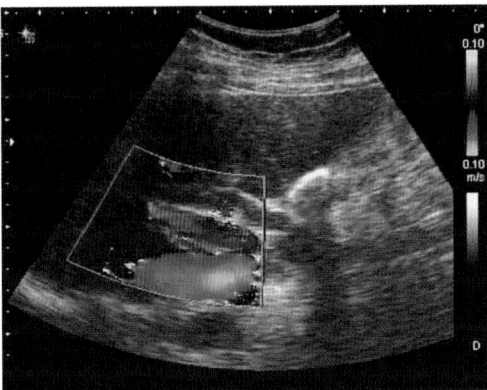

B

Figure 7-20. **A.** Dilated common bile duct (CBD) above the hepatic artery (*arrow*) and the portal vein (PV), producing an "olive sandwich" appearance. **B.** Color Doppler distinguishes structures with flow (PV, hepatic artery, and inferior vena cava [IVC]) from those without flow (dilated CBD).

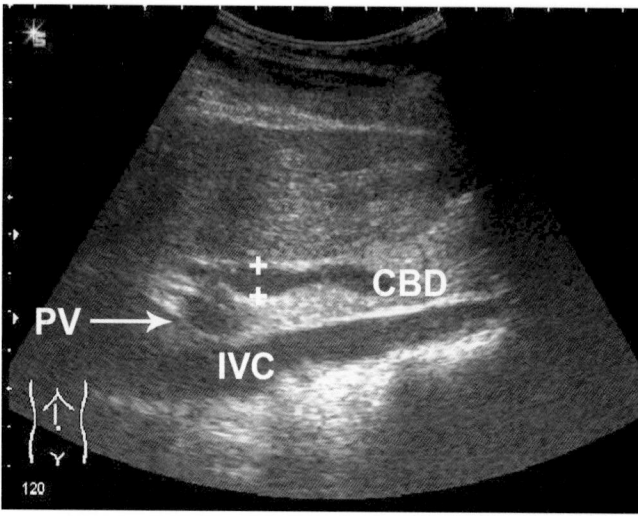

Figure 7-21. Choledocholithiasis. The common bile duct (CBD) of a patient with biliary colic measures 8 mm (*cursors*). A 4-mm stone was visualized in the distal CBD. IVC = inferior vena cava; PV = portal vein.

▶ ADDITIONAL FINDINGS

Liver Masses

See Figures 7-22 to 7-25.

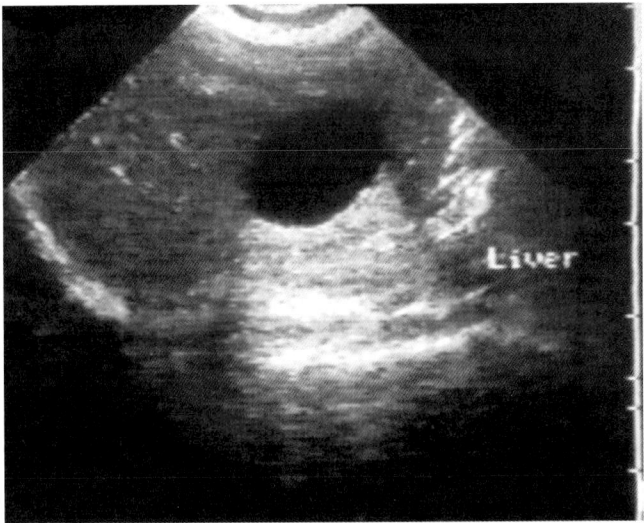

Figure 7-22. Liver cyst. Sharp margins, no internal echoes, and increased "through transmission" are demonstrated in this simple cyst of the right lobe of the liver. (Photo contributed by Lori Sens and Lori Green, Gulfcoast Ultrasound.)

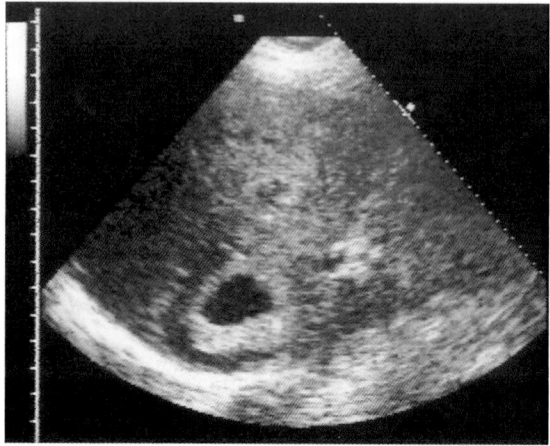

Figure 7-23. Liver abscess. An oblique view of the right lobe shows a fluid-filled cavity with thickened, poorly defined walls.

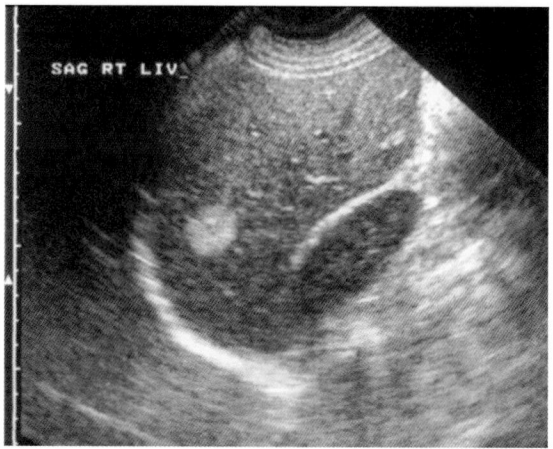

Figure 7-24. Hemangioma. Longitudinal view of the right lobe of the liver demonstrates the typical appearance. (Photo contributed by Lori Sens and Lori Green, Gulfcoast Ultrasound.)

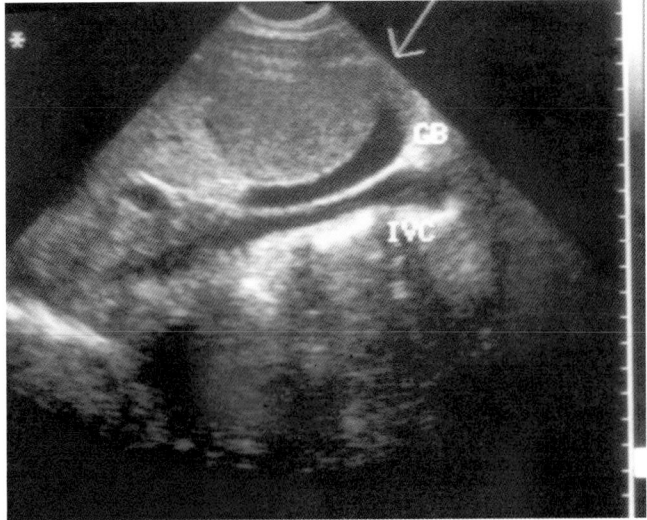

Figure 7-25. Hepatic adenoma. A hypoechoic mass (*arrow*) is seen compressing the gallbladder (Gb) in this long-axis view. IVC = inferior vena cava. (Photo contributed by Lori Sens and Lori Green, Gulfcoast Ultrasound.)

Other Common Abnormalities

See Figures 7-26 and 7-27.

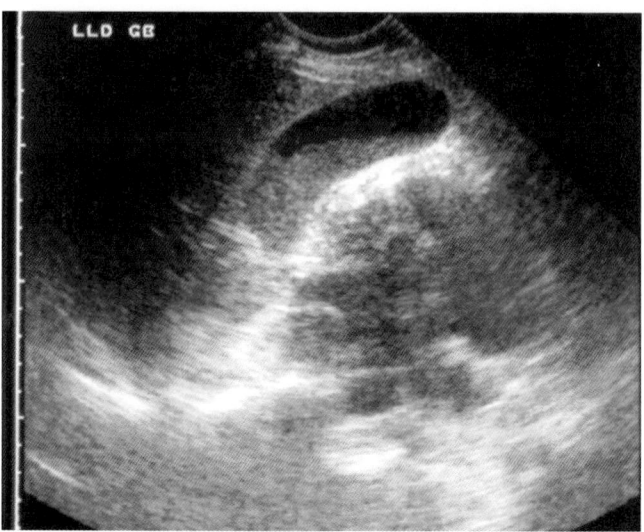

Figure 7-26. Biliary sludge is demonstrated as a dependent layer of nonshadowing midlevel echoes in this long-axis view of the gallbladder. (Photo contributed by Lori Sens and Lori Green, Gulfcoast Ultrasound.)

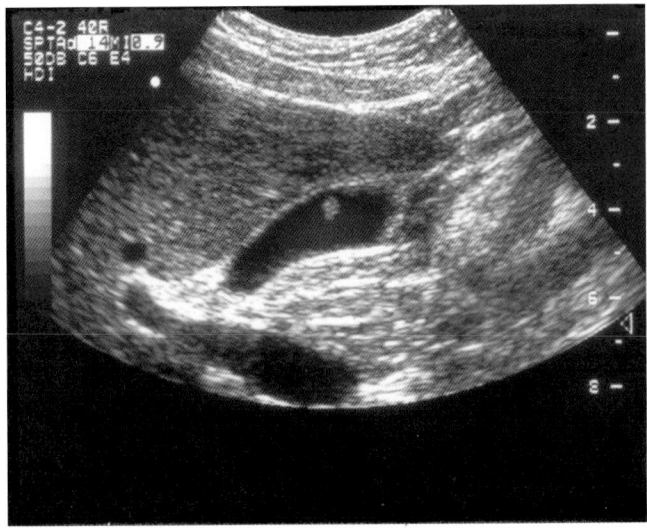

Figure 7-27. Longitudinal view of the gallbladder with a solitary small polyp attached to the anterior wall. There was no shadowing and no movement with patient positioning. (Photo contributed by Lori Sens and Lori Green, Gulfcoast Ultrasound.)

▶ PITFALLS

- Missing gallstones, especially in the gallbladder neck, usually because of inadequate patient positioning
- Misidentifying bowel as the gallbladder (confusing bowel with the wall echo shadow)
- Inadequate visualization of the gallbladder and ducts
- Confusion with shadowing, especially in the neck and at the periphery of the gallbladder
- Misdiagnosing cholecystitis in patients with ascites (Figure 7-28)
- Misidentifying shadowing from edge artifact as gallstones
- Neglecting to use color Doppler to differentiate ducts from vessels
- Missing cystic duct or common duct stones
- Misdiagnosis of biliary colic in patients with incidental cholelithiasis

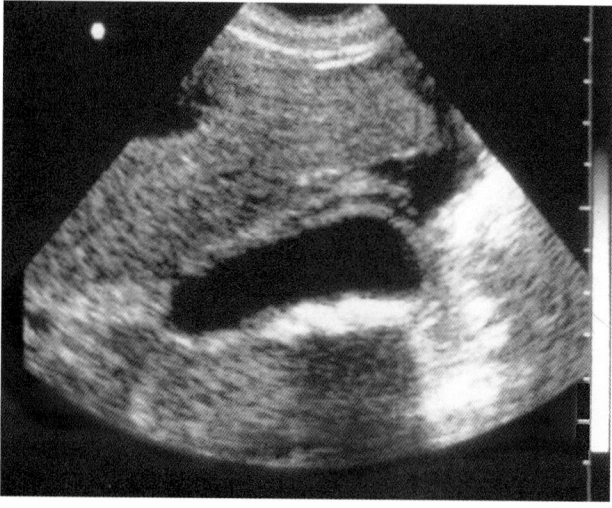

A

Figure 7-28. **A.** Long-axis view of the gallbladder shows typical ultrasound signs of cholecystitis: stones, a thickened wall, and pericholecystic fluid.

(Figure 7-28B continued on next page)

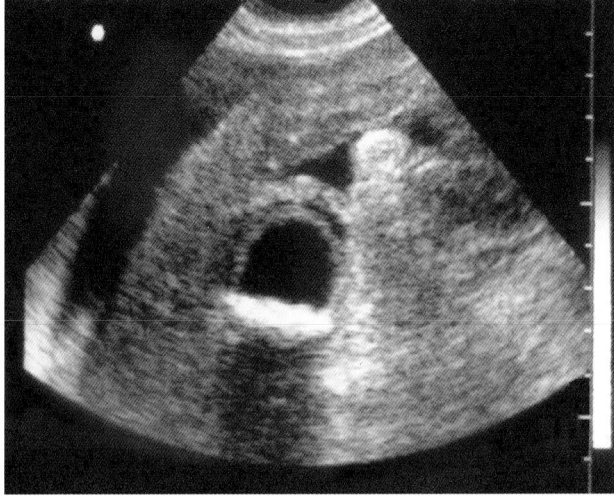

B

Figure 7-28. **B.** Transverse views of the same patient demonstrate ascites as the cause of wall thickening. The patient did not have cholecystitis on further clinical evaluation.

For more detailed information go to the comprehensive textbook Ma and Mateer's Emergency Ultrasound, 3rd edition, Chapter 10 "Hepatobiliary," by Resa Lewiss, MD and Daniel Theodore, MD.

CHAPTER 8
Renal

▶ CLINICAL CONSIDERATIONS

- The kidney and bladder are very accessible for sonography.
- The primary focus of renal ultrasound in the acute care setting is to identify hydronephrosis.
- Unilateral hydronephrosis in the setting of flank pain and hematuria is very sensitive for the presence of a ureteral stone.
- Severe hydronephrosis should prompt urgent consultation, close follow-up, and consideration of further work-up.

▶ CLINICAL INDICATIONS

- Acute flank pain or suspected renal colic
- Acute urinary retention and bladder size estimation
- Acute renal failure
- Acute pyelonephritis and renal abscess
- Possible renal mass
- Trauma

▶ ANATOMIC CONSIDERATIONS

- There is significant asymmetry in the position of the kidneys (Figure 8-1).
- The right kidney is inferior to the left kidney.
- The right kidney is easier to image because the liver is an excellent acoustic window.
- The kidneys are composed of the outer cortex, inner medulla, and renal sinus (Figure 8-2).

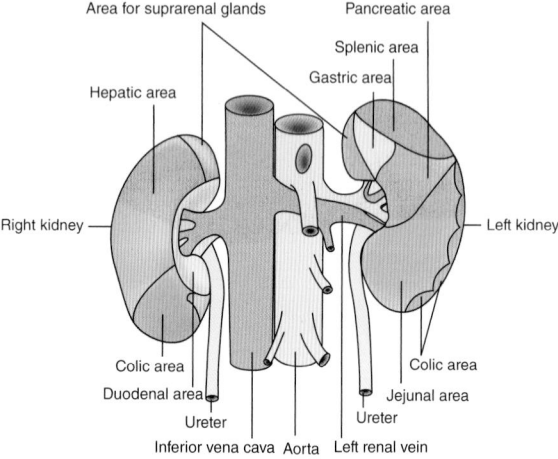

Figure 8-1. Anatomic relationship of the kidneys.

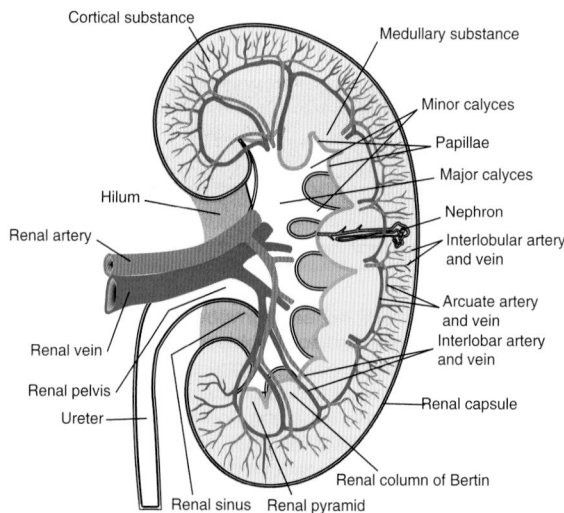

Figure 8-2. Gross anatomy of the kidney.

▶ TECHNIQUE AND NORMAL FINDINGS

Longitudinal View of the Right Kidney

- Place the probe in the subcostal or intercostal position (Figures 8-3 to 8-5).
- Images can be obtained from several different positions using the liver as a window.
- Point the indicator toward the patient's head or posterior axilla.

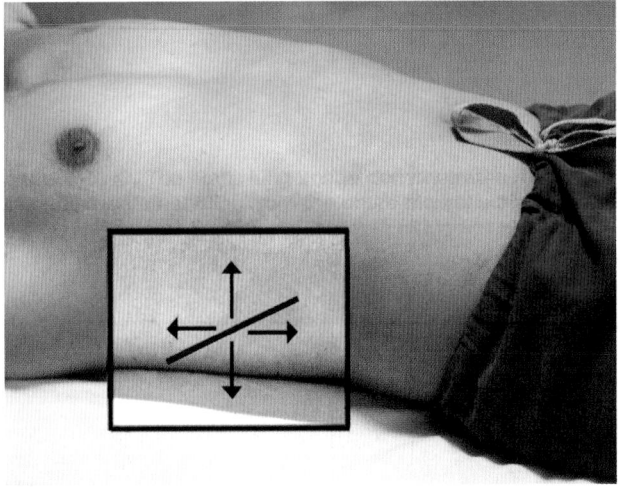

Figure 8-3. Transducer placement for imaging the right kidney. The *central line* represents the longitudinal axis of the kidney.

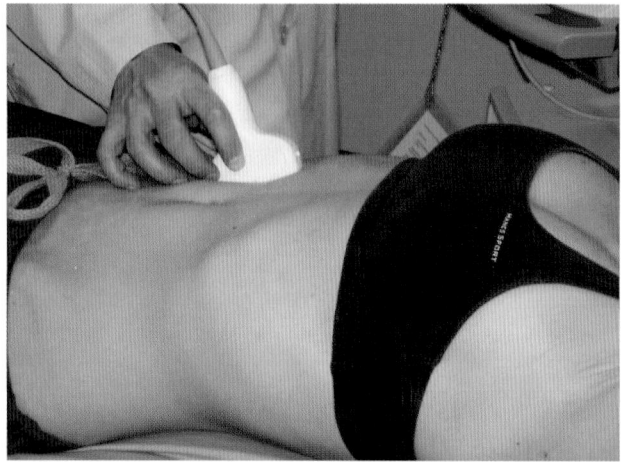

A

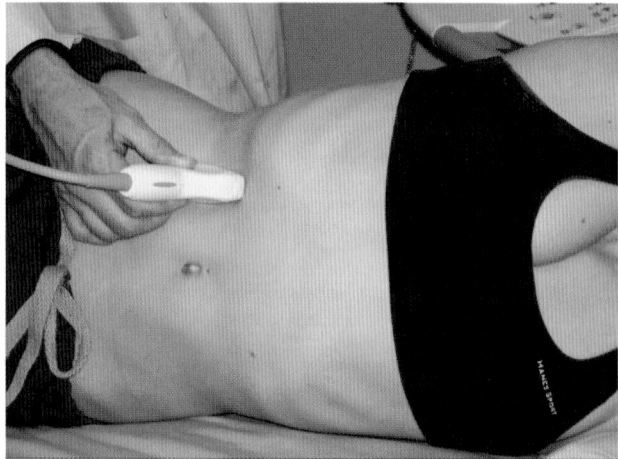

B

Figure 8-4. Subcostal longitudinal view of the normal right kidney. **A.** Probe position for a supine patient. **B.** Probe position for a patient in the left lateral decubitus position.

(Figure 8-4C continued on next page)

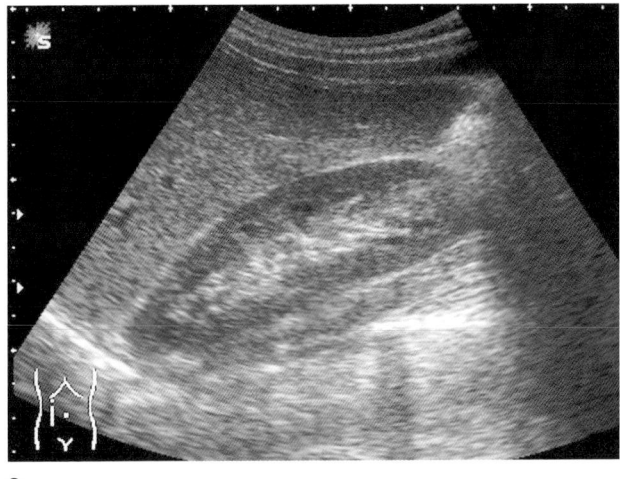

C

Figure 8-4. **C.** Corresponding ultrasound image. The model is holding a deep breath for improved kidney imaging.

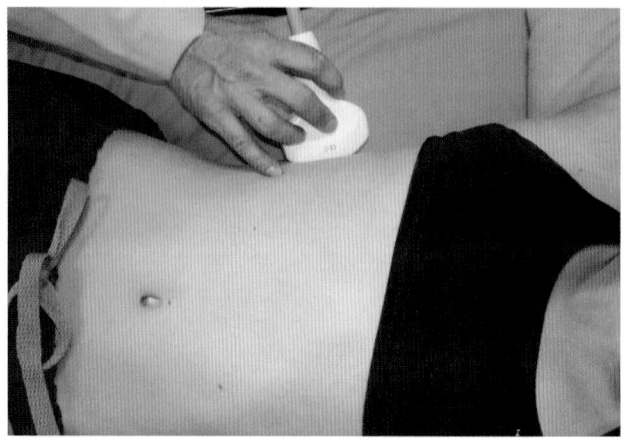

A

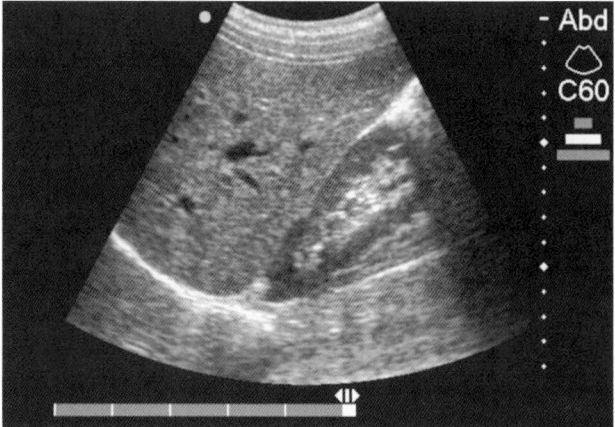

B

Figure 8-5. Intercostal oblique view of the normal right kidney.
A. Probe position. **B.** Corresponding longitudinal coronal
ultrasound image.

Transverse View of the Right Kidney

- Rotate the probe 90 degrees counterclockwise from the best longitudinal view (Figure 8-6).
- Sweep superiorly and inferiorly to obtain images of the entire kidney.

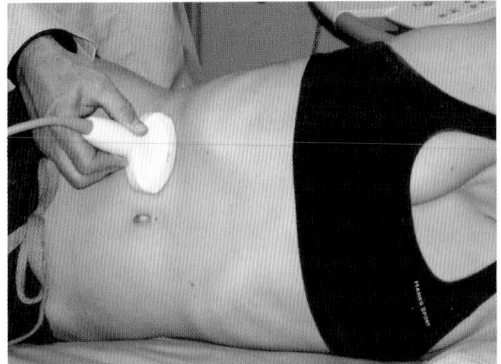

A

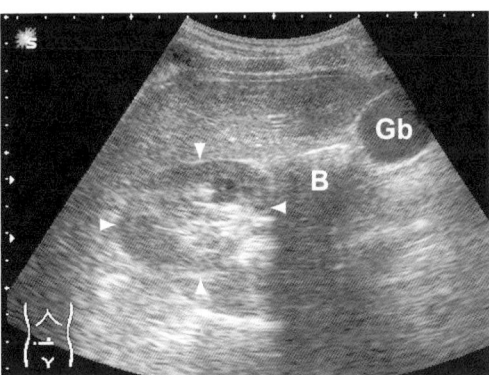

B

Figure 8-6. Transverse ultrasound view of the normal right kidney. **A.** Probe position. **B.** Corresponding ultrasound image with the kidney border outlined (*arrowheads*). B = bowel with posterior shadowing; Gb = gallbladder.

Longitudinal View of the Left Kidney

- Place the probe in an intercostal or posterior position (Figures 8-7 and 8-8).

- Point the indicator toward the posterior axilla.

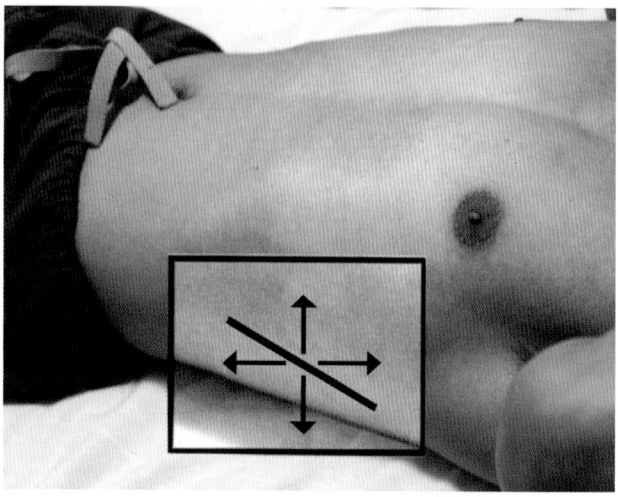

Figure 8-7. Transducer placement for imaging the left kidney. The *central line* represents the longitudinal axis of the kidney.

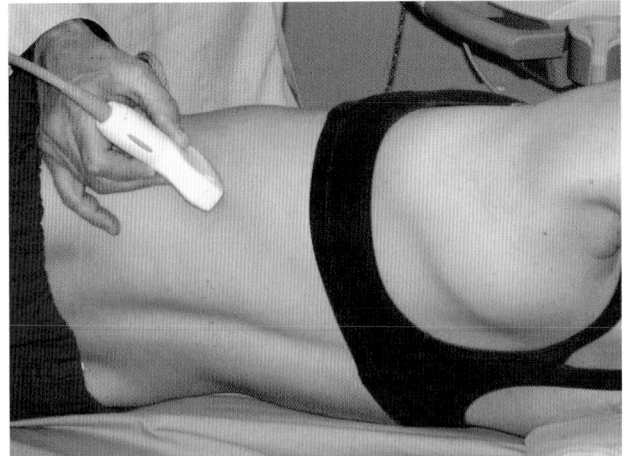

A

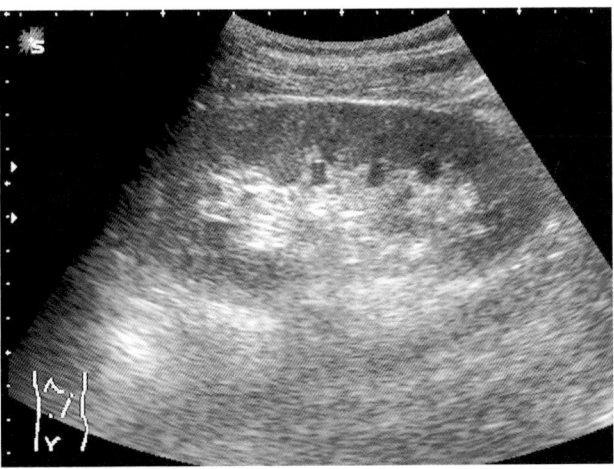

B

Figure 8-8. Intercostal oblique view of the normal left kidney.
A. Probe position. **B.** Corresponding longitudinal coronal
ultrasound image.

Transverse View of the Left Kidney

- Rotate the probe 90 degrees counterclockwise from the best longitudinal view (Figure 8-9).

- Sweep superiorly and inferiorly for images of the entire kidney.

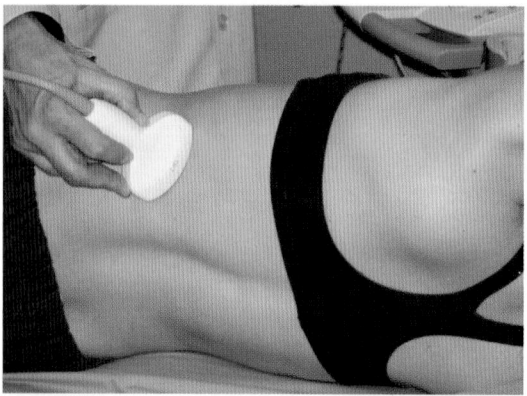

A

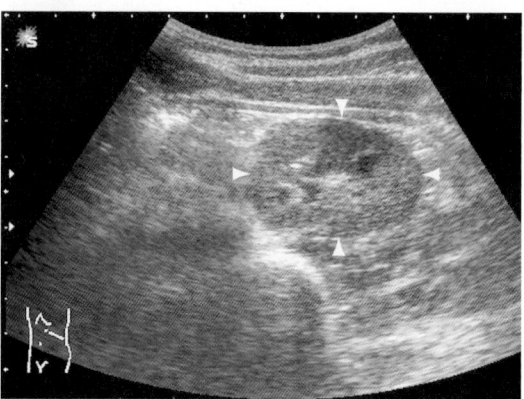

B

Figure 8-9. Transverse view of the normal left kidney. **A.** Probe position. **B.** Corresponding short-axis ultrasound image with the kidney border outlined (*arrowheads*).

Longitudinal View of the Bladder

- Probe placement is suprapubic in the anterior midline.
- Place the indicator toward the patient's head and angle the probe inferiorly.
- In females, the uterus lies posterior/cephalad to the bladder (Figure 8-10).
- In males, the prostate and seminal vesicles lie posterior/caudad to the bladder (Figure 8-11).

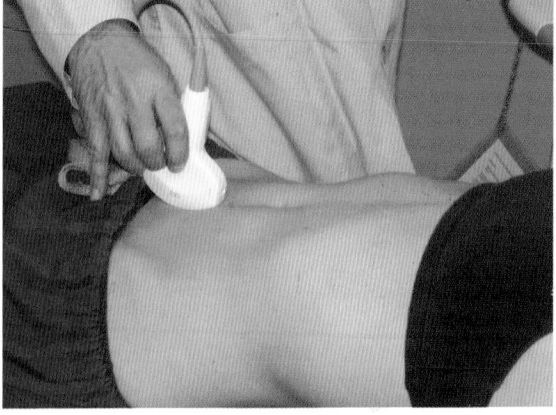

A

Figure 8-10. Normal filled urinary bladder. **A.** Longitudinal probe position.

(Figure 8-10B continued on next page)

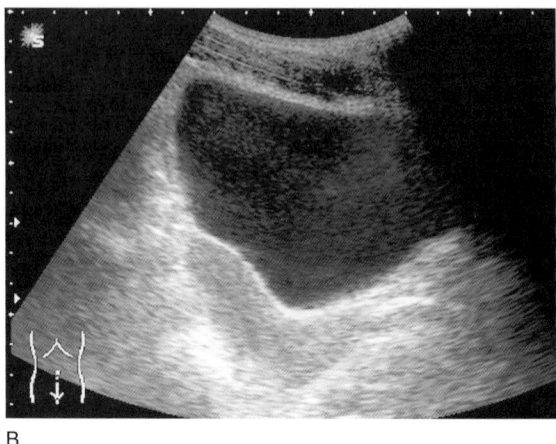

B

Figure 8-10. **B.** Long-axis ultrasound image of the bladder in a female. Note the uterus posterior to the bladder.

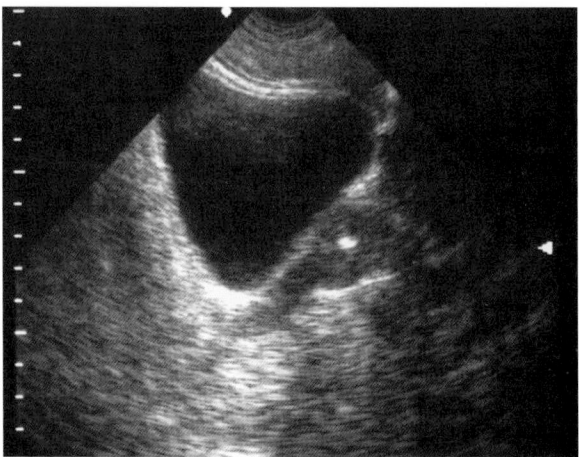

Figure 8-11. Longitudinal view of the male bladder reveals the prostate posteriorly, which contains a small central calcification.

Transverse View of the Bladder

- Rotate the probe 90 degrees counterclockwise from the longitudinal view (Figure 8-12).

- Position the probe just cephalad to the pubic bone and angle inferiorly.

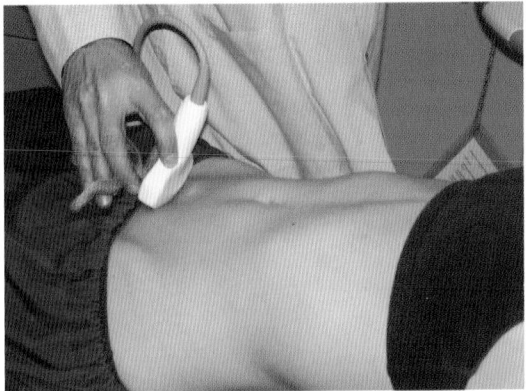

A

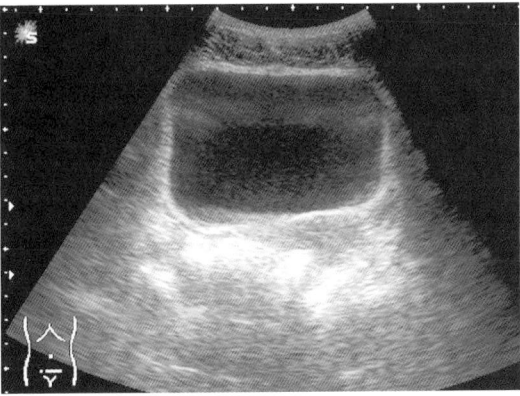

B

Figure 8-12. Normal filled urinary bladder. **A.** Transverse probe position. **B.** Short-axis ultrasound image of the bladder.

▶ TIPS TO IMPROVE IMAGE ACQUISITION

- Use the liver as a window when scanning the right kidney.
- Use a more posterior approach when scanning the left kidney.
- Place the patient in the right decubitus or left decubitus position if needed.
- Have the patient take a deep breath and hold it.
- Start with the longitudinal view when scanning the bladder.

▶ COMMON AND EMERGENT ABNORMALITIES

Obstructive Uropathy

See Figures 8-13 to 8-18.

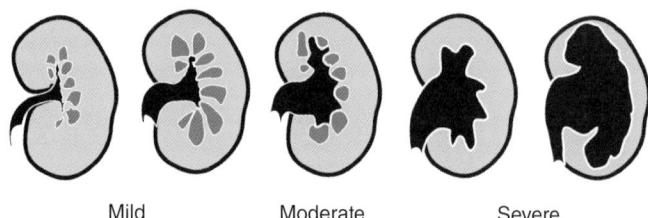

Mild   Moderate   Severe

Figure 8-13. Grades of hydronephrosis.

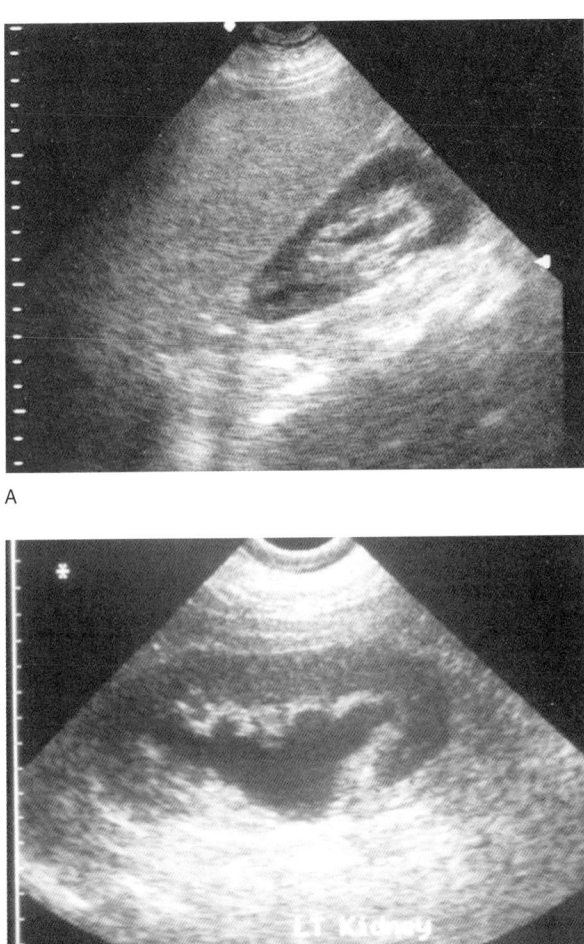

A

B

Figure 8-14. Long-axis ultrasound images of the stages of hydro-nephrosis. **A.** Mild hydronephrosis. **B.** Moderate hydronephrosis.

(Figure 8-14 C continued on next page)

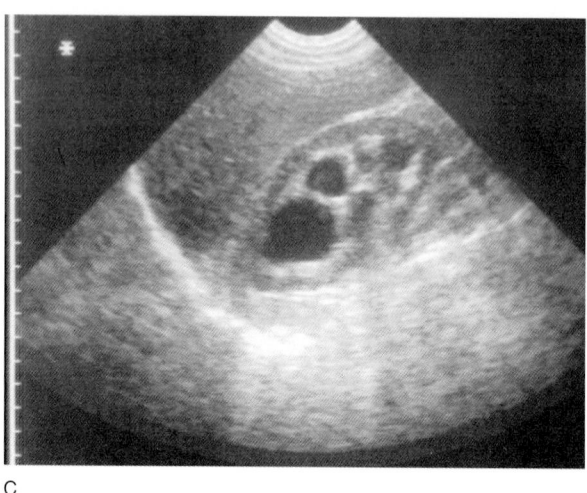

C

Figure 8-14. **C.** Severe hydronephrosis with cortical thinning. (Photos B, C contributed by Lori Sens and Lori Green, Gulfcoast Ultrasound.)

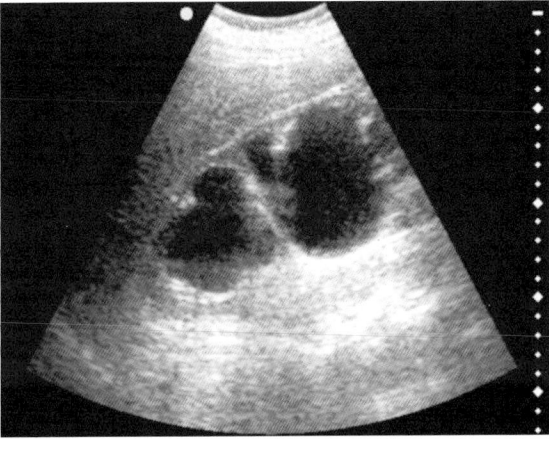

A

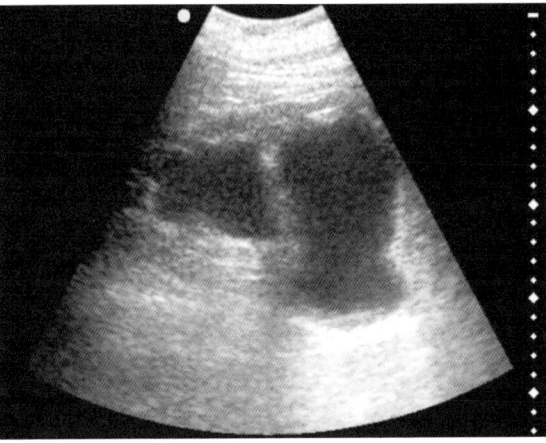

B

Figure 8-15. Chronic severe hydronephrosis. **A.** Coronal views of the kidney show severe hydronephrosis and cortical atrophy. **B.** Another view of the same kidney demonstrating severe urinary distension of the renal pelvis.

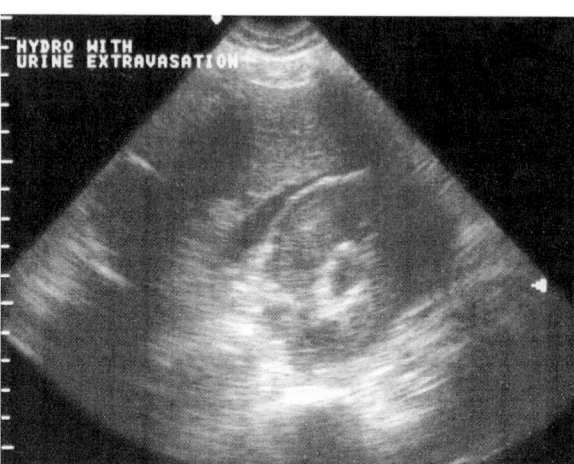

Figure 8-16. Hydronephrosis with acute calyceal rupture. Transverse view of the right kidney (outlined by rib shadows) with hydronephrosis and urinary extravasation into the perirenal space.

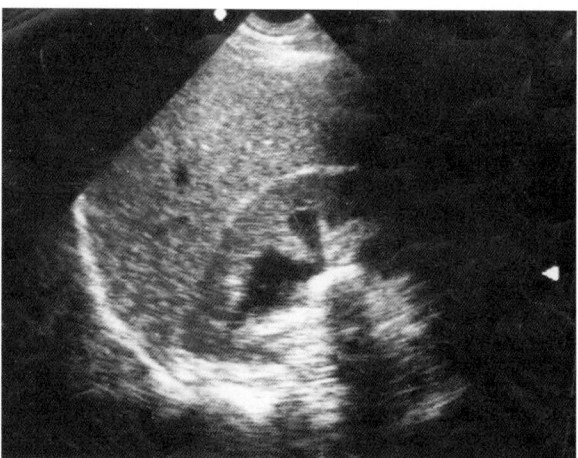

Figure 8-17. Longitudinal view of the right kidney shows moderate hydronephrosis and a large stone within the renal pelvis.

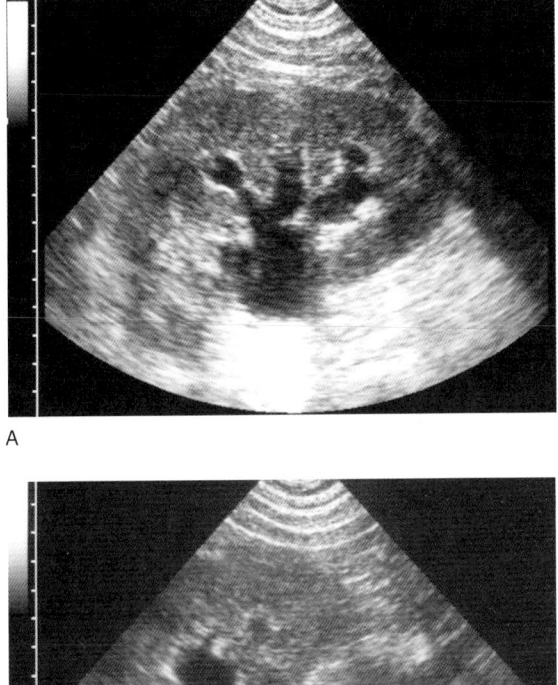

A

B

Figure 8-18. Ureteropelvic junction stone. **A.** Coronal view of the kidney shows moderate hydronephrosis. **B.** A slightly different angle of the same kidney demonstrates a ureteropelvic junction stone (with posterior shadowing) as the cause of the urinary obstruction.

Bladder Volume Measurement

See Figure 8-19.

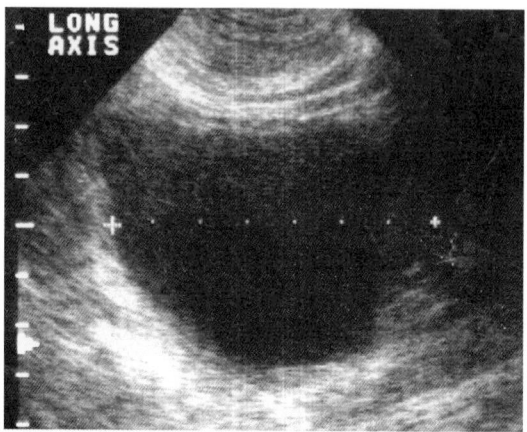

A

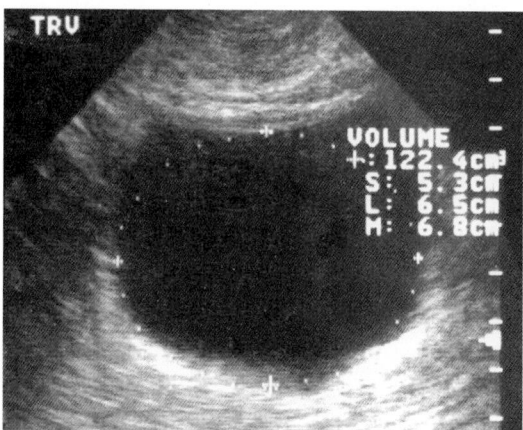

B

Figure 8-19. Use of a software calculation program to determine bladder volume. **A.** Longitudinal view of the bladder. **B.** Transverse view of the bladder.

▶ ADDITIONAL FINDINGS

Bladder Outlet Obstruction

See Figure 8-20.

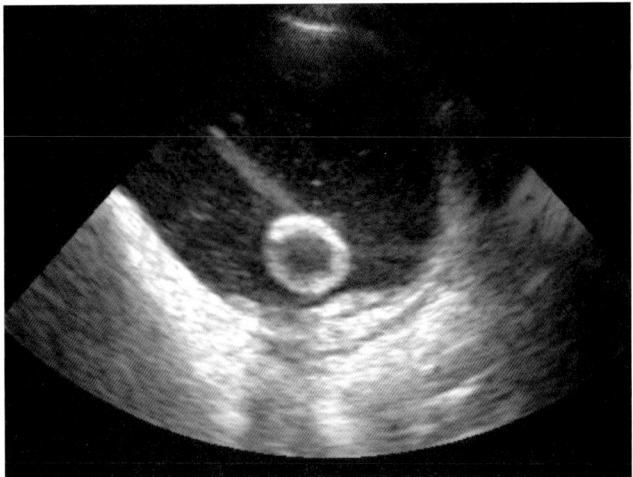

Figure 8-20. Longitudinal view of the bladder in an unconscious febrile patient. This image shows that the patient's chronic indwelling Foley catheter is correctly placed but not emptying the bladder. There is diffuse echogenic debris within the bladder, which is more obvious in real time (see video at www.hqmeded.com/foley-catheter-with-debris-2/). Replacement of the Foley catheter resulted in immediate output of 1 liter of thick urine resembling frank pus. The patient was ultimately diagnosed with urosepsis.

Renal Cell Carcinoma

See Figure 8-21.

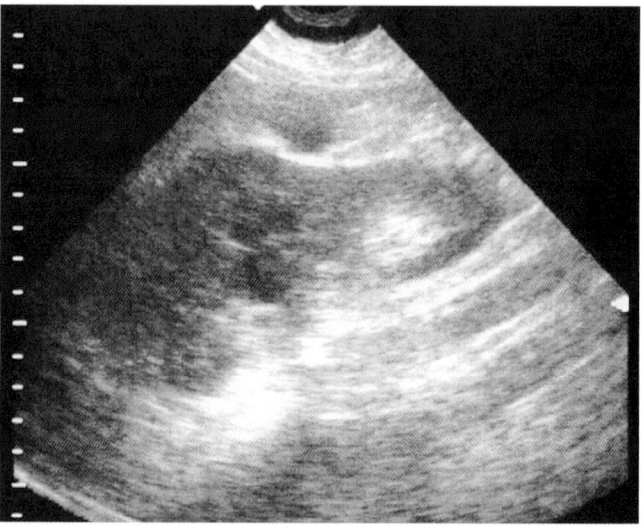

Figure 8-21. Renal cell carcinoma. Long-axis view through the right kidney shows renal cell carcinoma with enlargement of the upper pole, including both solid and cystic elements.

Renal Cyst

See Figures 8-22 and 8-23.

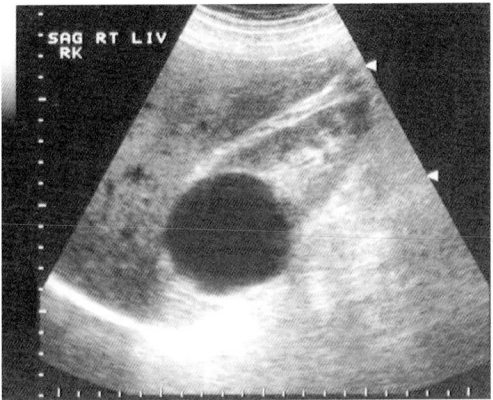

A

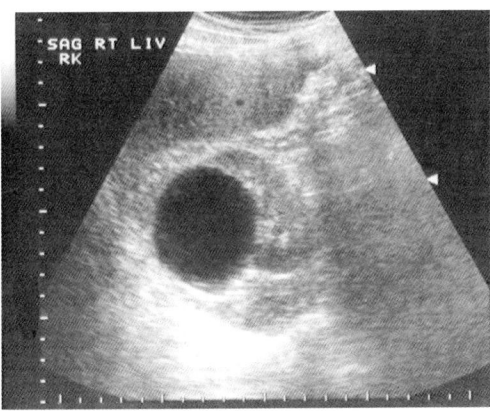

B

Figure 8-22. Renal cyst. **A.** Longitudinal view of the right kidney. **B.** Transverse view of the right kidney. Both views demonstrate the usual features of a simple cyst. (Photos contributed by Lori Sens, Gulfcoast Ultrasound.)

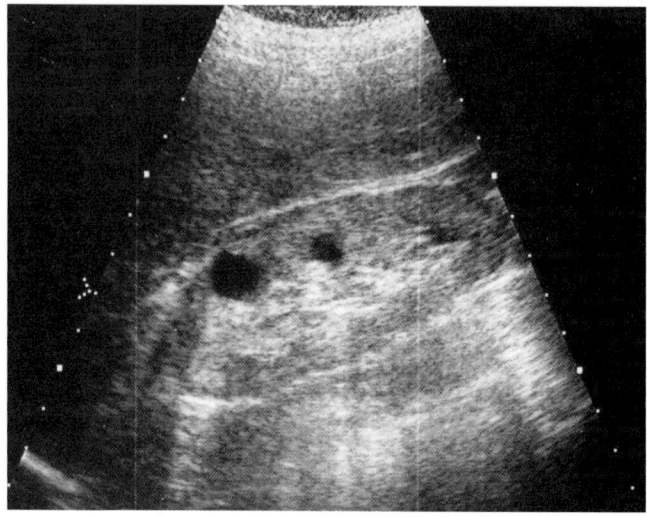

Figure 8-23. Longitudinal view of the right kidney with two small, simple-appearing cysts within the middle and upper poles.

Polycystic Kidneys

See Figure 8-24.

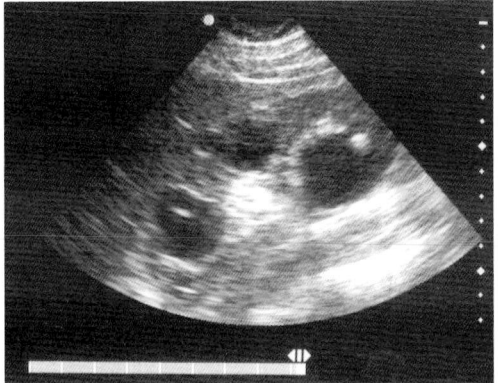

A

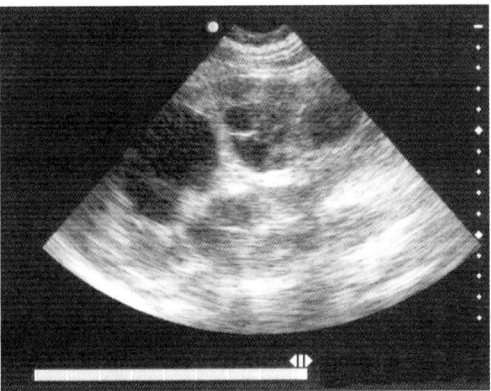

B

Figure 8-24. Polycystic kidneys. **A.** Coronal view of the right kidney demonstrates adult polycystic kidney disease. **B.** Coronal view of the left kidney also demonstrating adult polycystic kidney disease.

(Figure 8-24C continued on next page)

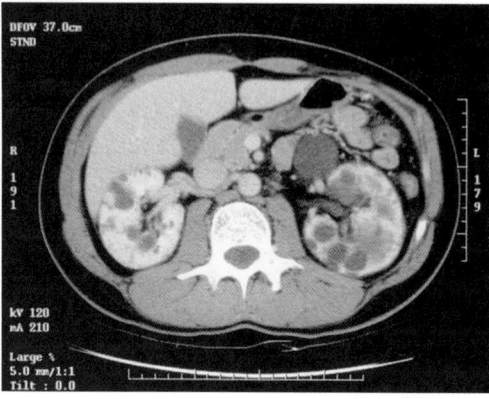

C

Figure 8-24. C. Computed tomography scan of the same patient for comparison.

Bladder Mass

See Figure 8-25.

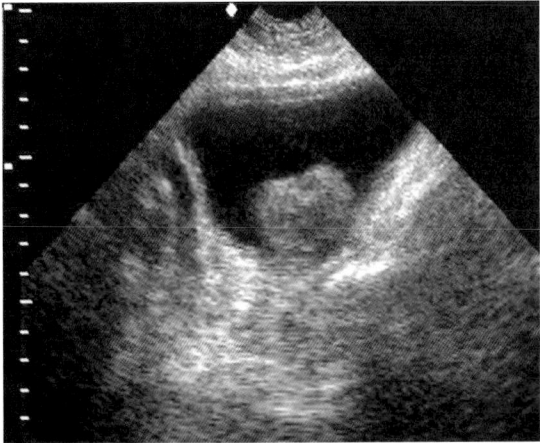

Figure 8-25. A large polypoid bladder mass noted in the posterior bladder on an oblique view.

▶ PITFALLS

- Bedside ultrasound is limited in scope. Additional findings (eg, possible abnormal renal masses) require close follow-up.
- Hydronephrosis may be mimicked by prominent pyramids, renal cysts, bladder overdistension, and pregnancy.
- Hydronephrosis may be masked by dehydration.
- The absence of hydronephrosis does not rule out a ureteral stone.
- Patients with a ruptured abdominal aortic aneurysm (AAA) often present with flank pain. A large AAA may cause hydronephrosis.
- A bladder mass may be a hematoma.

For more detailed information go to the comprehensive textbook Ma and Mateer's Emergency Ultrasound, 3rd edition, Chapter 12 "Renal," by Dina Seif, MD and Stuart Swadron, MD.

CHAPTER 9

Obstetric and Gynecologic

▶ CLINICAL CONSIDERATIONS

- In early pregnancy, bedside ultrasound is used to differentiate intrauterine pregnancy from ectopic pregnancy.
- In late pregnancy, it is used to evaluate the fetus after trauma and before emergency delivery and to detect placenta previa in patients with vaginal bleeding.
- Ultrasound is used to evaluate for ovarian torsion, pelvic masses, and signs of infection in nonpregnant women presenting with pelvic pain.

▶ CLINICAL INDICATIONS

- Potential ectopic pregnancy
- Trauma during pregnancy
- Vaginal bleeding in late pregnancy
- Impending emergency delivery
- Unexplained pelvic pain or mass

► ANATOMIC CONSIDERATIONS

- The uterus is the main landmark, and other pelvic structures are identified based on their positions relative to the uterus.

- The cervix is always found in the same location, behind the posterior angle of the bladder, regardless of pregnancy status (Figure 9-1).

- The position of pelvic structures is altered with changes in bladder filling.

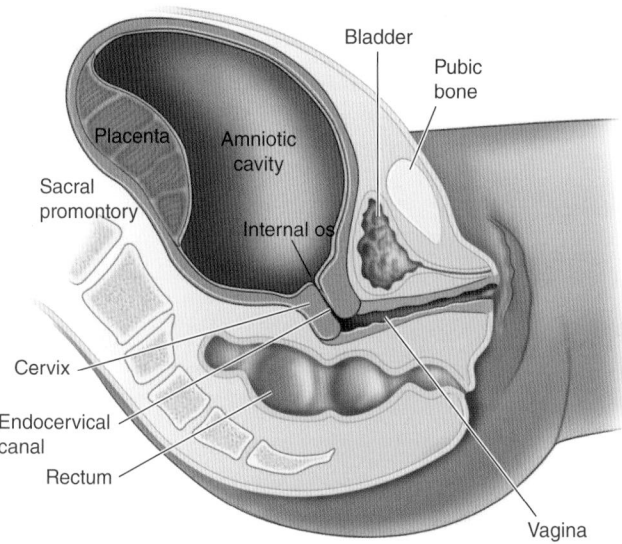

Figure 9-1. Diagram of the cervix and surrounding structures, sagittal view.

▶ TECHNIQUE AND NORMAL FINDINGS

Transabdominal Midline Sagittal View

- Start in the suprapubic region in the midline longitudinal orientation and identify the uterus (Figures 9-2 to 9-4).

- Place the probe indicator toward the patient's head.

- Note that the cervix lies immediately posterior to the lowest point of the bladder.

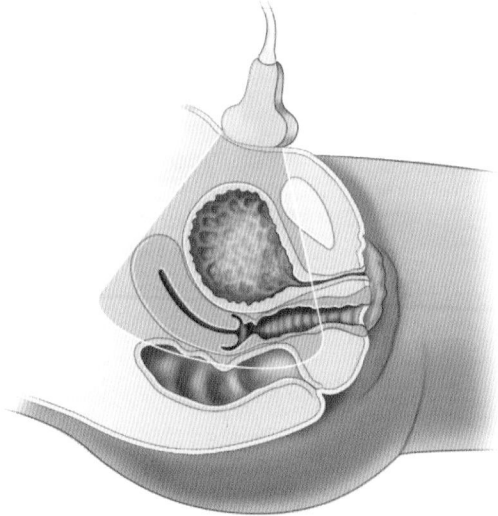

Figure 9-2. Scan plane for the transabdominal midline, sagittal view. The marker dot is pointed cephalad.

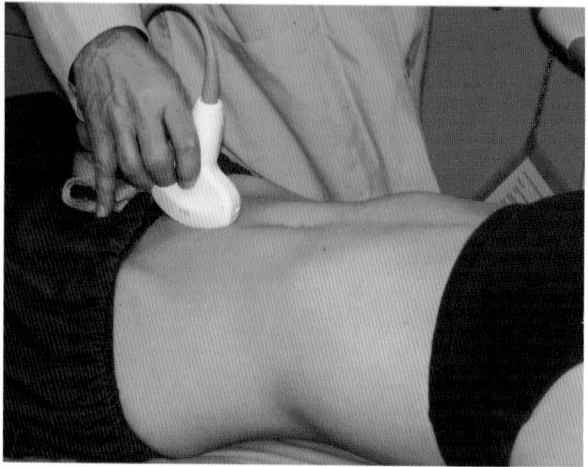

A

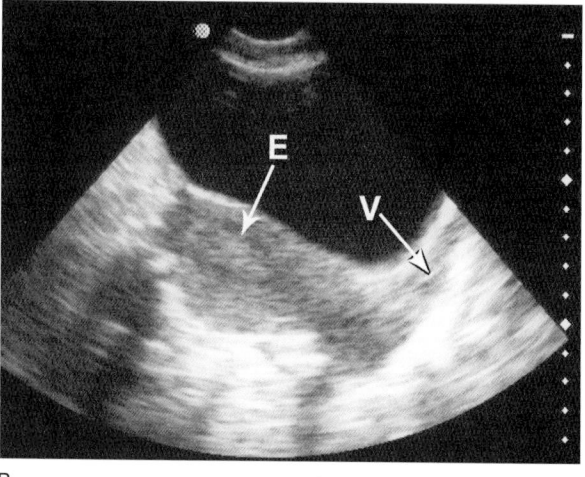

B

Figure 9-3. Transabdominal longitudinal view of the pelvis.
A. Probe position. **B.** Ultrasound image. E = endometrial stripe;
V = vaginal stripe.

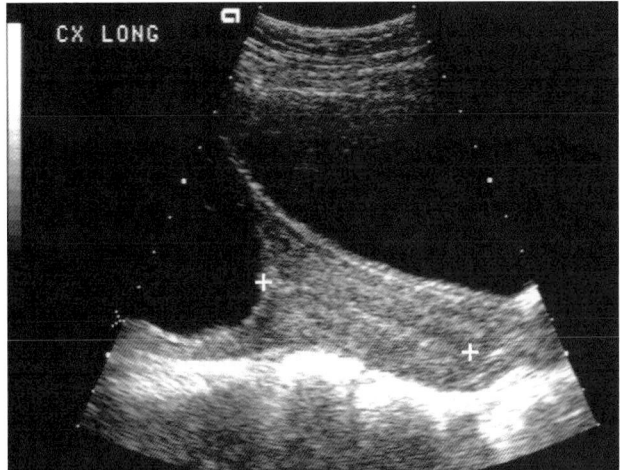

Figure 9-4. Normal cervix with no placenta previa (cursors mark the internal and external os). Transabdominal midline sagittal view.

Transabdominal Transverse View

- Center the transducer over the uterine fundus and rotate it 90 degrees counterclockwise (Figures 9-5 to 9-7).

- Place the probe indicator toward the patient's right side.

- One or both ovaries may be identified adjacent to the fundus.

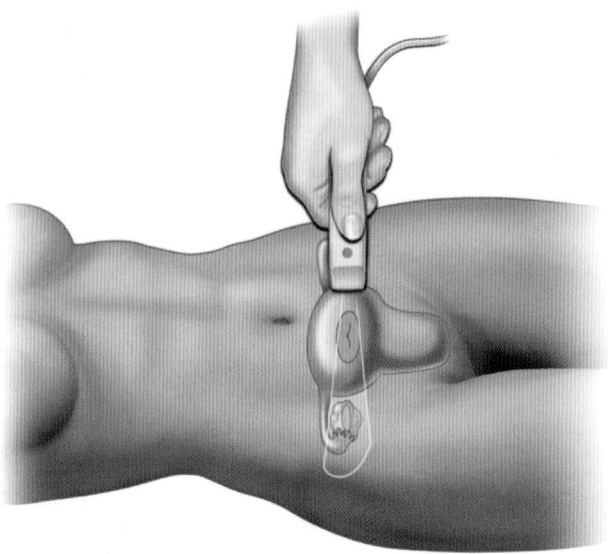

Figure 9-5. Scan plane for the transabdominal transverse view. The marker dot is pointed toward the patient's right side.

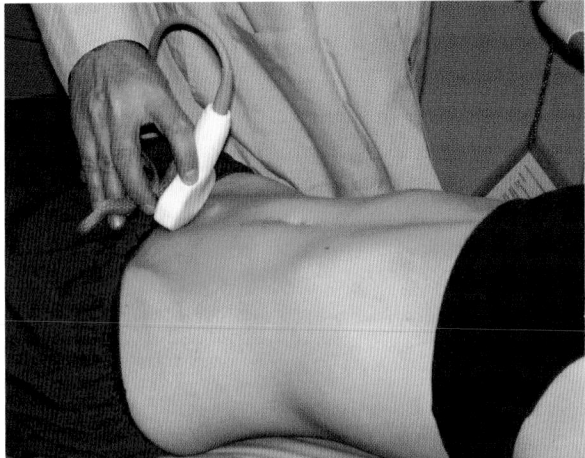

A

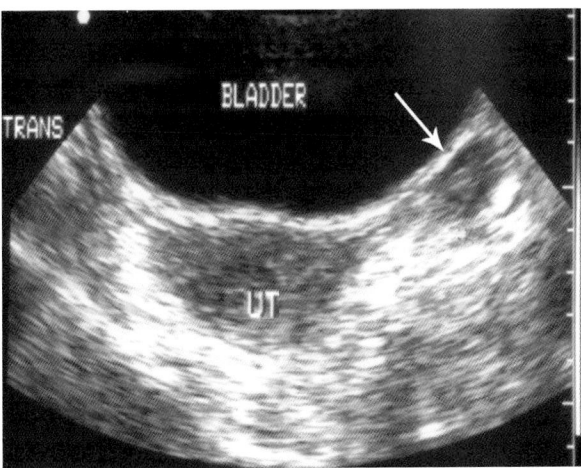

B

Figure 9-6. Transabdominal transverse view of the pelvis. **A.** Probe position. **B.** Ultrasound image. The *arrow* indicates the left ovary. UT = uterus.

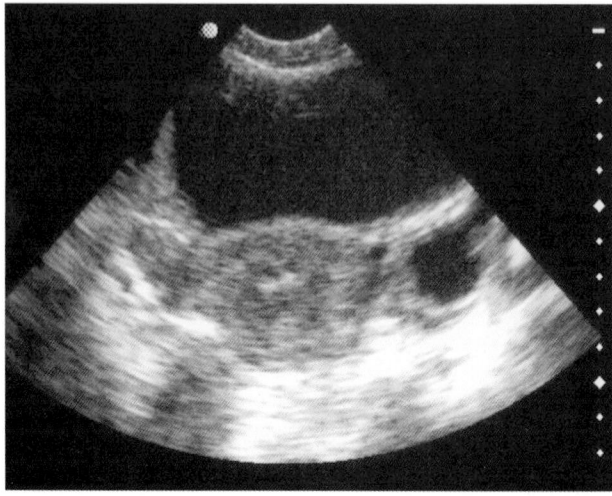

Figure 9-7. Transverse ultrasound view of the uterus and both ovaries. The right ovary is small and of similar echogenicity as the uterus; the left ovary is more prominent because it contains a cyst.

Transvaginal Midline Sagittal View

- Insert the transvaginal probe 4 to 5 cm into the vagina with the indicator pointed toward the ceiling (Figure 9-8).
- Find the midline of the uterus by angling the probe from side to side (Figures 9-9 and 9-10).
- The fundus is visualized by angling the probe upward (Figure 9-11).
- The cervix is visualized by angling the probe downward (Figure 9-12).
- About 10% of women have a retroverted uterus (Figure 9-13).

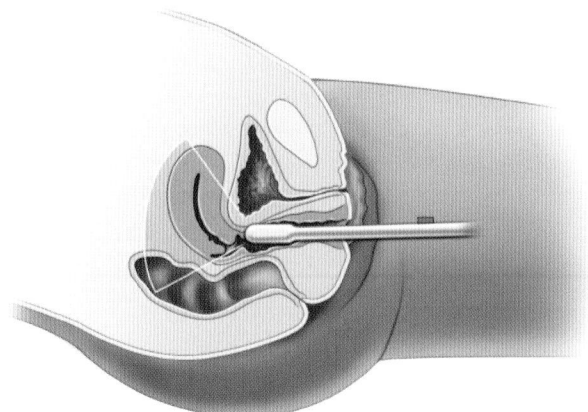

Figure 9-8. Scan plane for the transvaginal sagittal view (sagittal perspective). The marker dot is pointed toward the ceiling.

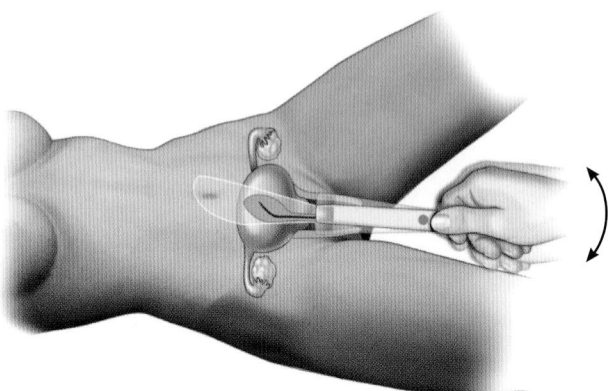

Figure 9-9. Scan plane for the transvaginal sagittal view (frontal perspective). The marker dot is pointed toward the ceiling.

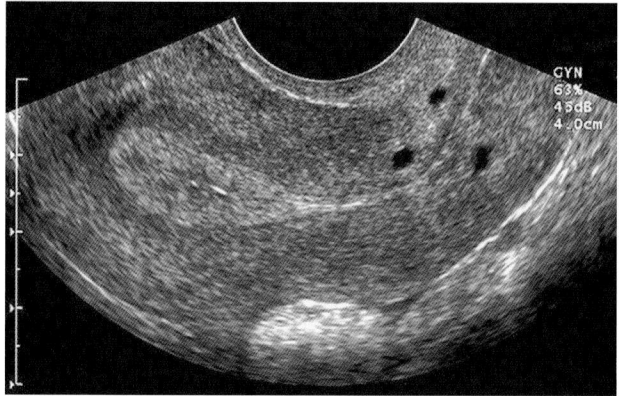

Figure 9-10. Transvaginal midline sagittal ultrasound image of the uterus during the secretory menstrual phase. The endometrium is thickened and echogenic. Three nabothian cysts are seen in the cervix.

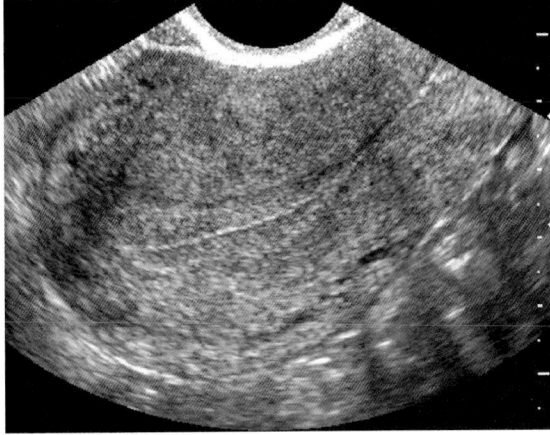

Figure 9-11. Transvaginal midline sagittal ultrasound image of the uterus during the late proliferative menstrual phase. The endometrial stripe is slightly thickened but not very echogenic.

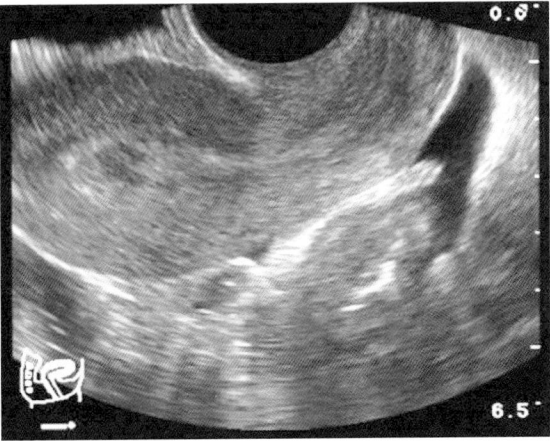

Figure 9-12. Transvaginal sagittal view of the uterine body and cervix. A small (physiologic) fluid collection is present in the posterior cul-de-sac.

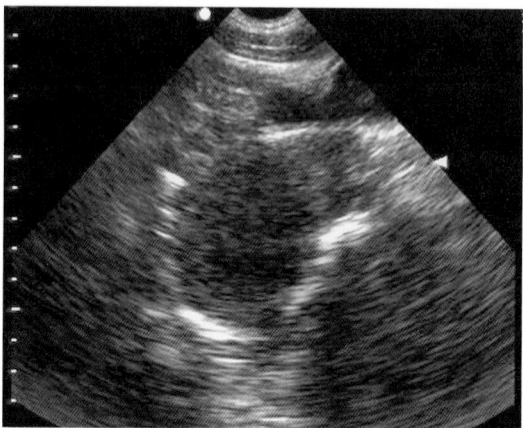

A

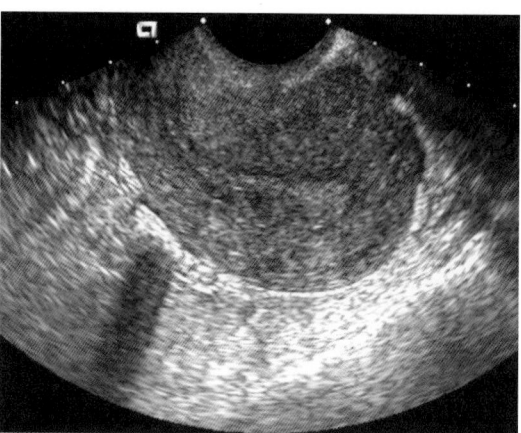

B

Figure 9-13. Retroverted uterus. **A.** Transabdominal sagittal view of a retroverted uterus. The uterine body and fundus are not well visualized because of the uterine position and empty bladder. **B.** Transvaginal longitudinal view of the uterus provides improved resolution. Note that with a retroverted uterus, the fundus is projected to the right side of the image and the cervix to the left.

Transvaginal Coronal View

- Center the uterine fundus on the monitor and then rotate the probe 90 degrees counterclockwise (Figures 9-14 and 9-15).
- Scan through the entire uterus by angling the probe up or down (Figure 9-16).
- To find the ovaries, first search the region lateral to the widest portion of the uterus and then scan up and down in this region while maintaining the coronal orientation (Figures 9-17 to 9-19).

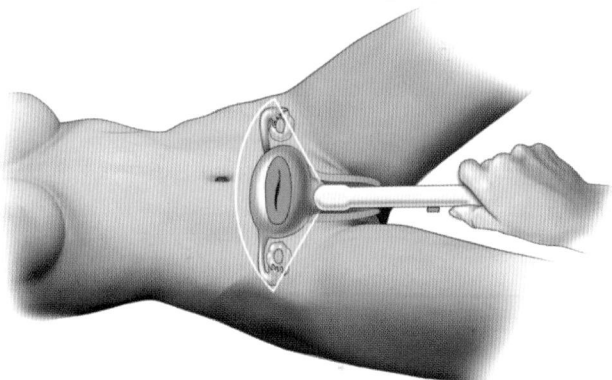

Figure 9-14. Scan plane for the transvaginal coronal view (frontal perspective). The marker dot is pointed toward the patient's right side.

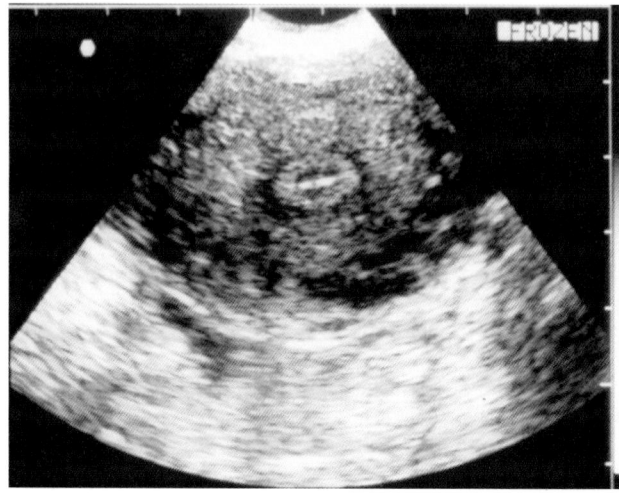

Figure 9-15. Transvaginal coronal ultrasound image of the uterus. Note the prominent arcuate venous plexus in the peripheral myometrium.

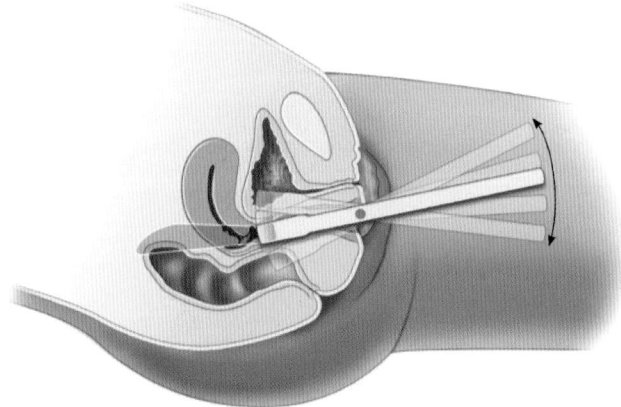

Figure 9-16. Scan plane for the transvaginal coronal view (sagittal perspective). The marker dot is pointed toward the patient's right side.

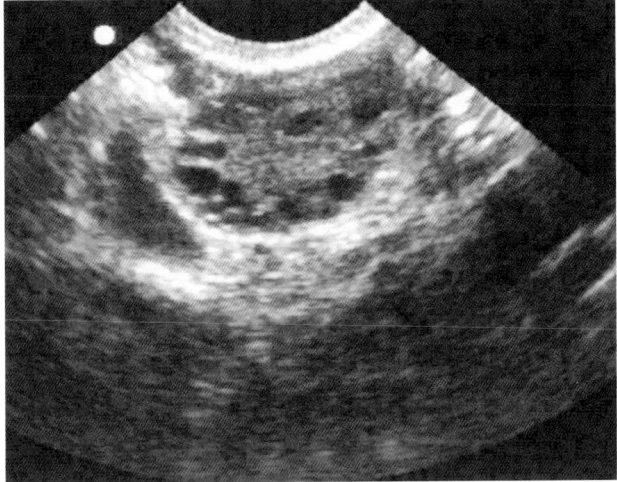

Figure 9-17. Transvaginal ultrasound image of the left ovary containing normal follicles.

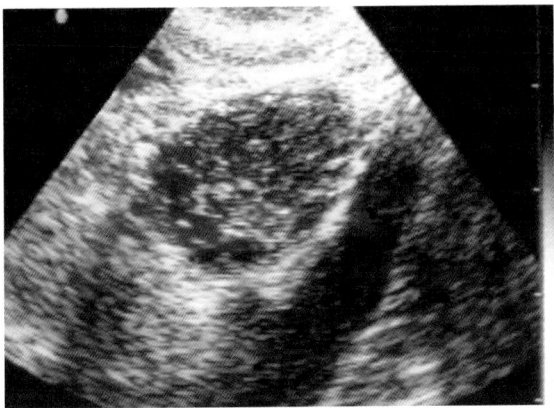

Figure 9-18. Transvaginal view of a normal left ovary. The ovary is recognized by the oval shape, peripheral follicles, and echogenicity similar to the myometrium of the uterus. This ovary is adjacent to the iliac vein.

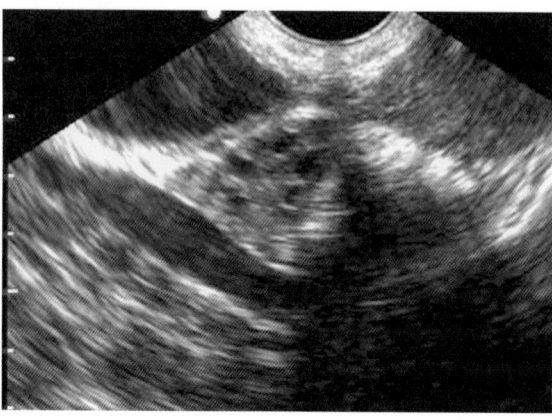

Figure 9-19. Transvaginal view of a normal ovary. This ovary (center of the image) is surrounded by the bladder (*above left*), iliac vein (*below*), intestine with gas and shadows (*below right*), and uterus (*above right*).

▶ TIPS TO IMPROVE IMAGE ACQUISITION

- The patient's bladder should be full for transabdominal pelvic sonography.

- The patient's bladder should be empty for transvaginal pelvic sonography.

- Always start in the longitudinal orientation and identify the uterus and cervix.

- The midline of the uterus is not always in the midline of the pelvis.

- Look for the ovaries adjacent to the widest portion of the uterus in the transverse (coronal) plane.

- Bowel may be repositioned with steady pressure or with the patient in the Trendelenburg position.

- Touch the ovaries (or other adnexal masses) with the tip of the transvaginal probe to improve image quality and to assess for tenderness.

- The ovaries will be located between the lateral wall of the uterus and iliac vessels.

▶ COMMON AND EMERGENT ABNORMALITIES

- Intrauterine pregnancy (IUP) (Figures 9-20 to 9-25).

- Ectopic pregnancy (Table 9-1 and Figures 9-26 to 9-37).

- Pregnancy loss (Figures 9-38 to 9-41).

- Fetal heart rate, gestational age, and fetal position (Figures 9-42 to 9-44).

- Placenta previa (Figures 9-45 to 9-47).

- Placental abruption (Figure 9-48): Ultrasound has poor sensitivity for abruption; bleeding in late pregnancy is assumed to be from abruption if placenta previa is not present.

- Adnexal masses (Figures 9-49 to 9-55).

- Pelvic inflammatory disease (PID) (Figures 9-56 and 9-57).

- Ovarian torsion (Figures 9-58 and 9-59): Doppler flow studies have poor accuracy for ruling out and diagnosing ovarian torsion. Regardless, this is the only test available, and it is important to know that torsion is more likely when no flow is detected and when the ovary is large (>5 cm) and tender.

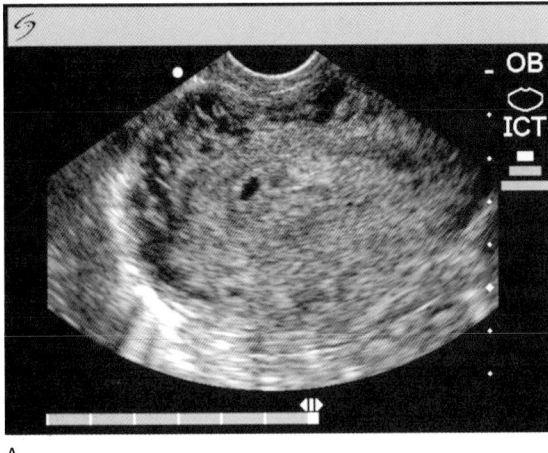

A

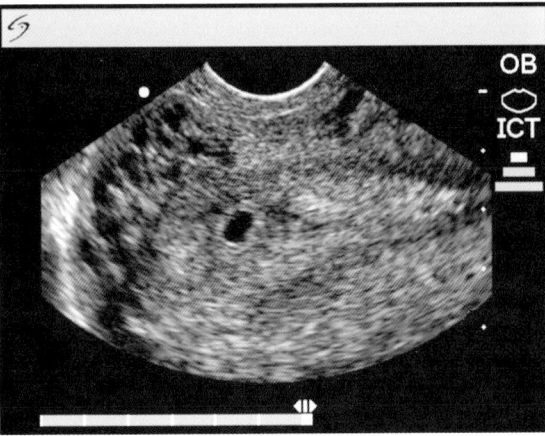

B

Figure 9-20. IUP. Intradecidual sign. **A.** Longitudinal transvaginal view of the uterus at 7.5 MHz. **B.** Magnified long-axis view of the endometrium shows a 5-mm gestational sac within a slightly thickened endometrium.

(Figure 9-20C continued on next page)

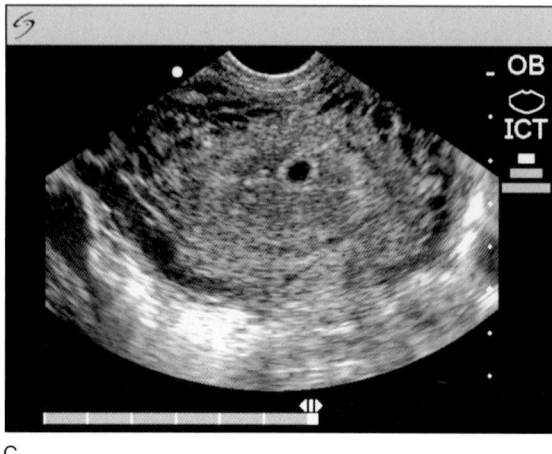

C

Figure 9-20. **C.** Transvaginal coronal view of the same patient demonstrates the location within the upper endometrium and the lack of deformation of the midline stripe. All views show a prominent arcuate venous plexus (a variant of normal) within the myometrium of the uterus for this patient.

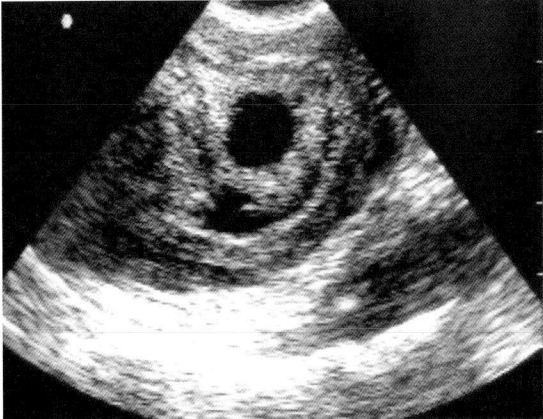

Figure 9-21. IUP. Double decidual sign surrounding an intrauterine gestational sac. Normal early pregnancy. Transvaginal image. This sign is often subtle and usually only noticeable along one side of the gestational sac but is very distinct in this example.

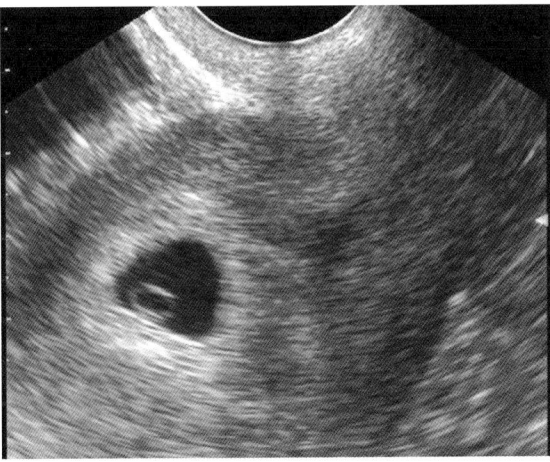

Figure 9-22. IUP. Yolk sac within an intrauterine gestational sac. Normal early pregnancy. Transvaginal image.

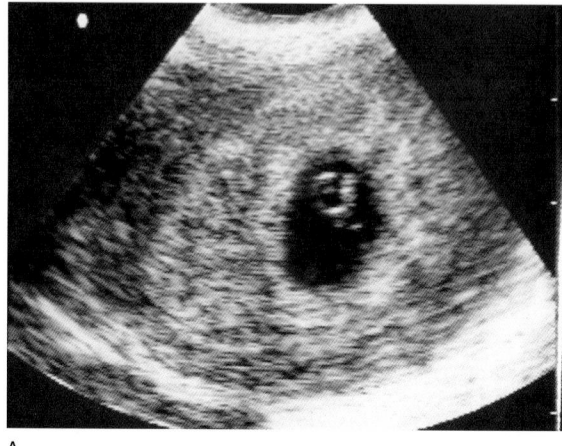

A

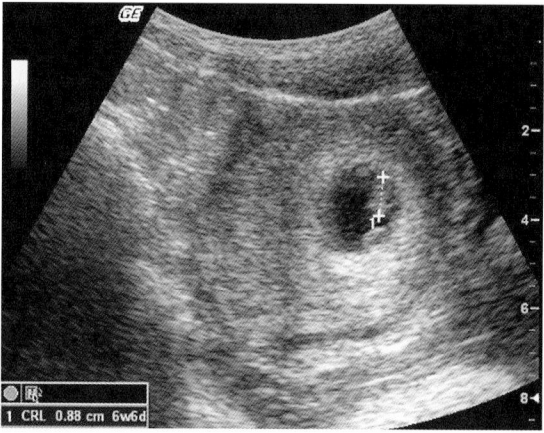

B

Figure 9-23. IUP. **A.** Small embryo and yolk sac within an intra-uterine gestational sac. The 5-mm embryo is positioned along the right side of the yolk sac in this image; cardiac pulsations were visible during real-time sonography. Transvaginal image at 7.5 MHz. **B.** The embryonic pole is separated from the yolk sac and measures 6 weeks, 6 days via crown-rump length. Trans-abdominal longitudinal view with an empty bladder.

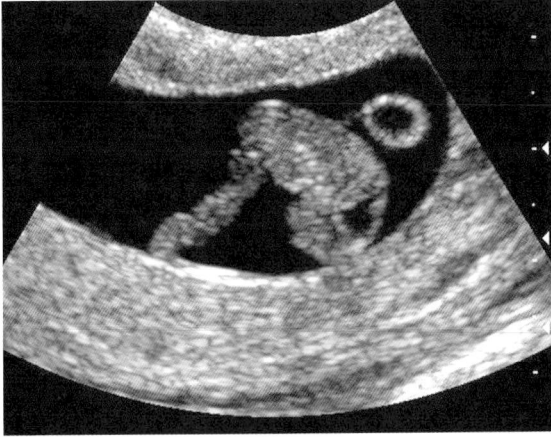

Figure 9-24. IUP. Intrauterine embryo and yolk sac. Normal pregnancy at 8 weeks. Transvaginal image.

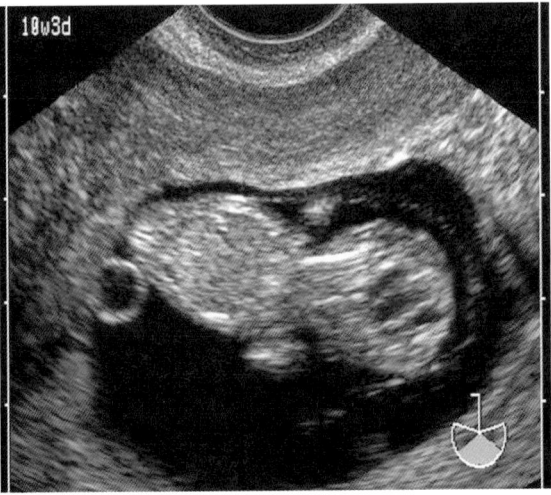

Figure 9-25. IUP. Intrauterine fetus and yolk sac with amnion surrounding the embryo. Normal pregnancy at 10 weeks. Transvaginal image.

▶ **TABLE 9-1.** **NONSPECIFIC SONOGRAPHIC SIGNS OF ECTOPIC PREGNANCY**

Sonographic Finding	Likelihood of Ectopic Pregnancy (%)
Any free pelvic fluid	52
Complex pelvic mass	75
Moderate or large free pelvic fluid	86
Tubal ring	>95
Mass and free fluid	97
Hepatorenal free fluid	~100

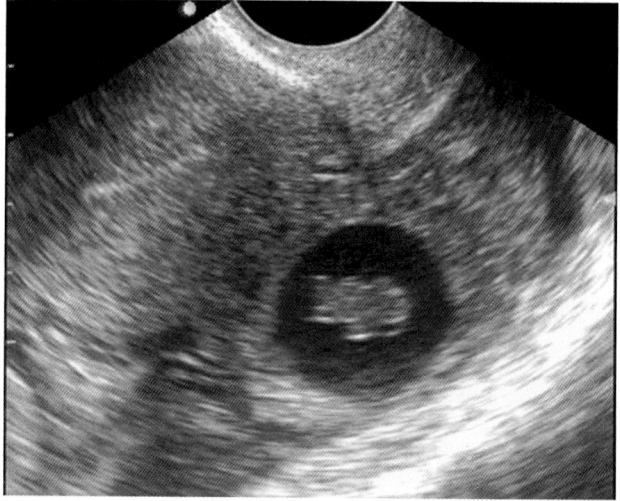

Figure 9-26. Ectopic pregnancy. Living embryo in the adnexa and empty uterus (endometrial echo is visible in the left upper portion of the image). Embryonic cardiac activity was present on real-time imaging. Transvaginal image.

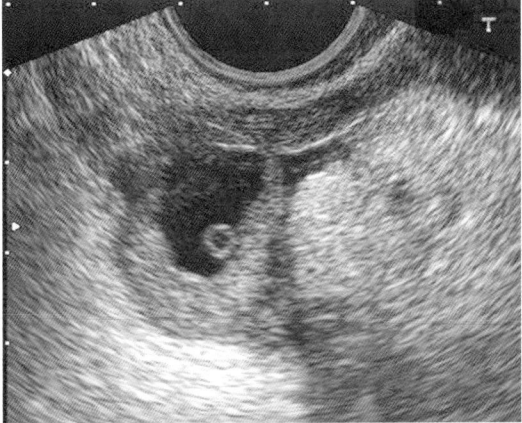

A

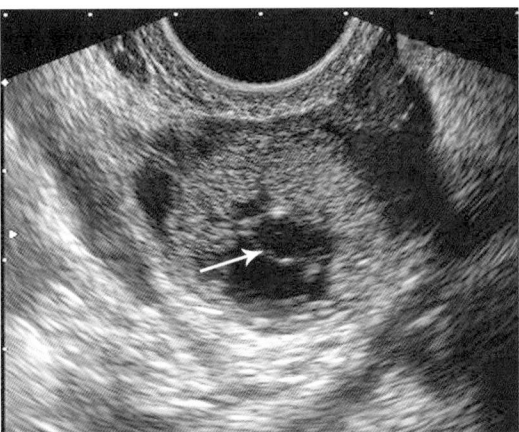

B

Figure 9-27. Ectopic pregnancy. Transvaginal images.
A. Extrauterine gestational sac with a thick echogenic ring and a yolk sac within. A small stripe of free fluid is present as well as bowel gas artifact surrounding the structure. **B.** A thick concentric echogenic ring in the adnexa is surrounded by free fluid. A subtle yolk sac is contained within the structure (*arrow*).

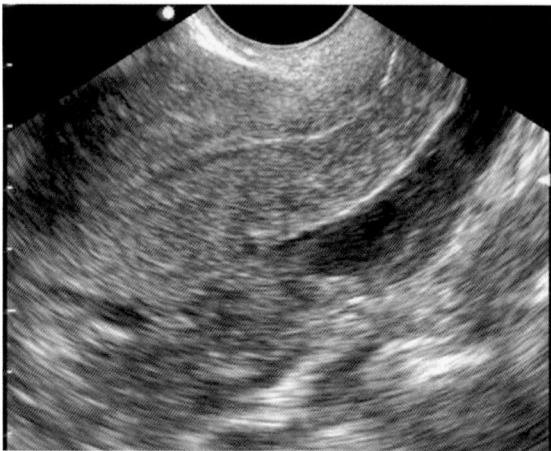

Figure 9-28. Ectopic pregnancy. Empty uterus and free fluid in the posterior cul-de-sac. Transvaginal sagittal image.

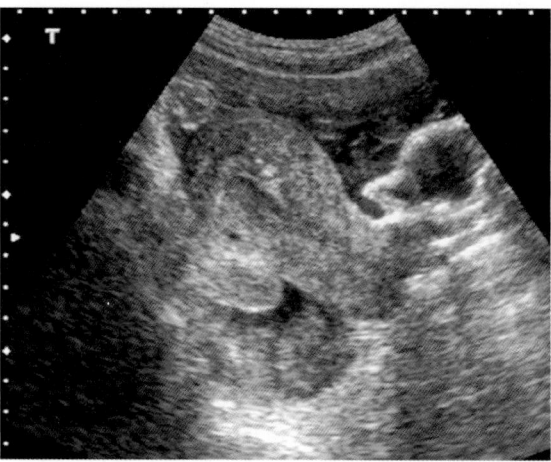

Figure 9-29. Ectopic pregnancy. Transabdominal longitudinal view shows an empty uterus. Complex fluid from liquid and clotted blood is present in both the anterior and posterior cul-de-sac areas. The bladder is collapsed around a Foley catheter balloon.

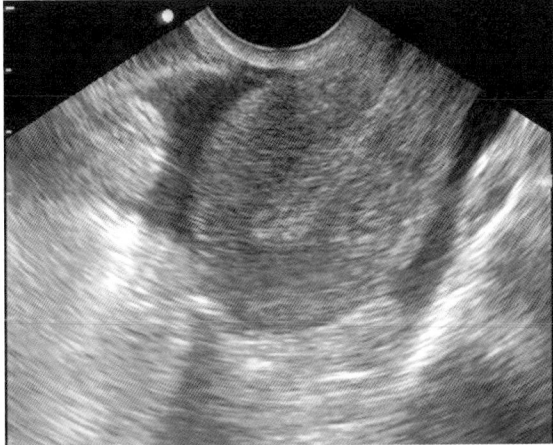

Figure 9-30. Ectopic pregnancy. Free fluid surrounding an empty uterus. Transvaginal image.

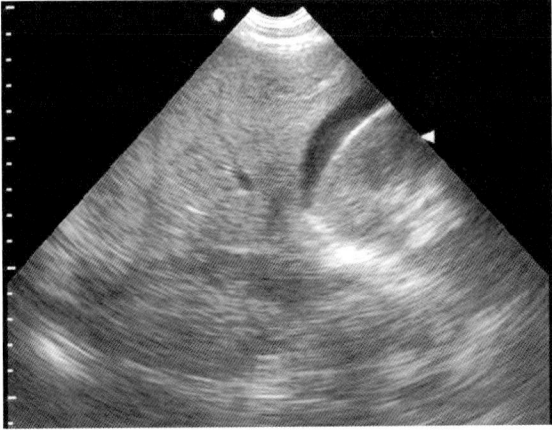

Figure 9-31. Ectopic pregnancy (Morison's pouch). Free fluid in the hepatorenal space. Transabdominal image.

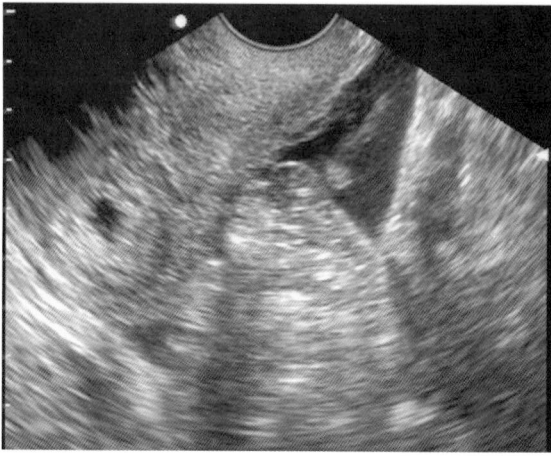

Figure 9-32. Ectopic pregnancy. Tubal ring (2 cm). Free pelvic fluid with floating bowel. Transvaginal image.

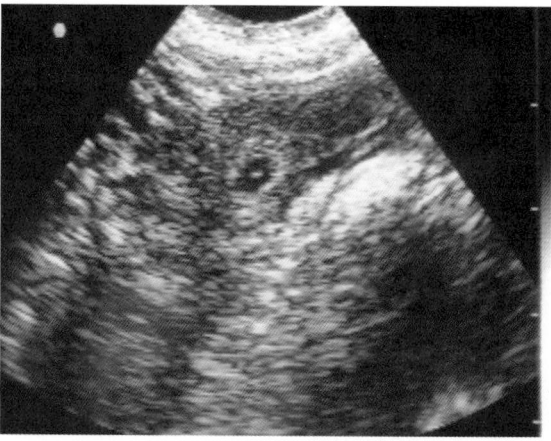

Figure 9-33. Ectopic pregnancy. Tubal ring. Transvaginal view of the right adnexa shows a tiny (7 mm), brightly echogenic ring-like structure. This was determined to be a very early ectopic pregnancy.

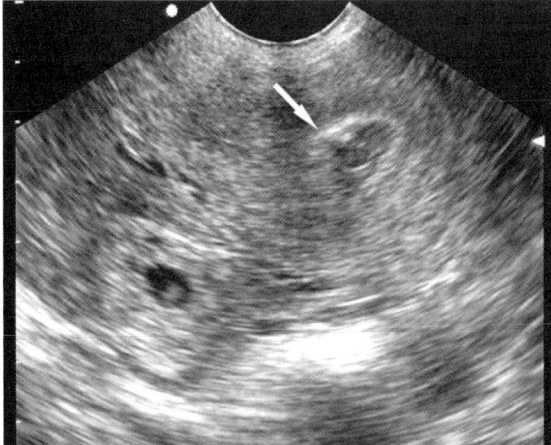

Figure 9-34. Ectopic pregnancy. Pseudogestational sac in the uterus (*arrow*) and 2.5-cm brightly echogenic tubal ring in the adnexa. Transvaginal image.

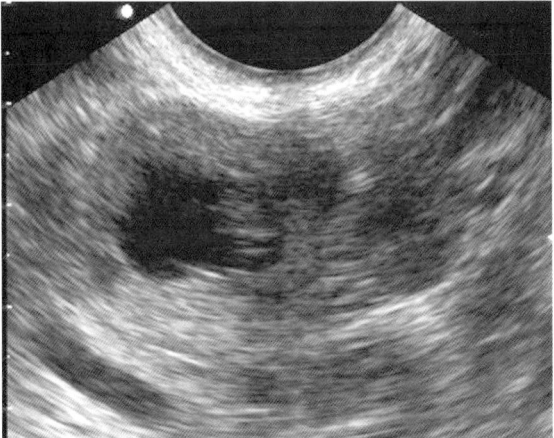

Figure 9-35. Ectopic pregnancy. Complex right adnexal mass located above the iliac vein on the image. Transvaginal technique.

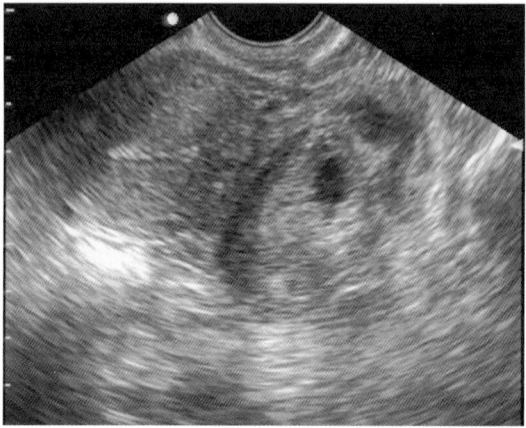

Figure 9-36. Ectopic pregnancy. An empty uterus is seen in the coronal transvaginal view and is identified by the endometrial stripe. The complex mass is in the left adnexa and adjacent to the uterus.

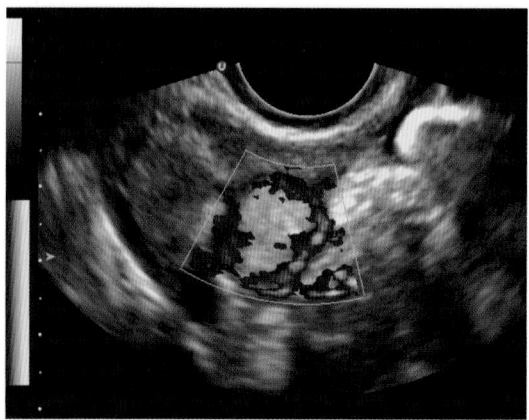

Figure 9-37. Ectopic pregnancy. Ring of fire. Transvaginal ultrasound of the adnexa demonstrates an ectopic mass with the surrounding power Doppler signal. (Photo contributed by J. Christian Fox, MD.)

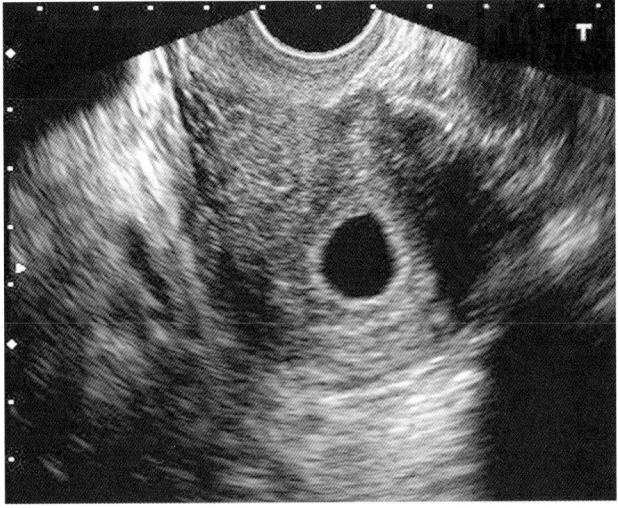

Figure 9-38. Early embryonic demise. An empty intrauterine sac consistent with a 6.5-week gestational sac size contains no yolk sac or embryo. Transvaginal image.

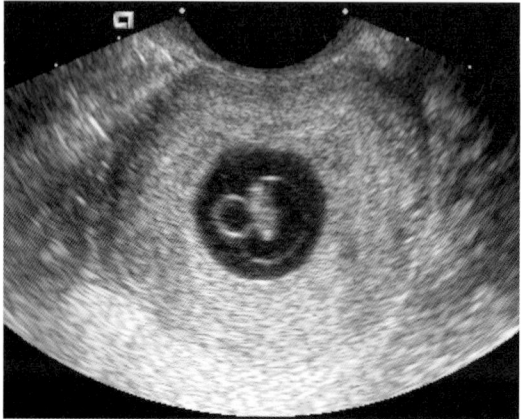

A

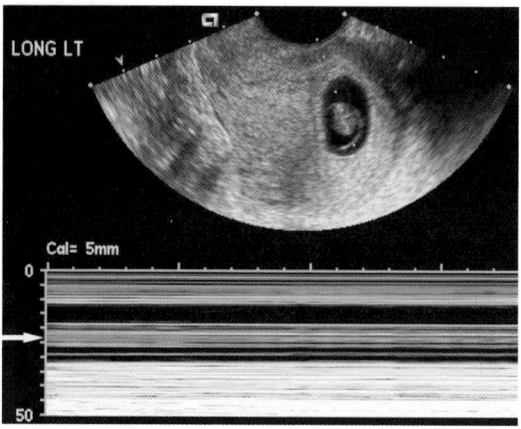

B

Figure 9-39. Embryonic demise. **A.** Transvaginal image of the fetal pole, which measured 7 weeks via crown-rump length. The yolk sac appears slightly enlarged, and the amnion is clearly visible. **B.** There was no cardiac activity on real-time sonography, and this was documented by the M-mode examination. Note the lack of any motion in the fetal band (*arrow*).

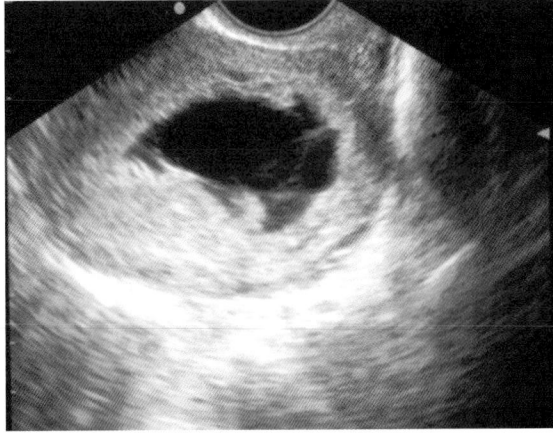

Figure 9-40. Embryonic demise. Distorted gestational sac. Transvaginal image.

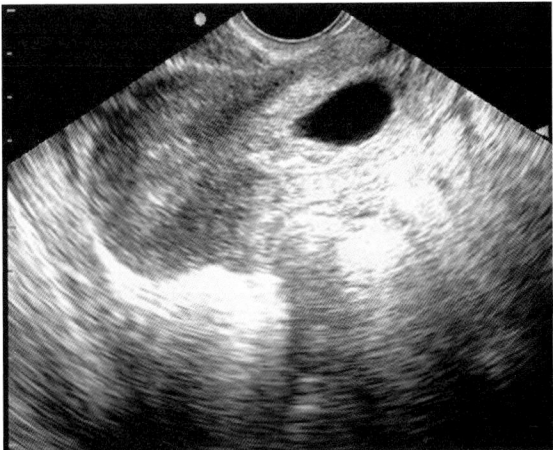

Figure 9-41. Inevitable abortion. The fundus is on the left of the image, and the gestational sac is approaching the cervical portion of the uterus. Transvaginal image.

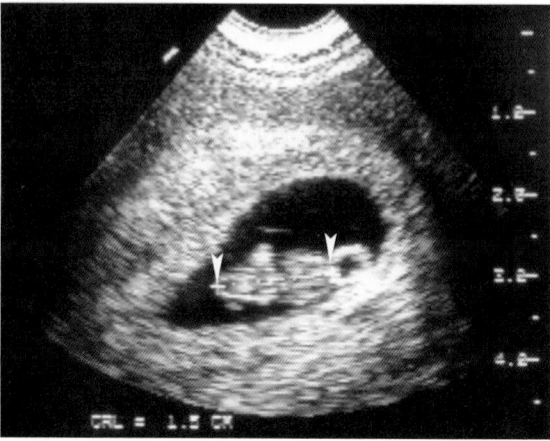

A

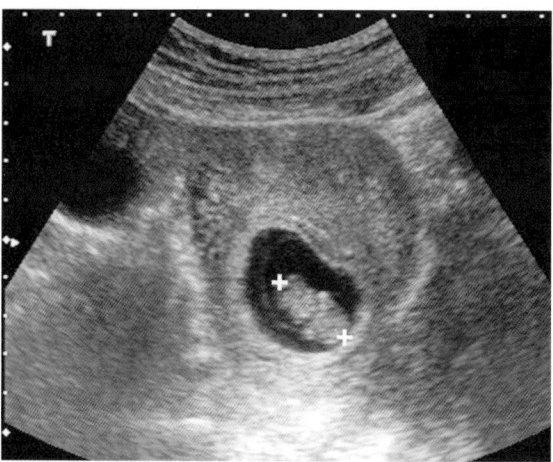

B

Figure 9-42. Crown-rump length (CRL). **A.** Transvaginal ultrasound shows proper placement of cursors for CRL measurement. The maximal embryo length, excluding the yolk sac, should be measured. **B.** Transabdominal transverse ultrasound of a 9-week intrauterine pregnancy.

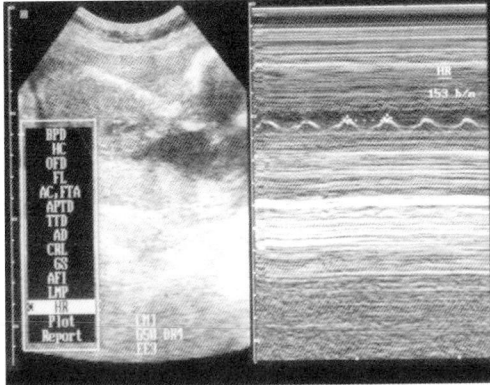

Figure 9-43. Fetal heart rate determination. The B-mode image and M-mode tracing are simultaneously displayed. The Doppler cursor passes through the fetal heart. Cardiac oscillations are evident on the M-mode tracing. With the image frozen, a cardiac cycle length is automatically calculated and displayed with obstetrics measurement software.

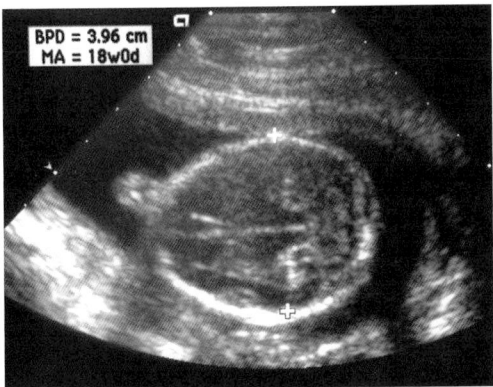

Figure 9-44. Biparietal diameter to estimate gestational age. Measurement is taken from the outer wall of the calvarium to the inner wall (see marker cursors) in a line that crosses the paired thalami and third ventricle. In the plane shown, the cavum septi pellucidi is seen.

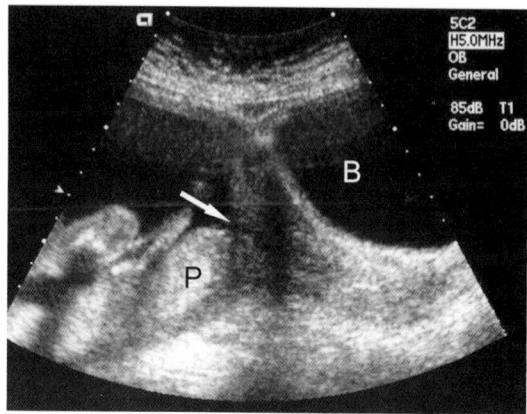

Figure 9-45. Posterior marginal placenta previa (P). Trans-abdominal approach, sagittal plane. The endocervical canal (*arrow*) is obscured by an edge artifact emanating from the bladder (B).

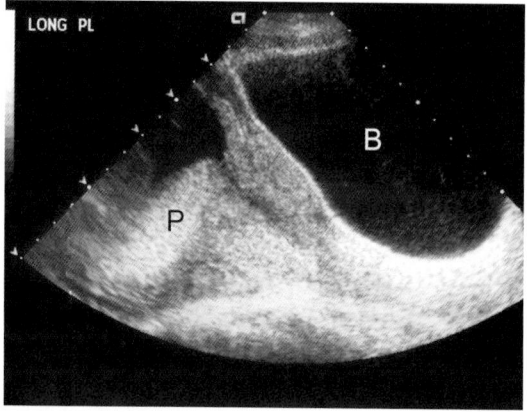

Figure 9-46. Posterior marginal placenta previa (P). Trans-abdominal approach, sagittal plane. In this case, an overdistended bladder (B) may be compressing the lower uterine segment, causing a false-positive impression of placenta previa.

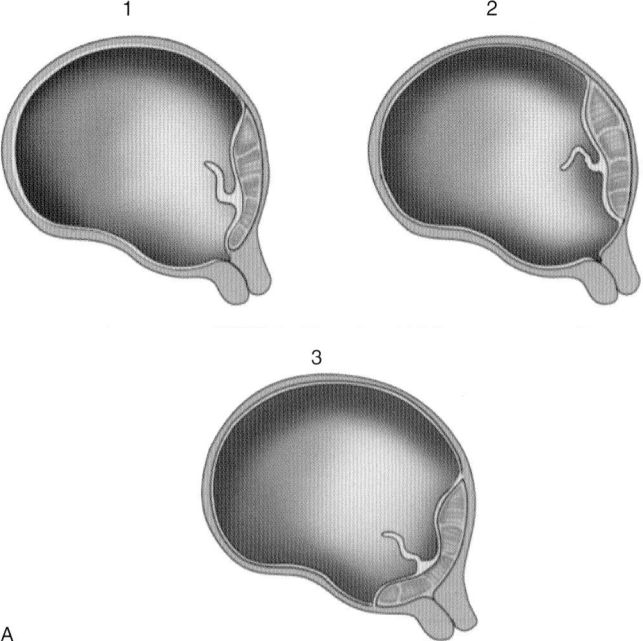

Figure 9-47. **A.** Classification of placenta previa: 1 = marginal; 2 = low lying; 3 = complete.

(Figures 9-47B and C continued on next page)

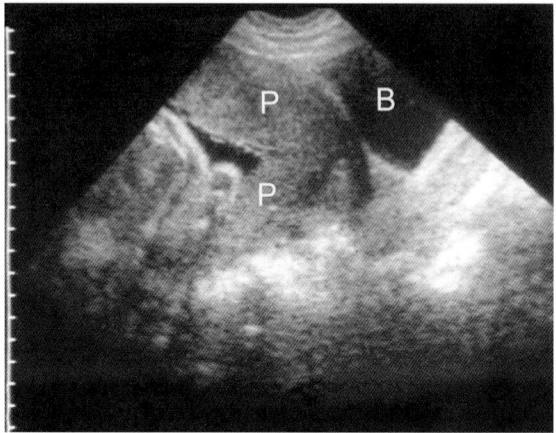

B

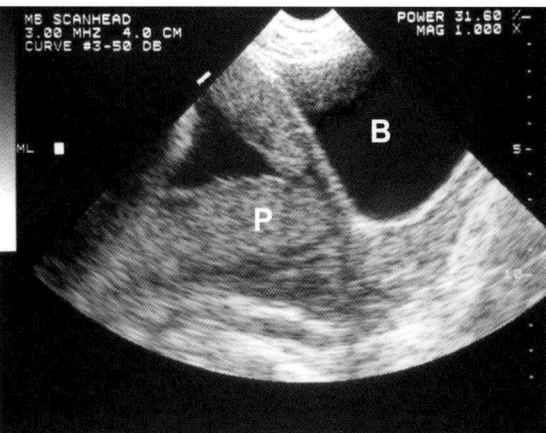

C

Figure 9-47. **B.** Transabdominal longitudinal ultrasound demonstrates complete placenta previa. **C.** Transabdominal longitudinal ultrasound demonstrates partial placenta previa. B = bladder; P = placenta. (Sonograms contributed by Lori Sens and Lori Green, Gulfcoast Ultrasound.)

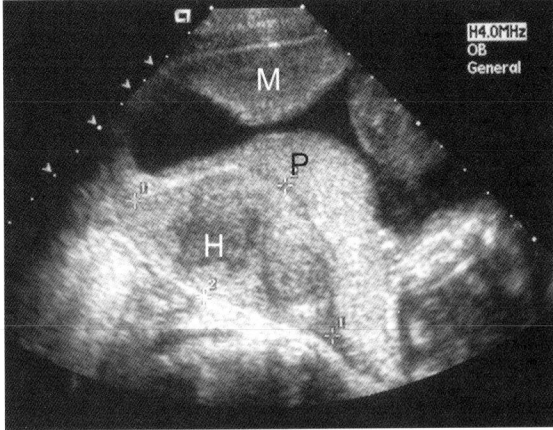

Figure 9-48. Placental abruption. Transabdominal scan, sagittal plane, demonstrates retroplacental hematoma (H) in an 18-week pregnancy. The placenta (P) is located on the posterior wall. A myometrial contraction (M) of the anterior wall is evident.

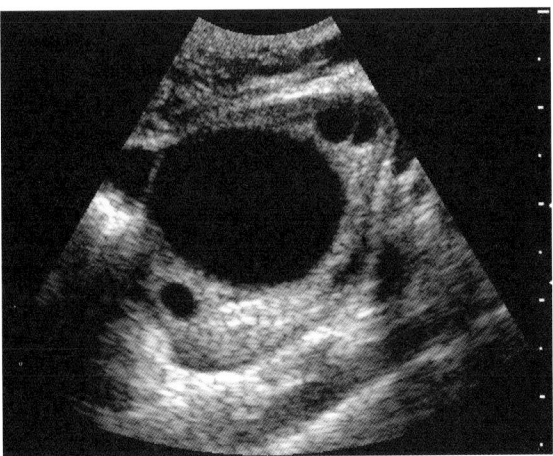

Figure 9-49. "Simple" ovarian cyst. Transvaginal image.

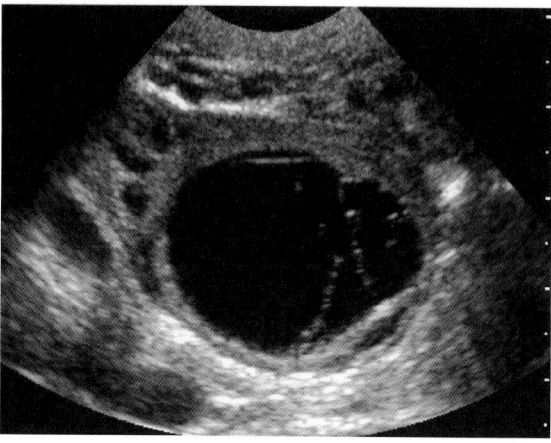

Figure 9-50. Ovarian cyst (mostly "simple") with a few fine septations from a small amount of internal hemorrhage. Transvaginal image.

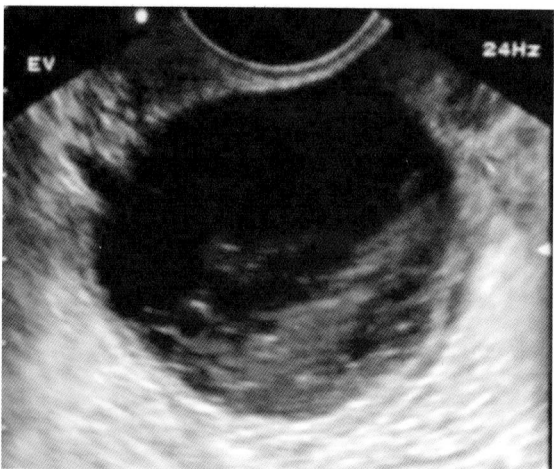

Figure 9-51. Hemorrhagic ("complex") ovarian cyst. Transvaginal image.

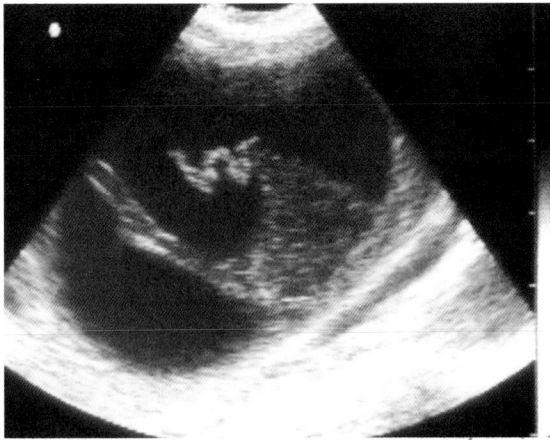

Figure 9-52. Hemorrhagic ("complex") ovarian cyst. Transvaginal image.

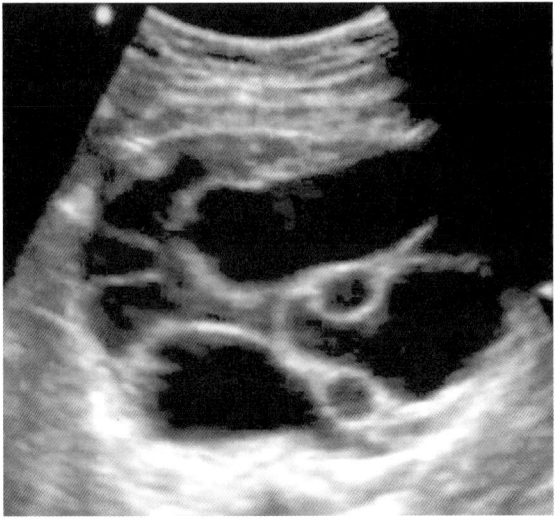

Figure 9-53. Multiseptated ("complex") ovarian cyst. Transvaginal image.

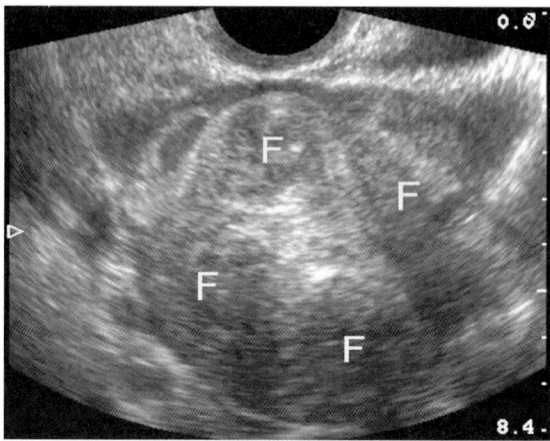

A

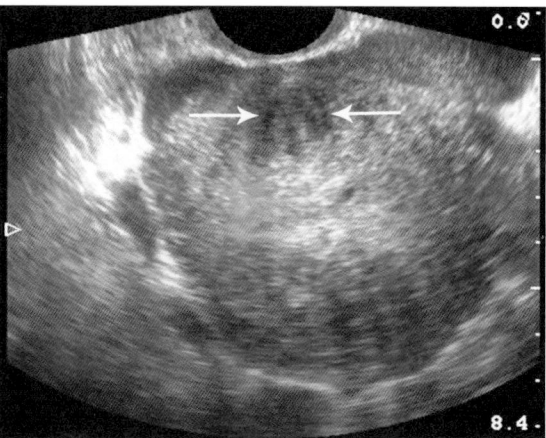

B

Figure 9-54. Fibroid uterus. **A.** Transvaginal ultrasound image reveals multiple isoechoic discrete masses embedded in the uterine wall. **B.** A single hypoechoic fibroid is outlined (*arrows*). F = fibroids.

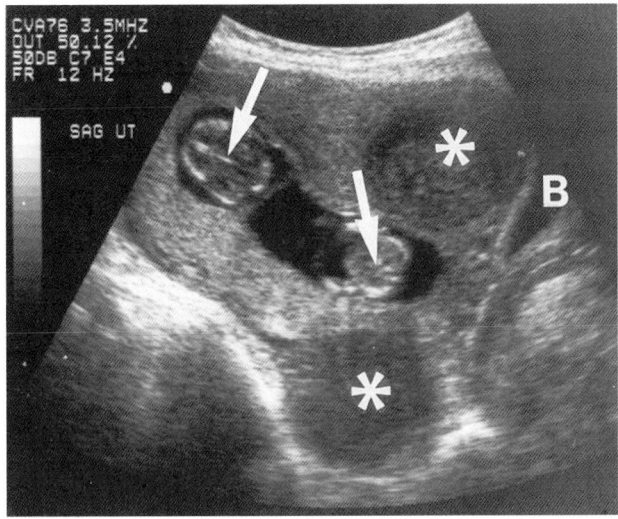

Figure 9-55. Uterine fibroids (*asterisks*) with pregnancy (*arrows*). Transabdominal midline sagittal image. B = bladder. (Reproduced with permission from *Williams Obstetrics*, 21st ed. New York: McGraw-Hill, 2001: Figure 35-13, p. 929.)

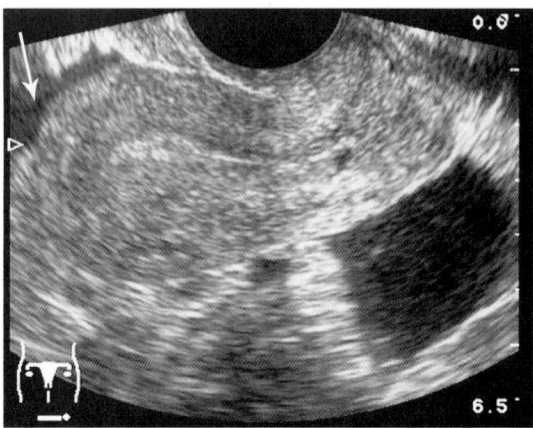

A

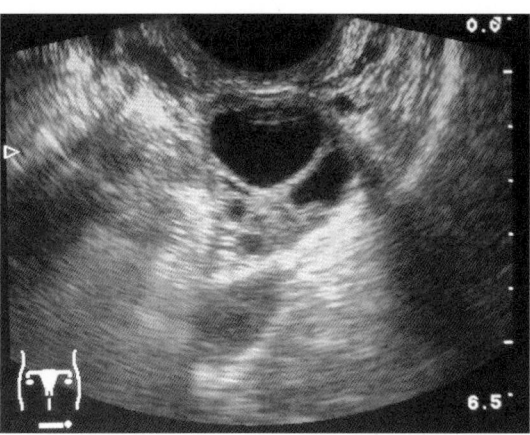

B

Figure 9-56. PID. Four markers of pelvic inflammatory disease. Transvaginal views. **A.** Longitudinal ultrasound image showing significant free fluid in the posterior cul-de-sac (pouch of Douglas) and a small amount of fluid in the anterior cul-de-sac. **B.** Endovaginal ultrasound image demonstrating a multicystic ovary.

(Figures 9-56C and D continued on next page)

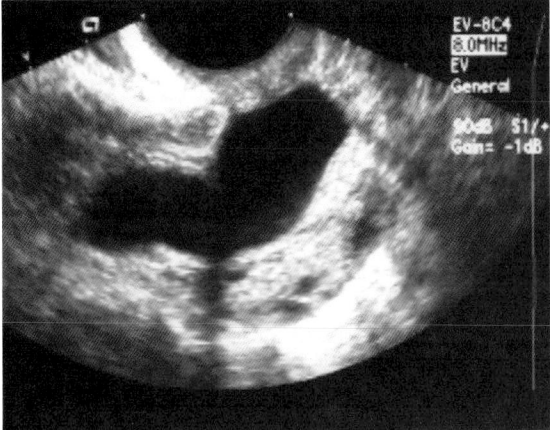

C

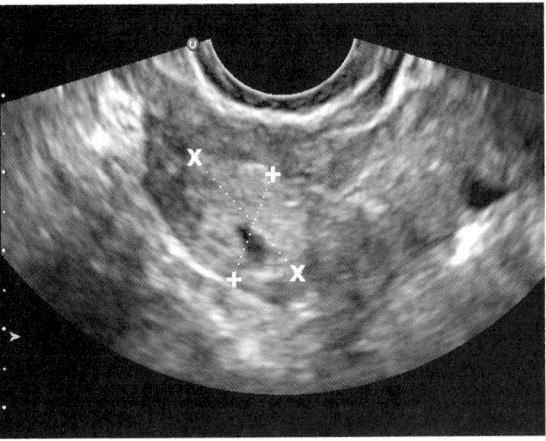

D

Figure 9-56. **C.** Hydrosalpinx. Fluid-filled fallopian tube adjacent to the ovary. **D.** A small adnexal mass is outlined by the measurement cursors.

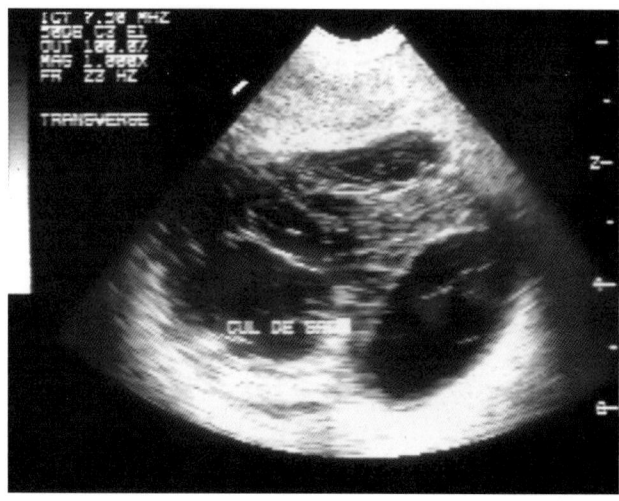

Figure 9-57. Tubo-ovarian abscess (TOA). Transvaginal coronal view of the cul-de-sac area shows a complex septated cystic mass 4 × 6 cm in size, which proved to be a TOA.

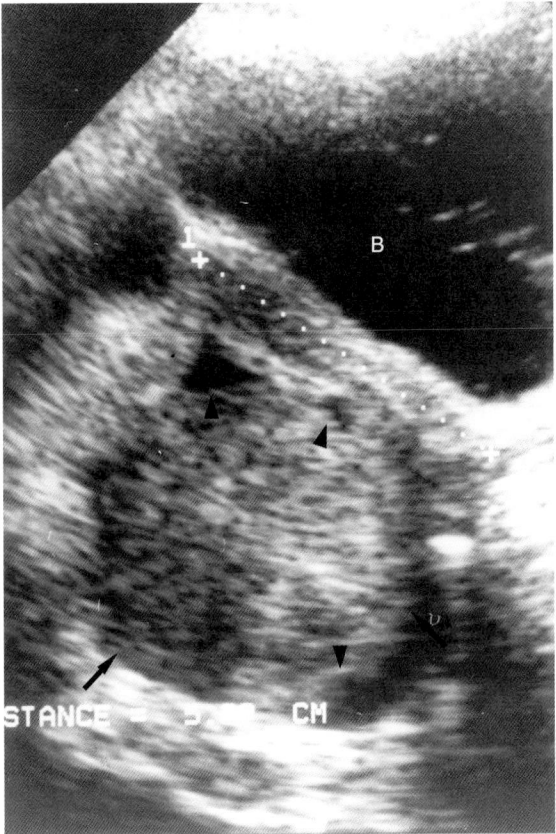

Figure 9-58. Ovarian torsion. Transabdominal sagittal view. The uterus is marked off by calipers and is 5 cm in length. Posterior to it is a large solid mass (*arrows*) with a few peripheral cysts (*arrowheads*). This is a relatively classic image for ovarian torsion, although the echogenicity of the ultrasound image is related to the variable internal contents of the torsed ovary. This mass, which is the patient's torsed left adnexa, was much larger than the patient's normal right adnexa. B = bladder. (Reproduced with permission from Cohen HL, Sivit CJ. *Fetal and Pediatric Ultrasound*. New York: McGraw-Hill, 2001:516.)

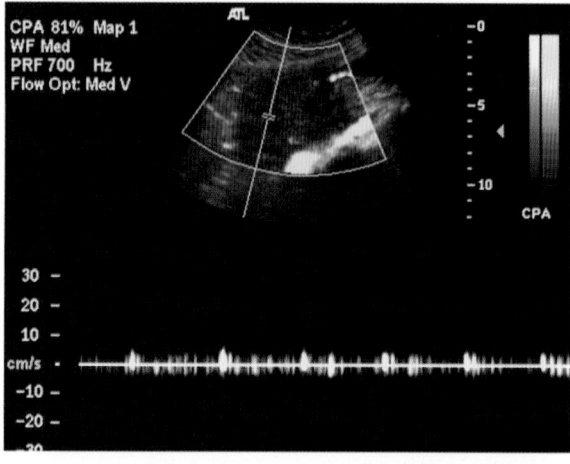

A

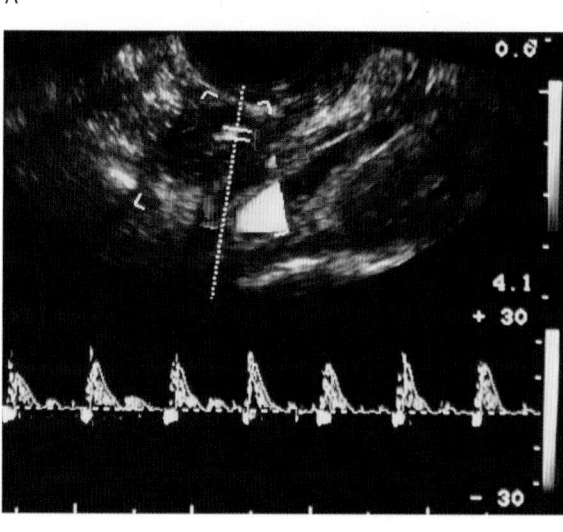

B

Figure 9-59. **A.** Inadequate ovarian arterial flow seen on spectral wave Doppler. **B.** Normal ovarian arterial flow seen on spectral wave Doppler.

▶ ADDITIONAL FINDINGS

- Intrauterine devices (Figures 9-60 and 61)

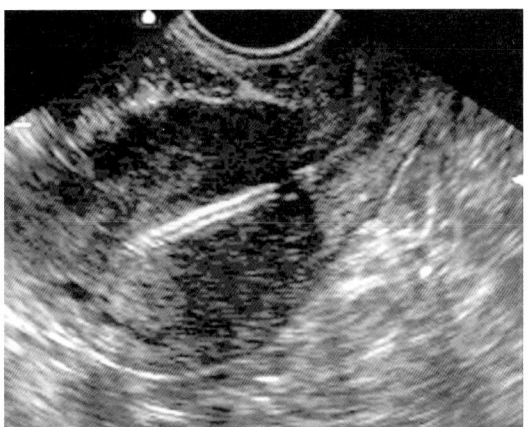

Figure 9-60. Intrauterine device (IUD). An IUD is strongly reflective and easily identified on transvaginal views.

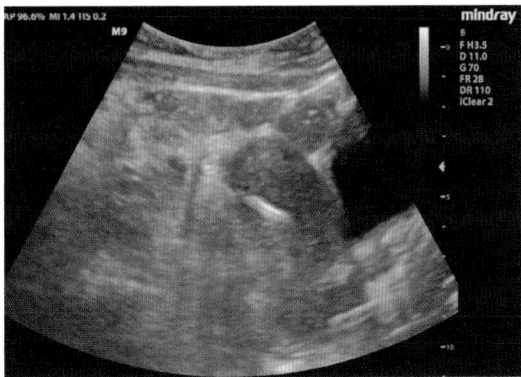

Figure 9-61. Uterine perforation from IUD. The IUD can be seen going through the myometrium and entering the abdominal cavity.

▶ PITFALLS

- Neglecting to look for free fluid in Morison's pouch when evaluating for ectopic pregnancy.

- Neglecting to look for an ectopic pregnancy because of a low β-human chorionic gonadotropin level.

- Attributing an empty uterus to an early intrauterine pregnancy or missed spontaneous abortion.

- Making the diagnosis of an intrauterine pregnancy without seeing a yolk sac or embryo within the uterus (Figure 9-62).

- Mistaking an interstitial pregnancy for an intrauterine pregnancy (Figure 9-63).

- Failure to diagnose a heterotopic pregnancy (especially in a patient on fertility drugs).

- Missing adnexal or ovarian torsion, especially during pregnancy.

- Doppler ultrasound is not accurate for diagnosing or ruling out ovarian torsion.

- A full bladder and myometrial contraction may confuse the exam for placenta previa.

- Placental abruption cannot be excluded by ultrasound.

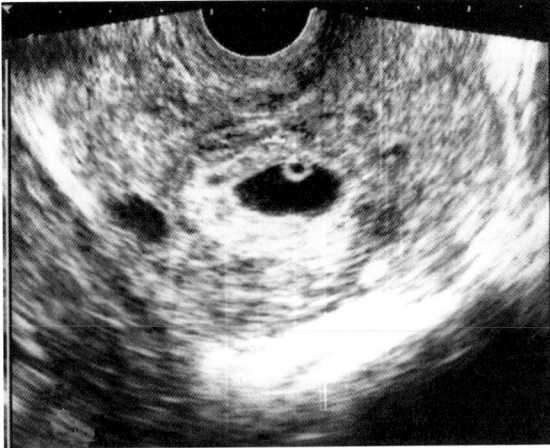

Figure 9-62. Ectopic pregnancy. Extrauterine gestational sac with a bright thick echogenic ring and a yolk sac within. A cursory examination could mistake the surrounding mid-level echoes as uterine tissue, but note the absence of any endometrial echo. Transvaginal image.

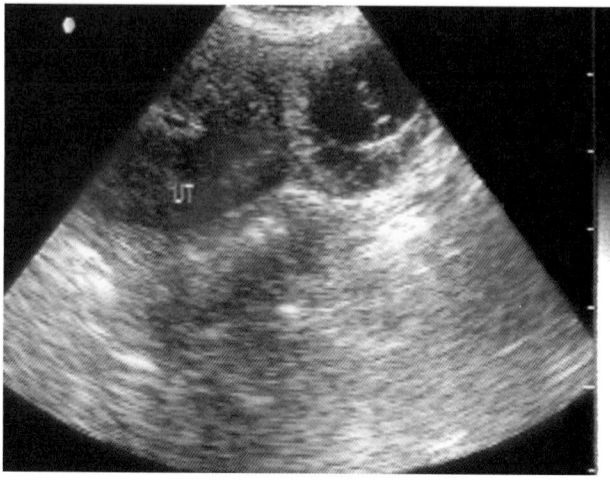

Figure 9-63. Interstitial ectopic pregnancy. Coronal transvaginal ultrasound image reveals a small fluid collection within the endometrium of the uterus (UT). The round echogenic ectopic ring was partially embedded within the uterine myometrium.

For more detailed information go to the comprehensive textbook Ma and Mateer's Emergency Ultrasound, 3rd edition, Chapter 14 "First Trimester Pregnancy" by Robert Reardon, MD, Jamie Hess-Keenan, MD, Chad Roline, MD, Liberty Caroon, RDMS and Scott Joing, MD; Chapter 15 "Second and Third Trimester Pregnancy" by Donald Bears, MD and Barry Knapp, MD; and Chapter 16 "Gynecological Concepts" by Christian Fox, MD and Michael Lambert, MD.

CHAPTER 10

Pediatrics

▶ CLINICAL CONSIDERATIONS

- Children are more sensitive to ionizing radiation than adults.

- Many of the ultrasound applications used in adults can be applied to children. Most anatomic structures are easier to visualize in children because of their smaller body habitus.

- Significant abnormalities, such as hemoperitoneum, pneumothorax, and pericardial effusion can be easily visualized in the pediatric trauma patient.

- In children presenting to the emergency department (ED) with head trauma, the finding of a skull fracture on ultrasound can prompt the decision to obtain a head computed tomography (CT) in a child who otherwise would be observed.

- In infants and children, ultrasound should be used initially to evaluate for any intra-abdominal pathology in order to minimize exposure to ionizing radiation.

- An inferior vena cava (IVC)/aorta ratio is better at determining dehydration in children than the World Health Organization dehydration scale or IVC inspiratory collapse.

- Ultrasound guidance can be used for many procedures in the pediatric patient.

▶ CLINICAL INDICATIONS

- Blunt or penetrating trauma
- Skull fracture
- Suspicion of appendicitis
- Suspicion of pyloric stenosis
- Suspicion of intussusception
- Volume status
- Urine collection

▶ ANATOMIC CONSIDERATIONS

- Children's small size and relatively less body fat make it easier to visualize intra-abdominal organs, including the bowel.

▶ TECHNIQUE AND NORMAL FINDINGS

Blunt or Penetrating Trauma

- The EFAST exam is carried out in the same fashion as it is in adults (see Chapter 2). See Figure 10-1.

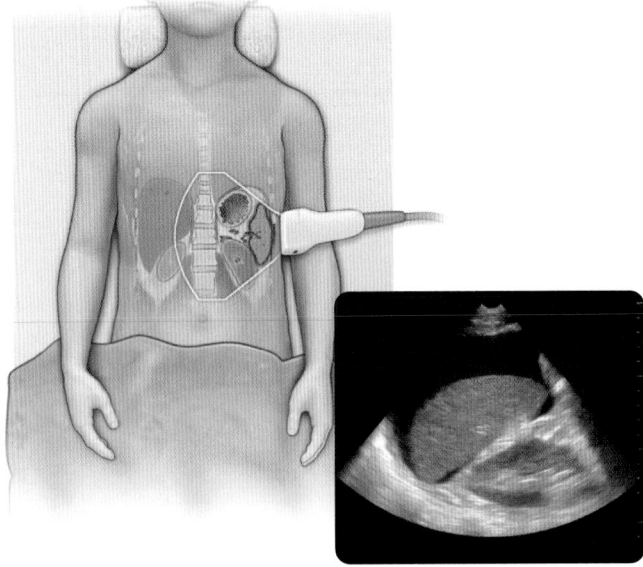

Figure 10-1. Hemoperitoneum-perisplenic free fluid. Details of the trauma ultrasound exam can be found in Chapter 2.

Skull Fracture

- Place the linear transducer on the skull over the area of injury (Figures 10-2 and 10-3).

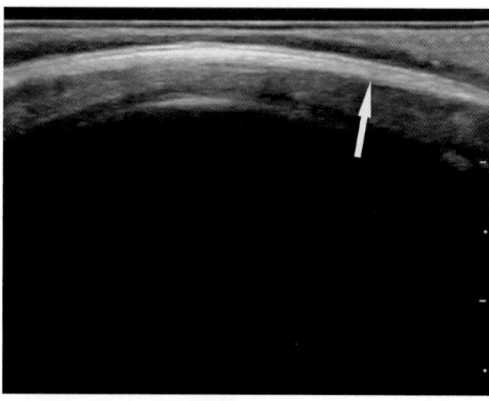

Figure 10-2. Normal skull. The cortex of the skull appears as a hyperechoic curvilinear line (*arrow*).

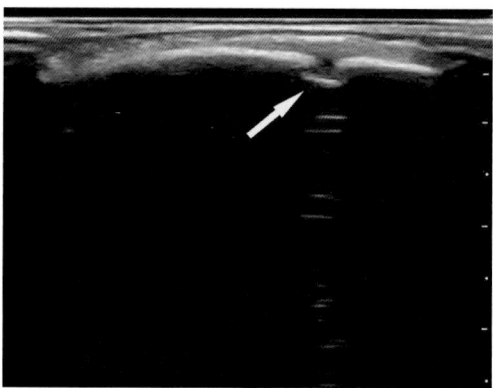

Figure 10-3. Normal cranial sutures may have an end-to-end appearance (*arrow*).

(See Figures 10-11 and 10-12 for abnormal findings.)

Suspicion of Appendicitis

- Use the linear transducer to evaluate the appendix.
- Scan the right lower quadrant in the transverse orientation using the bladder, iliac vessels, spoas muscle and cecum as landmarks (Figure 10-4A and B).
- Scan the cecum, ileum, and appendix in the transverse and sagittal planes.
- Appendix diameter of greater than 6 mm (outer wall-to-outer wall) is suspicious for appendicitis (Figure 10-4C).
- The appendix must be identified in two planes—as a circular target-like structure in the short axis and as a tubular structure with a blind end in the long axis.

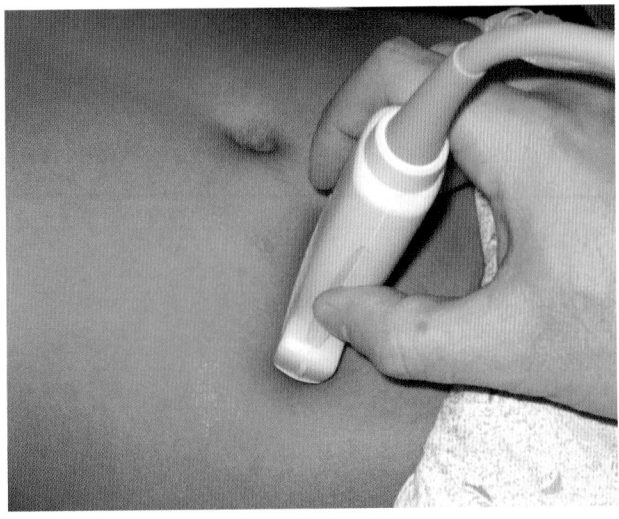

A

Figure 10-4. Ultrasound of appendix. **A.** Transducer positioning in transverse view.

(Figures 10-4B and C continued on next page)

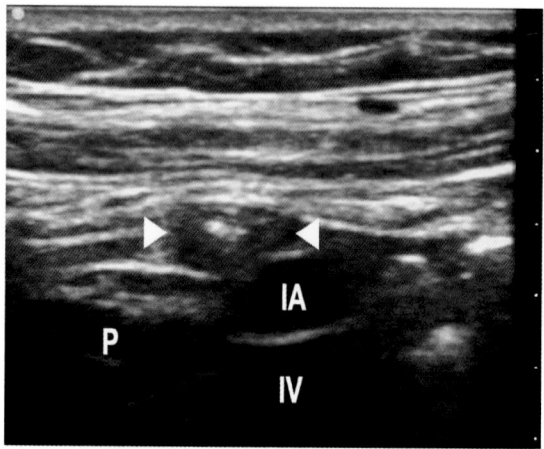

B

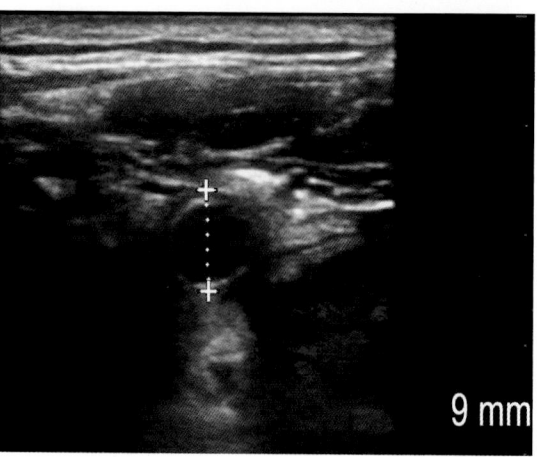

C

Figure 10-4. Ultrasound of appendix. **B.** Short-axis view with compression shows a normal appendix with targetoid appearance and diameter of 4 mm. P = psoas muscle; IA = iliac artery; IV= iliac vein; arrowheads = appendix. **C.** Short-axis view of appendix with diameter of 9 mm, suspicious for acute appendicitis.

Suspicion of Pyloric Stenosis

- Place the linear transducer in the epigastric region in the transverse orientation (Figure 10-5).

- The pylorus will be visualized through or adjacent to the left lobe of the liver (Figure 10-6).

- The normal pylorus is a ring of muscle with a muscle wall thickness of <3 mm and a length <17 mm.

- With pathologic hypertrophy it both thickens and lengthens.

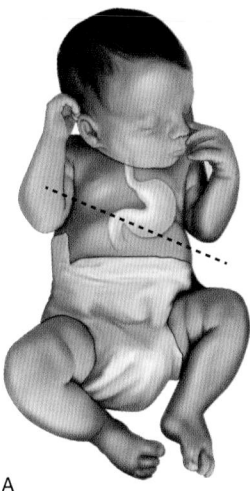

A

Figure 10-5. Transducer position for the pylorus. **A.** Orientation line for pylorus. The plane for imaging the pylorus along its length (represented by dotted line) is intermediate between the transverse and sagittal planes.

(Figure 10-5B continued on next page)

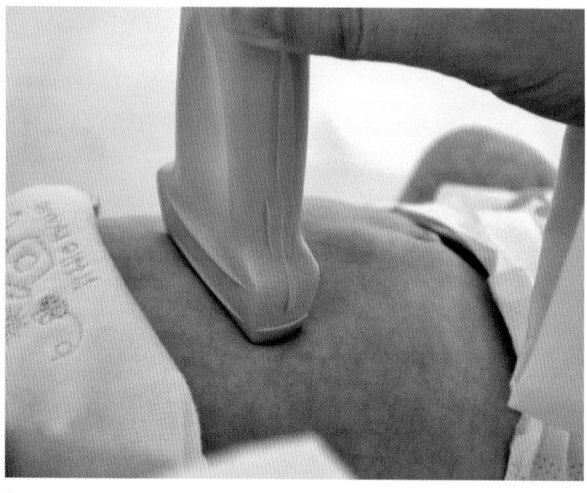

B

Figure 10-5. **B.** Initial probe position. A high-frequency linear array probe is started in the transverse body plane, and aligned with the long-axis view of the pylorus.

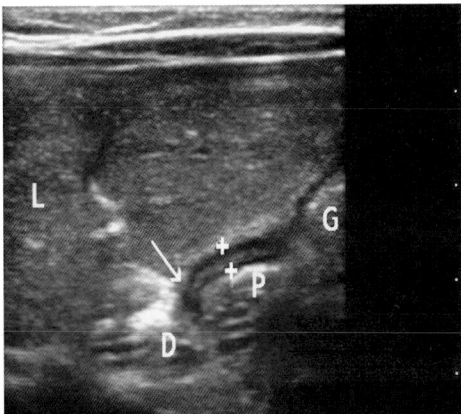

A

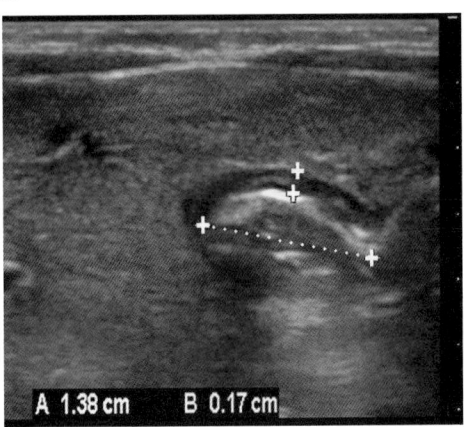

B

Figure 10-6. Normal pylorus. **A.** The pylorus (P) and pyloric sphincter (*arrow*) visualized using the liver (L) as an acoustic window. **B.** Pyloric channel length (calipers A), MWT (calipers B). The posterior pyloric wall is obstructed by gas within the canal. MWT = muscle wall thickness (calipers); G = gastrum; D = duodenum. Arrow points to the pyloric sphincter.

(See Figures 10-13 and 10-14 for abnormal findings.)

Suspicion of Intussusception

- Place the linear transducer in the transverse plane on the abdominal wall.

- An ileocolic intussusception is most commonly found in the right upper quadrant.

- Scan the transverse and ascending colon and cecum in both the transverse and longitudinal planes (Figure 10-7).

- If an abdominal mass is palpated, scan it in multiple planes.

- A segment of intussuscepted bowel will have multiple thick hypoechoic layers and look distinctly different from normal bowel.

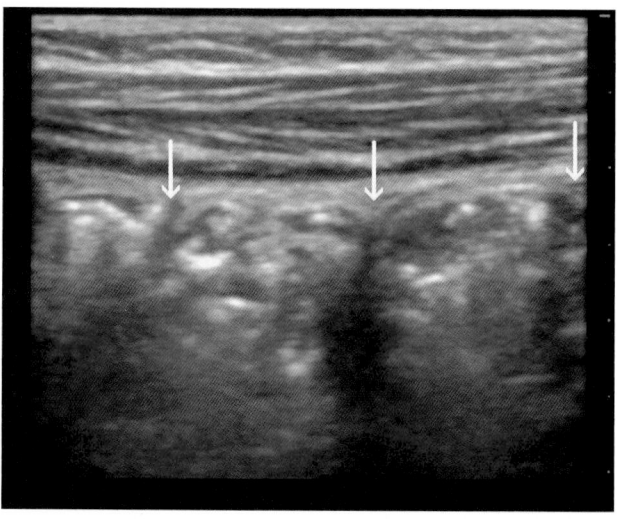

Figure 10-7. Normal ascending colon in sagittal view with regular haustral markings (*arrows*).

(See Figure 10-15 for abnormal findings.)

Volume Status

- Use an appropriate sized probe (usually curvilinear) and place in the transverse plane in the midline of the abdomen.
- Visualize both the IVC and aorta (Figure 10-8).
- Measure the AP diameter of both the IVC and aorta in the expiratory phase.
- An IVC/aorta ratio of less than or equal to 0.8 suggests significant dehydration.

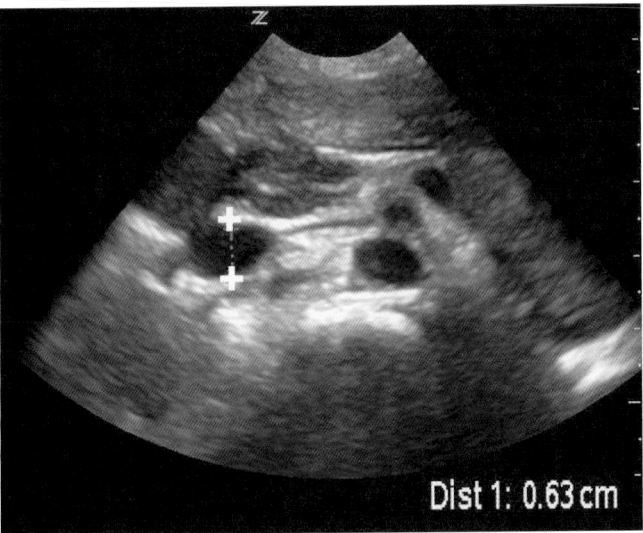

Figure 10-8. Transverse view IVC and aorta. Caliper measurements of the anterior-posterior diameter of the IVC.

Urine Collection

- Place either the linear or curvilinear transducer in the sagittal plane over the suprapubic region to visualize the bladder (Figure 10-9).

- If the bladder is not empty, urine may be collected by catheterization or suprapubic aspiration.

- For suprapubic urine aspiration, insert the needle directly over the bladder and visualize the needle entering the bladder (Figure 10-10).

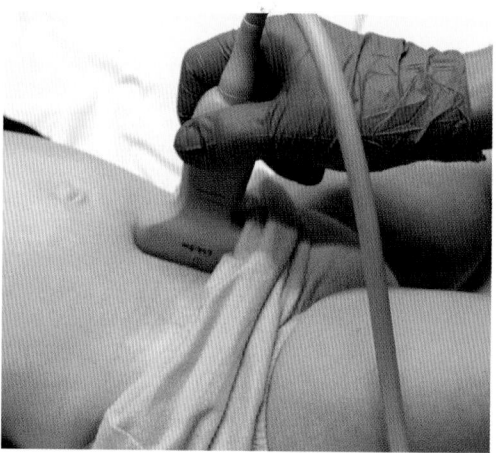

A

Figure 10-9. Urinary bladder. **A.** The transducer should be placed in a sagittal orientation, just above the symphysis pubis in the midline of the lower abdomen.

(Figures 10-9B continued on next page)

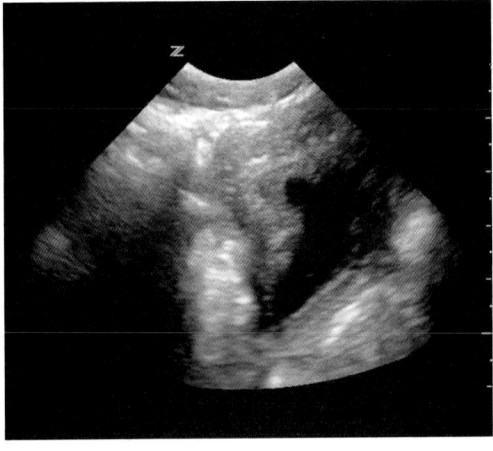

B

Figure 10-9. **B.** Corresponding longitudinal ultrasound image of a partially filled bladder.

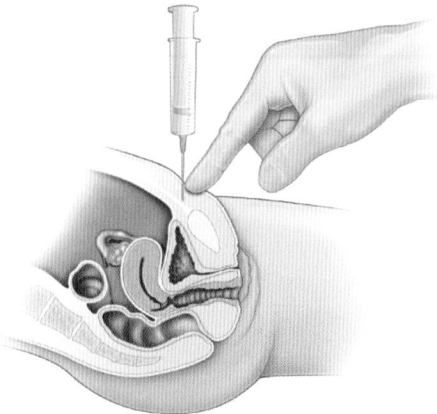

Figure 10-10. Suprapubic aspiration. The needle is generally inserted directly over the bladder and perpendicular to the skin, one fingerbreadth above the symphysis pubis. Ultrasound guidance (indirect or direct) provides a more accurate location for puncture.

► TIPS TO IMPROVE IMAGE ACQUISITION

- Choose the transducer with the highest frequency possible or a specialized pediatric transducer, as appropriate, for the size of the child.
- When imaging the bowel, graded compression with adequate pressure and patience is needed to push bowel gas out of the way.

► COMMON AND EMERGENT ABNORMALITIES

- Skull fracture (Figures 10-11 and 10-12)
- Suspicion of appendicitis
  - Obtain images
- Suspicion of pyloric stenosis (Figures 10-13 and 10-14)
- Suspicion of intussusception (Figure 10-15)

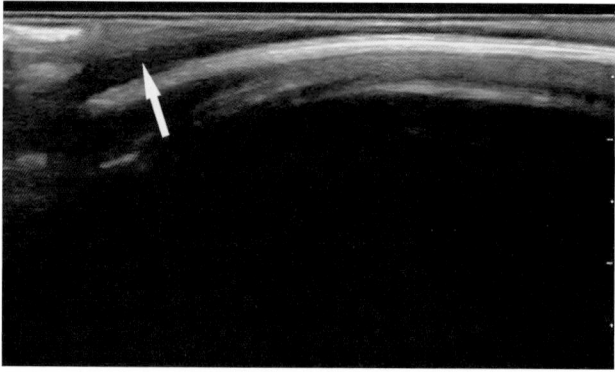

Figure 10-11. Overlying soft tissue may be edematous or demonstrate distinct hematoma formation (*arrow*) adjacent to the cortex.

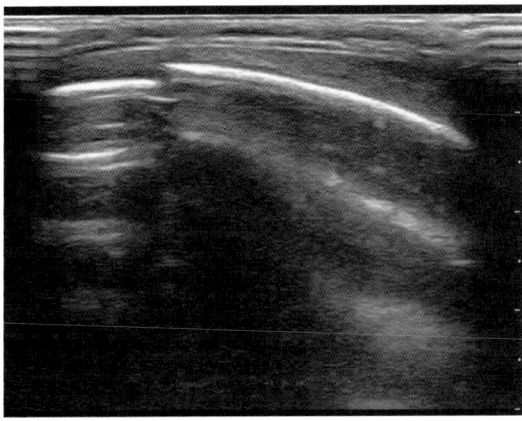

Figure 10-12. A skull fracture appears as a hypoechoic break in the contour of the hyperechoic skull.

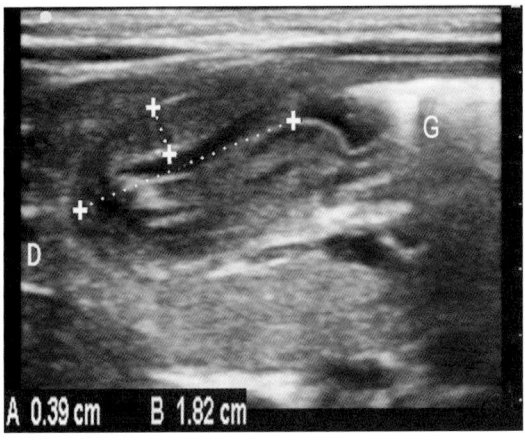

A

Figure 10-13. Hypertrophic pyloric stenosis. **A.** Long-axis view of thickened pyloric muscle wall (caliper A) and elongated channel (caliper B) situated between gastrum (G) and duodenum.

(Figure 10-13B continued on next page)

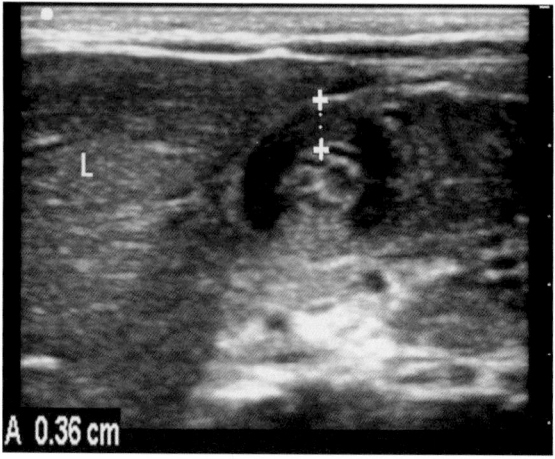

B

Figure 10-13. Hypertrophic pyloric stenosis. **B.** Short-axis view of thickened pyloric muscle wall (caliper). L = liver.

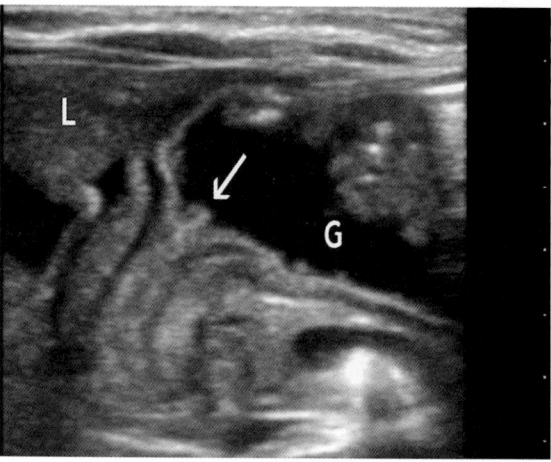

Figure 10-14. Hypertrophic pyloric stenosis. Antral nipple sign. The nipple-shaped mass (*arrow*) is protruding into the fluid-filled gastric antrum (G). L = liver.

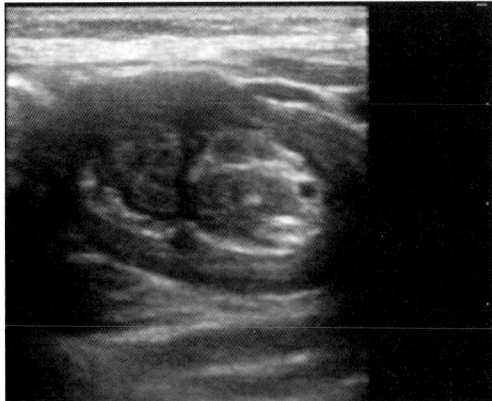

A

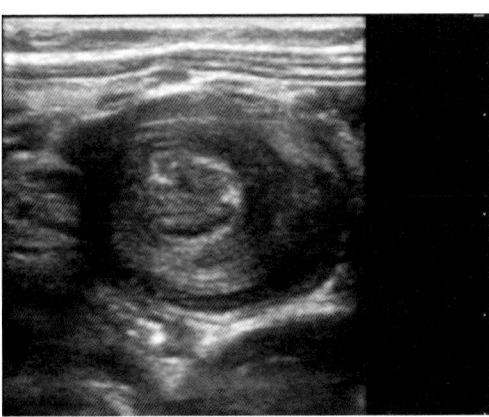

B

Figure 10-15. Intussusception. **A.** Longitudinal image of intussusception demonstrating the "pseudokidney sign." Hypodense areas of intussusception are edematous bowel wall. Hyperechoic central area is caused by bowel contents (and possibly intussuscepted mesenteric fat). **B.** Transverse scan through ascending colon demonstrates the "donut" appearance of intussusception. The outer ring is the intussuscipiens, while the central echoes are the intussusceptum.

▶ PITFALLS

- Using inappropriate depth settings, especially for providers who are used to scanning adults.

- Disorientation as a result of multiple organs being visualized in a single view due to the smaller size of children.

- Not being patient enough or applying adequate pressure to push bowel gas out of the way.

- Not realizing that in the severely dehydrated child it may be very difficult or impossible to visualize the IVC.

For more detailed information go to the comprehensive textbook Ma and Mateer's Emergency Ultrasound, 3rd edition, Chapter 20 "Pediatric Applications" by Jason Fischer, MD, Adam Sivitz, MD and Alyssa Abo, MD.

CHAPTER 11

Deep Venous Thrombosis

▶ CLINICAL CONSIDERATIONS

- Studies show that an abbreviated exam using simple compression of the proximal leg veins maintains accuracy for deep venous thrombosis (DVT) detection while decreasing the time required for the exam compared with comprehensive duplex sonography of the entire lower extremity.
- Considerable data demonstrate that emergency physicians can accurately use this method.
- Consider repeating the exam in 5 to 7 days to look for propagation of clots from the calf.

▶ CLINICAL INDICATION

- Suspicion of lower extremity DVT

▶ ANATOMIC CONSIDERATIONS

Limited compression sonography of the lower extremity deep veins includes scanning at the following anatomic locations:

- The junction of the common femoral vein (CFV) and great saphenous vein (GSV) just below the inguinal ligament (Figure 11-1)
- The CFV from the saphenous junction to the bifurcation of the superficial femoral vein (SFV) (see comment under Pitfalls) and the deep femoral vein (DFV)
- At the junction of the SFV (see comment under Pitfalls) and DFV
- The entire popliteal vein from the top of the popliteal fossa to the level of the trifurcation of the calf veins

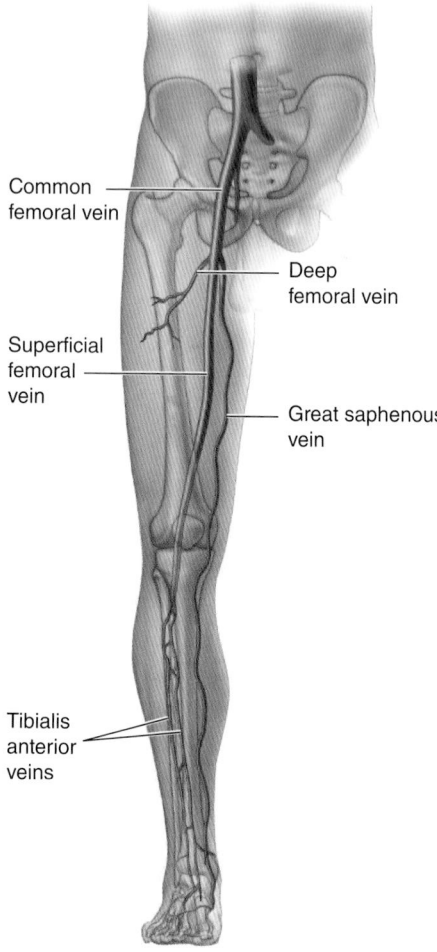

Common femoral vein

Deep femoral vein

Superficial femoral vein

Great saphenous vein

Tibialis anterior veins

Figure 11-1. The deep femoral vein and superficial femoral vein are seen to come together, forming the common femoral vein.

▶ TECHNIQUE AND NORMAL FINDINGS

- Use a high-resolution linear transducer.
- Position the patient with the head elevated (Figures 11-2 and 11-3).
- Image the vessels in the transverse orientation (Figures 11-4 and 11-5).
- Patent veins without thrombus should collapse completely.

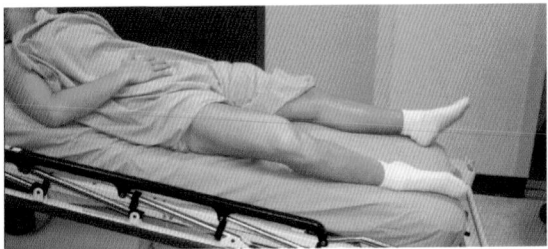

Figure 11-2. A bed angle of 30 to 45 degrees allows the lower extremity veins to fill and makes them easier to locate.

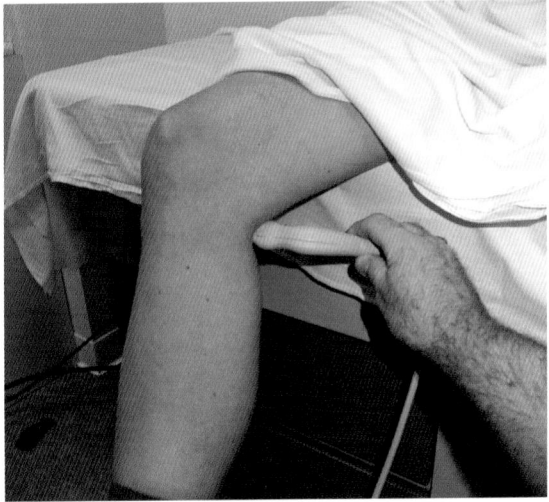

Figure 11-3. The leg is allowed to hang over the edge of the bed with the probe positioned in the popliteal fossa.

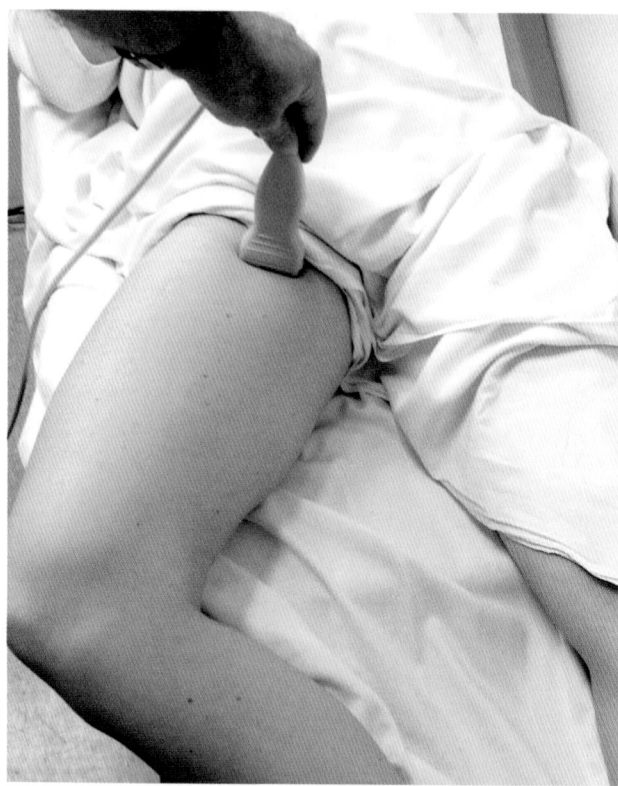

Figure 11-4. The approximate position of the linear probe is shown transversely over the common femoral vein. The probe handle is being held near the cord for demonstration.

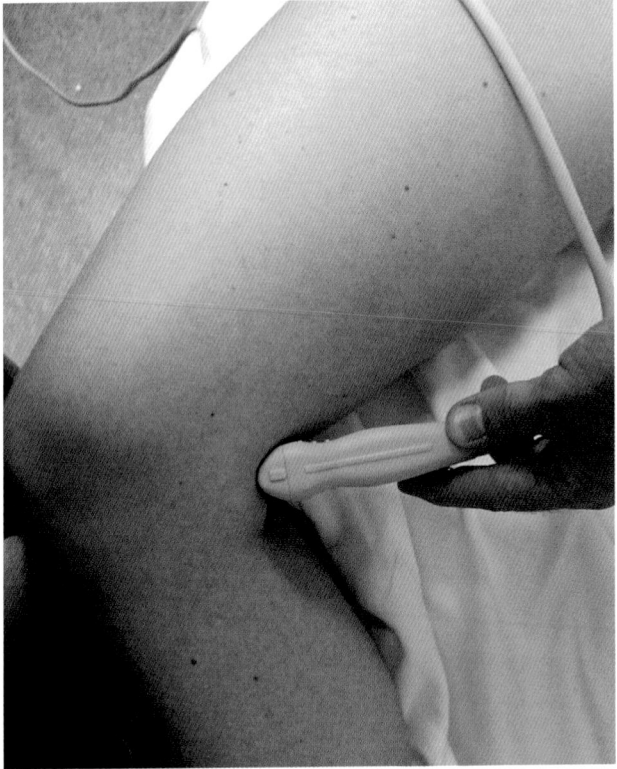

Figure 11-5. The probe is positioned in the popliteal fossa for visualization of the popliteal artery and vein.

Femoral Vein

- Start as proximal as possible, just below the inguinal ligament, and compress the CFV.

- Identify the junction of the CFV and GSV and compress both (Figure 11-6).

- Move distally and compress the CFV every 1 cm (Figure 11-7).

- Identify the junction of the SFV and DFV and compress both (Figure 11-8).

- The abbreviated exam does not require views of the SFV distal to the SFV/DFV junction.

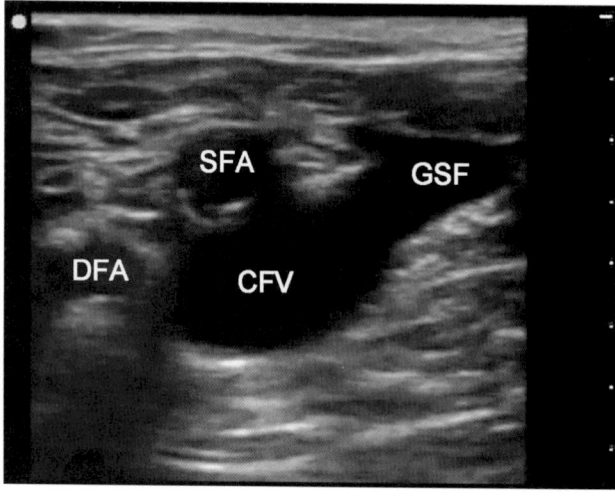

A

Figure 11-6. Transverse view of the common femoral vein (CFV) at the junction of the great saphenous vein (GSV). This is a common location for DVT formation. The CFV/GSF junction is often distal to the bifurcation of the common femoral artery into the deep femoral artery (DFA) and superficial femoral artery (SFA).

(Figure 11-6B continued on next page)

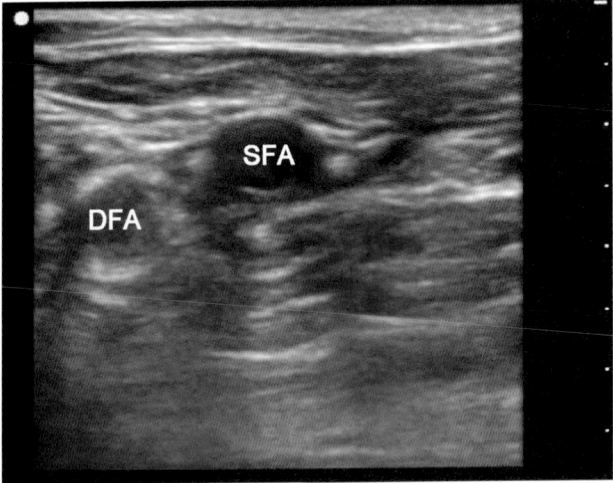

B

Figure 11-6. **B.** Compression view demonstrates complete collapse of the common femoral vein (CFV). The great saphenous vein can be seen branching anteromedially and is mostly collapsed in this view (slight probe repositioning and pressure should be applied to ensure complete collapse if subtle thrombus is to be excluded in this vessel). SFA = superficial femoral artery, DFA = deep femoral artery.

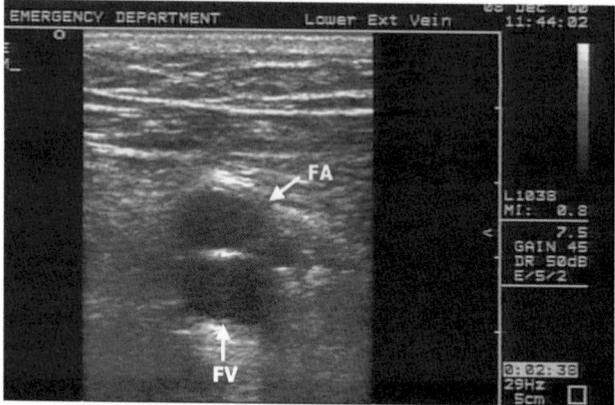

A

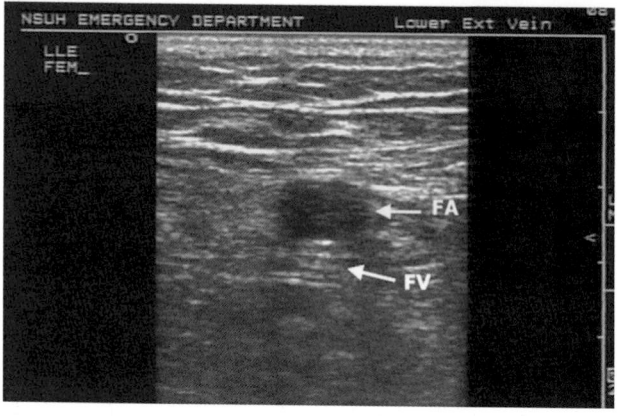

B

Figure 11-7. Normal (no DVT) common femoral vein (FV), a few centimeters below the inguinal ligament. **A.** With no transducer pressure. **B.** With moderate transducer pressure, resulting in complete compression of the femoral vein. FA = femoral artery.

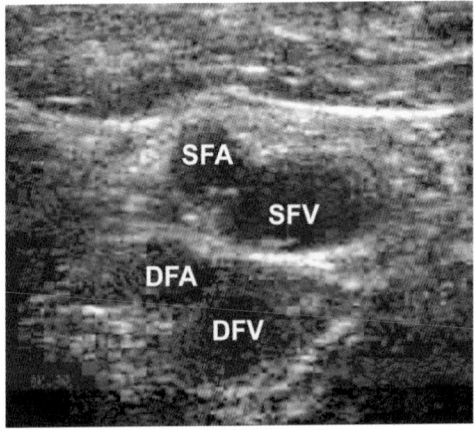

A

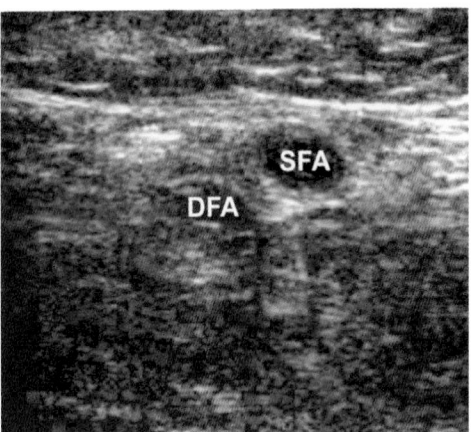

B

Figure 11-8. Normal (no DVT). The transducer is positioned just distal to the junction of the superficial and deep femoral veins (SFV and DFV, respectively). **A.** With no transducer pressure. **B.** With moderate transducer pressure, resulting in complete compression of the SFV and DFV. SFA = superficial femoral artery; DFA = deep femoral artery.

Popliteal Vein

- Start as proximal as possible in the popliteal fossa and compress the popliteal vein.
- Note that the popliteal vein is often duplicated.
- Move distally and compress the popliteal vein every 1 cm.
- Identify where the distal popliteal vein trifurcates and compress all three veins.
- The abbreviated exam does not require views of the distal calf veins.

▶ TIPS TO IMPROVE IMAGE ACQUISITION

- Position the patient as needed to maximally distend the leg veins.
- Decrease ultrasound frequency for deeper veins.
- Veins must be completely compressed to exclude the presence of thrombus.
- The front wall of the vein must touch the back wall to ensure complete compression.
- Press hard if needed to compress the veins.

▶ COMMON AND EMERGENT ABNORMALITY

Deep Vein Thrombosis

See Figures 11-9 to 11-11.

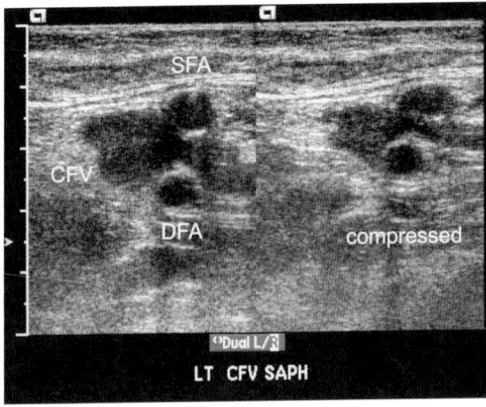

Figure 11-9. DVT in the left common femoral vein (CFV) near the saphenous junction. The CFV does not fully collapse with compression and contains internal echoes that represent clot. SFA = superficial femoral artery; DFA = deep femoral artery.

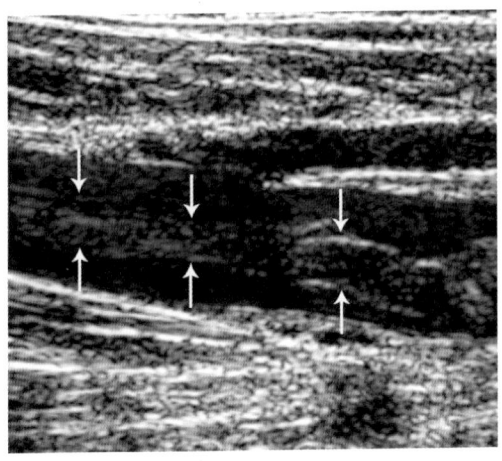

Figure 11-10. DVT. *Arrows* show a freely floating thrombus in the femoral vein. In this portion of the image, the clot does not come in contact with the anterior or posterior wall of the vein. The vein did not fully collapse with compression.

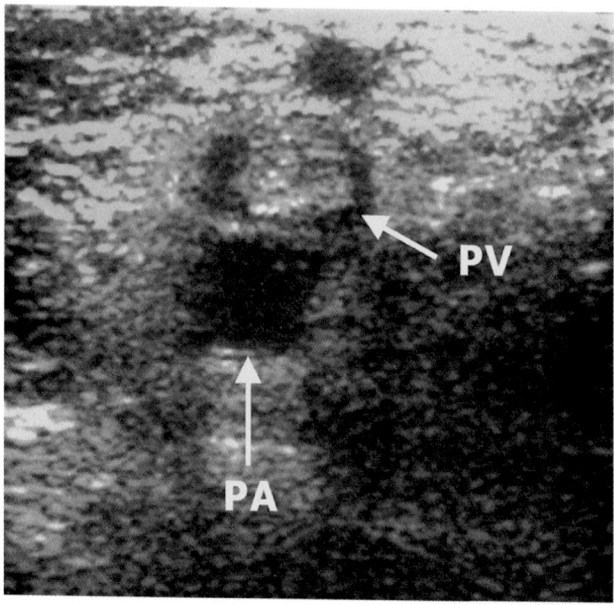

Figure 11-11. DVT. The popliteal vein (PV) is visualized above the popliteal artery (PA) and has a distinct echogenic thrombus within it. The PV did not collapse with compression.

► ADDITIONAL FINDINGS

Chronic Deep Vein Thrombosis with Recanalization

See Figures 11-12 to 11-14.

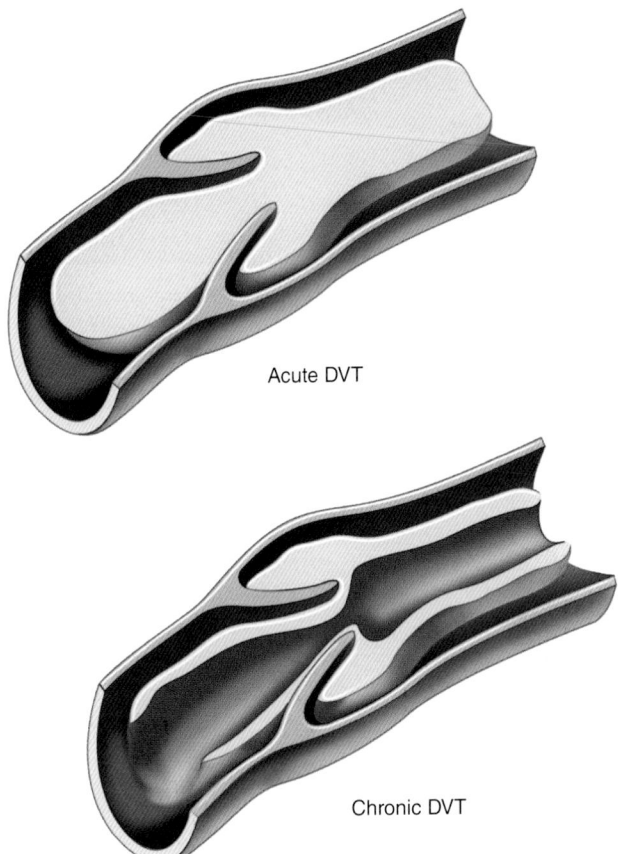

Acute DVT

Chronic DVT

Figure 11-12. The *bottom* illustration shows a recanalized, old thrombus. The *top* illustration demonstrates an early acute thrombus that can enlarge and obstruct flow completely.

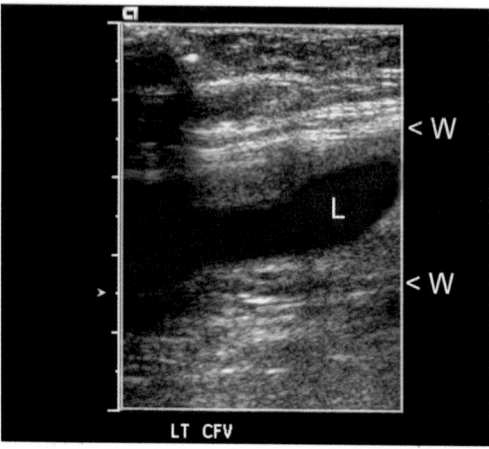

Figure 11-13. Longitudinal view of the common femoral vein shows chronic echogenic clot along the walls (W) with central recanalization of the lumen (L).

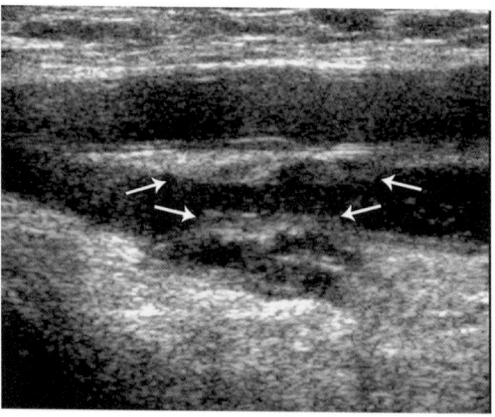

Figure 11-14. A chronic deep venous thrombosis (DVT) is seen in this deep femoral vein. *Arrows* point to areas of scarring that are echogenic and lie along the walls of the vein. A channel is open for blood flow in between the two areas of scar or chronic DVT.

Baker's Cyst

See Figures 11-15 to 11-17.

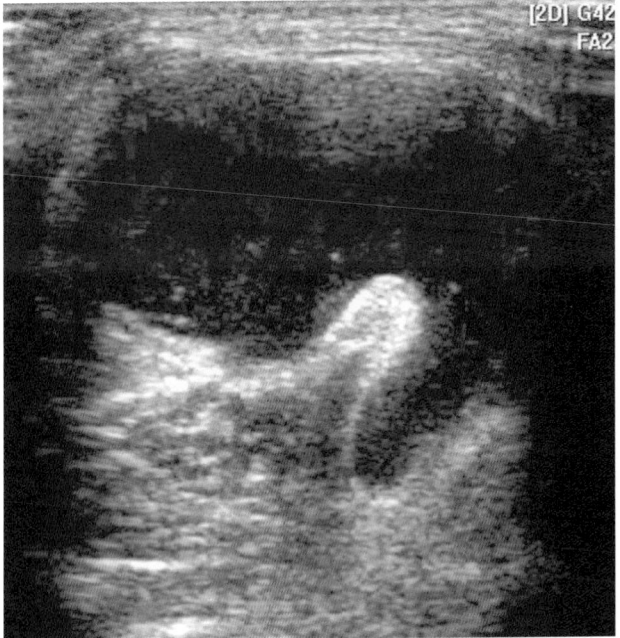

Figure 11-15. Longitudinal view of the posterior knee area demonstrates a large Baker's cyst.

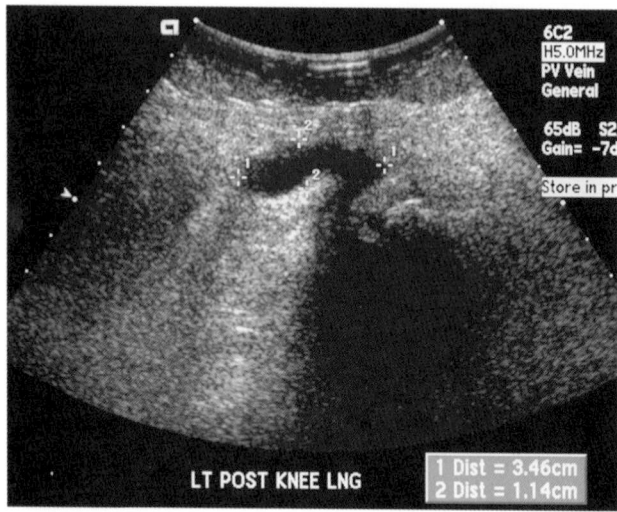

Figure 11-16. Longitudinal view of the posterior knee reveals a small Baker's cyst.

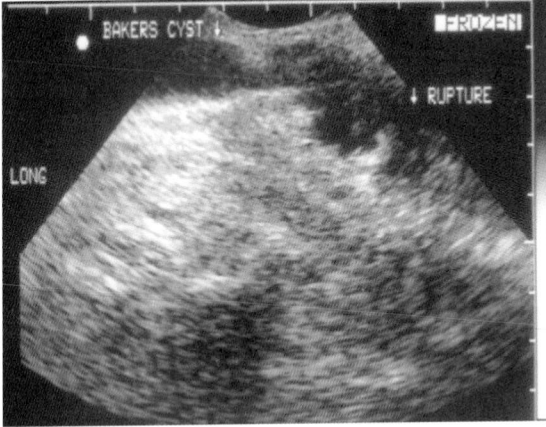

A

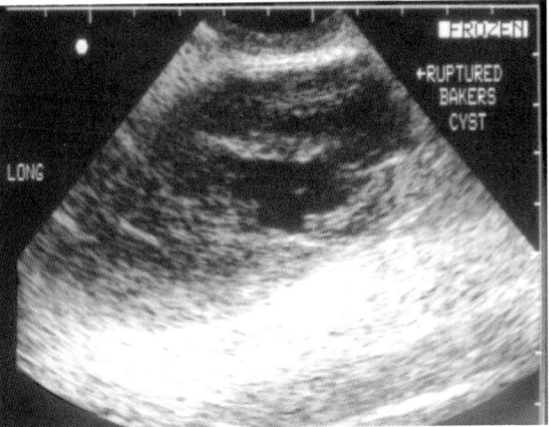

B

Figure 11-17. Ruptured Baker's cyst. **A.** Longitudinal view of the posterior knee shows a Baker's cyst (*left upper image*) communicating with subcutaneous fluid in the upper calf. **B.** Longitudinal view over the midcalf of the same patient shows a significant amount of subcutaneous fluid dissecting inferiorly.

▶ PITFALLS

- The SFV is actually a deep vein. To avoid confusion, some have renamed this the "femoral vein."

- Misunderstanding the limitations of simple compression ultrasound

- Do not rely on a difficult or incomplete exam (Figure 11-18).

- Missing a non-occlusive DVT with partial vein compression (Figure 11-19)

- Duplicated veins (especially popliteal)

- Segmental DVT (rare)

- Superficial vein thrombus in the great saphenous vein or the calf veins may propagate into the deep veins, so limited compression ultrasound exams should be repeated in 5 to 7 days if clinically indicated (Figure 11-20).

- Misidentifying an artery as a vein

- Mistaking femoral lymph nodes for DVT (Figure 11-21)

- Pelvic vein thrombosis: The abbreviated exam is not adequate to detect isolated iliac vein thrombosis; additional studies are required if pelvic vein thrombosis is suspected.

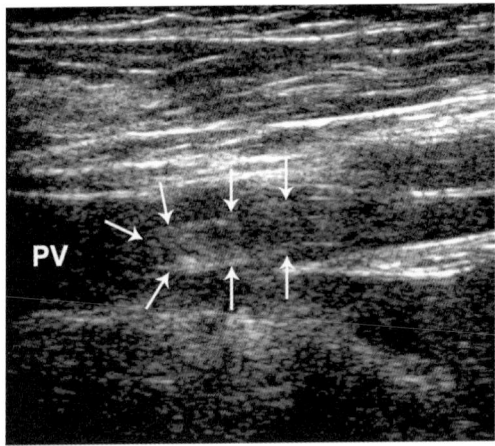

Figure 11-18. A longitudinal image of the popliteal vein (PV) on the left side of the image. On the right side, the PV is splitting. *Arrows* outline a free-floating thrombus coming out of a calf vein into the very distal portion of the PV. This clot would not have been caught if imaging had not included the proximal portion of the popliteal trifurcation. There was incomplete collapse of this vein with compression.

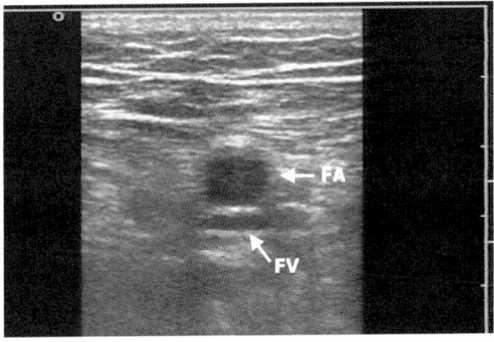

Figure 11-19. The femoral vein (FV) is not completely collapsed. If adequate pressure has been applied, a thrombus is likely present. FA = femoral artery.

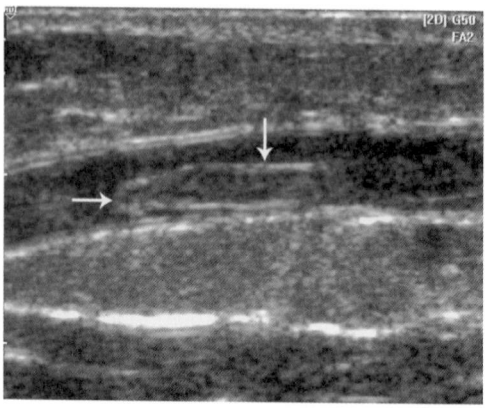

Figure 11-20. This thrombus (*arrows*) located in the great saphenous vein in the distal thigh was noted to travel to the upper thigh in just 2 days when the patient returned for follow-up. Scanning of this vein is not part of the limited exam. This case highlights the importance of repeating the evaluation of the deep veins in 5 to 7 days.

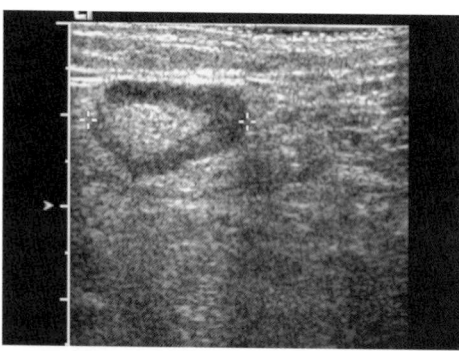

Figure 11-21. Typical appearance of an enlarged inguinal lymph node (2 cm). The thickened capsule is hypoechoic, and the central hilum is echogenic.

For more detailed information go to the comprehensive textbook Ma and Mateer's Emergency Ultrasound, 3rd edition, Chapter 17 "Deep Venous Thrombosis" by Thomas Costantino, MD, Harry Goett, MD and Michael Peterson, MD.

CHAPTER 12
Ocular

▶ CLINICAL CONSIDERATIONS

- Many serious ocular injuries are missed.
- Physical exam of the eye can be difficult and unreliable, especially after trauma and in patients who are unconscious or uncooperative.
- The eye is relatively easy to ultrasound because it is fluid filled.
- Optic nerve sheath measurements may be helpful in diagnosing elevated intracranial pressure (ICP).

▶ CLINICAL INDICATIONS

- Eye trauma
- Acute change in vision
- Elevated ICP

► ANATOMIC CONSIDERATIONS

- The anterior chamber consists of the cornea and lens.

- The cornea appears as a thin, hyperechoic structure attached to the sclera at the periphery.

- Echolucent aqueous humor fills the anterior chamber.

- The lens appears as a hyperechoic reflector, which is concave, and may show reverberation artifact at the anterior surface.

- The retina varies from 0.56 mm near the optic disk to 0.1 mm anteriorly. Its anterior surface is in contact with the vitreous body, and the posterior surface is strongly adherent to the choroid.

- The optic nerve and sheath may be seen posterior to the globe, traveling toward the optic chiasm.

- Measurement of the sheath is made 3 mm posterior to the globe. Normal measurements vary by age from 5 mm and smaller in adults, 4.5 mm in children 1 to 15 years of age, and 4 mm or smaller in children younger than 1 year of age.

► TECHNIQUE AND NORMAL FINDINGS

- Use a linear transducer with a frequency of 7 to 14 MHz.

- Apply a large amount of gel to fill the preorbital space (Figure 12-1).

- Float the transducer above the eyelid and obtain images in two orthogonal planes (Figure 12-2).

- Sweep the transducer from side to side or have the patient move the eye in order to identify the anterior structures and visualize the entire retina (Figure 12-3).

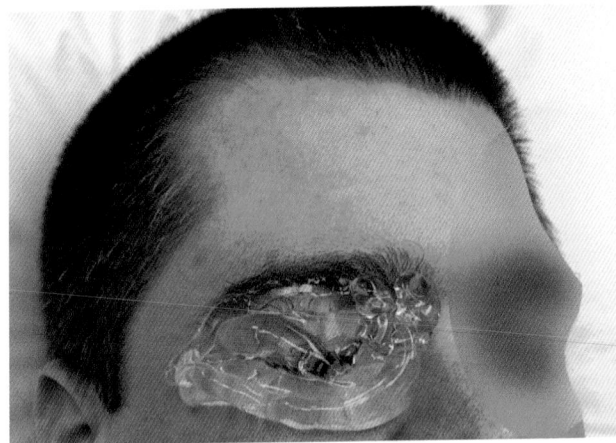

Figure 12-1. A generous amount of gel is placed on top of the closed eyelid. This much gel allows the sonologist to make no direct contact between the transducer and the eyelid itself.

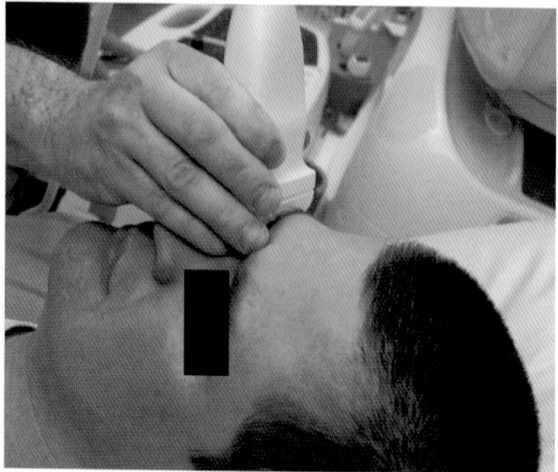

A

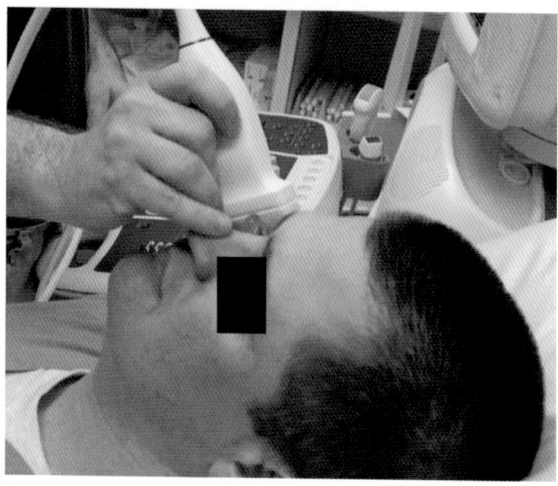

B

Figure 12-2. **A.** Longitudinal view probe position. **B.** Short-axis view probe position.

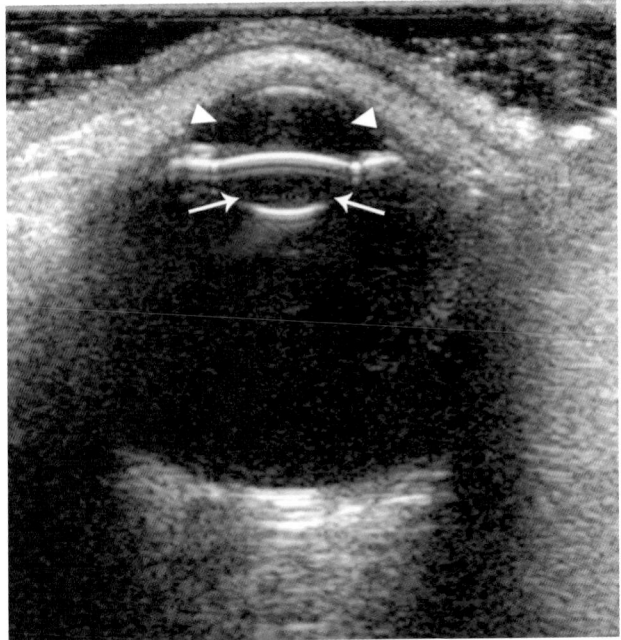

Figure 12-3. Normal ultrasound image of the eye. The anterior chamber (*arrowheads*) and the lens (*arrows*) are clearly seen. The vitreous appears black.

▶ TIPS TO IMPROVE IMAGE ACQUISITION

- Have the patient keep both eyes closed during the exam.
- Adjust gain up and down over a wide range to eliminate artifacts and identify subtle findings.
- Eye movement during the exam may unmask subtle pathology.

▶ COMMON AND EMERGENT ABNORMALITIES

- Retinal detachment (Figures 12-4 and 12-5)
- Vitreous detachment (Figure 12-6)
- Vitreous hemorrhage (Figure 12-7)
- Globe perforation (Figure 12-8)

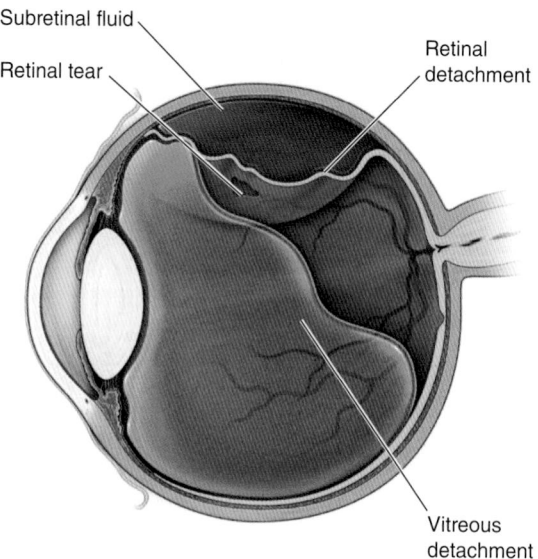

Subretinal fluid

Retinal tear

Retinal detachment

Vitreous detachment

Figure 12-4. Eye with retinal and posterior vitreous detachment.

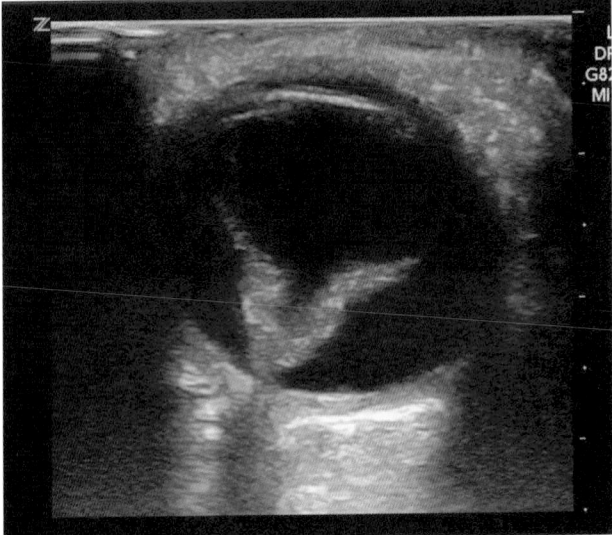

Figure 12-5. Complete retinal detachment. Characteristic
V-shaped membrane attached at the optic disc.

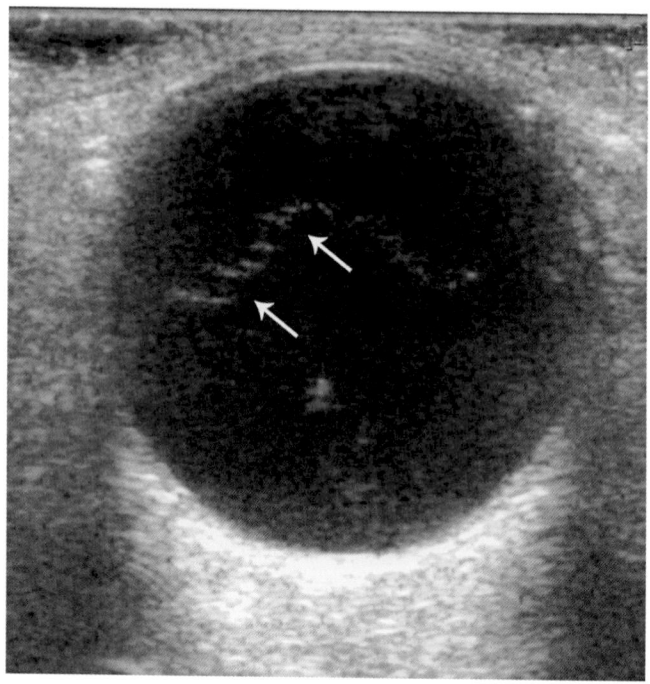

Figure 12-6. A web-like structure (*arrows*), representing the detached vitreous membrane.

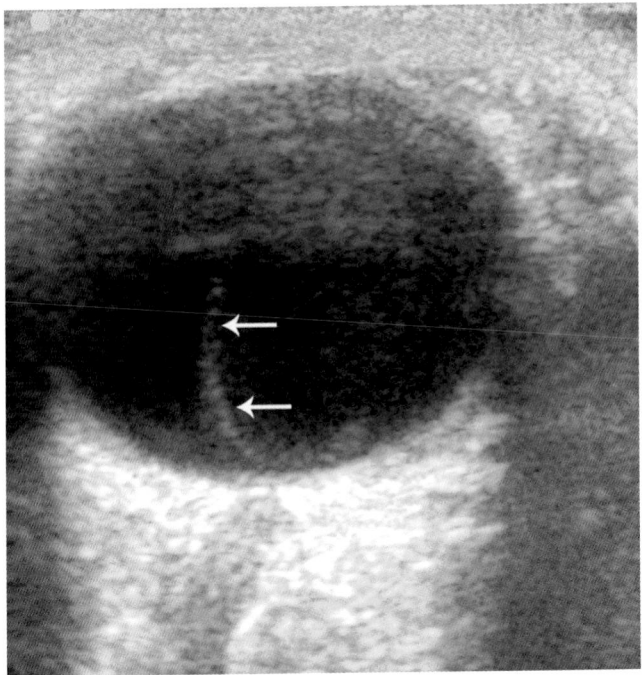

Figure 12-7. This vitreous hemorrhage could not be seen at normal gain settings. Turning the gain up significantly helped identify this strand of hemorrhage (*arrows*), which moved to and fro with eye movements.

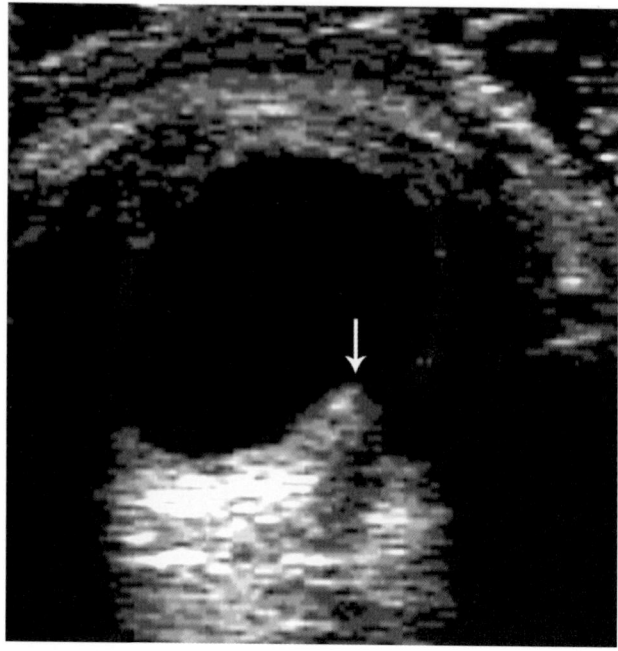

Figure 12-8. A collapsed globe from a penetrating injury showing a posterior fold (*arrow*).

► ADDITIONAL FINDINGS

- Elevated ICP (Figures 12-9 and 12-10)

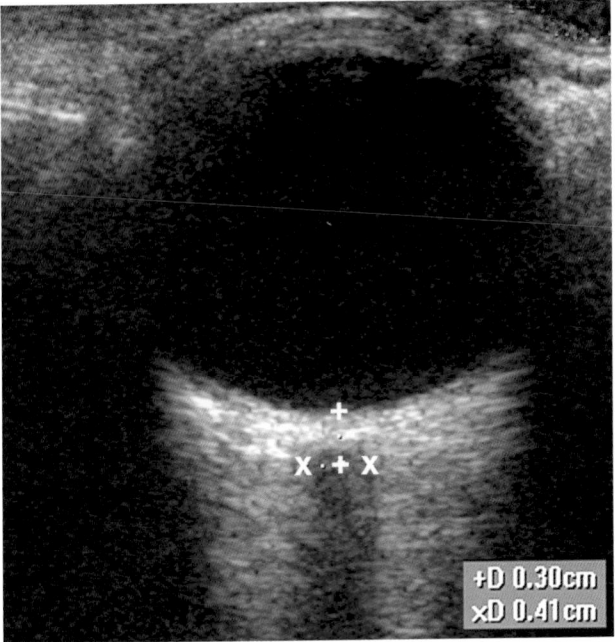

Figure 12-9. Normal measurement of the optic nerve sheath. The measurement should be taken 3 mm behind the globe.

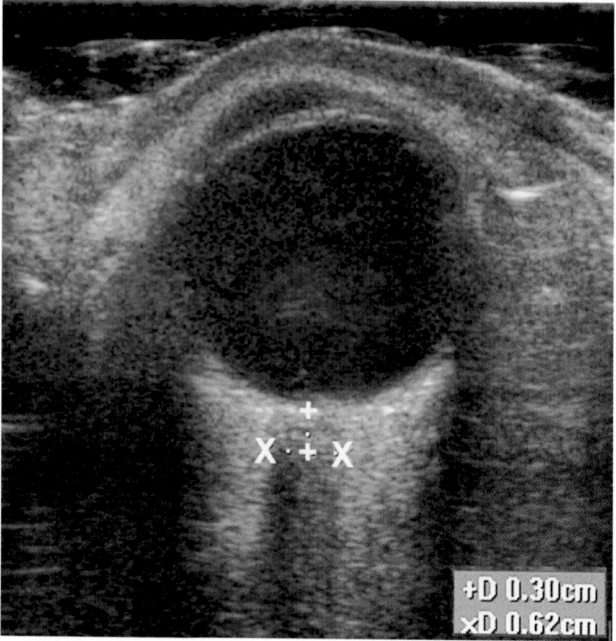

+D 0.30cm
xD 0.62cm

Figure 12-10. Abnormally wide optic nerve sheath (0.63 cm) in a patient with elevated intracranial pressure. Normal maximum measurements are 5 mm for adults, 4.5 mm for children ages 1 to 15 years, and 4 mm for children age less than 1 year.

▶ PITFALLS

• Touching a ruptured globe; the transducer should touch only the gel when a ruptured globe is possible.

• Over-reliance on ultrasound when worrisome symptoms or exam findings are present

• Misjudging artifacts or subtle abnormalities due to improper gain settings

For more detailed information go to the comprehensive textbook Ma and Mateer's Emergency Ultrasound, 3rd edition, Chapter 19 "Ocular" by Matthew Lyon, MD and Dietrich Jehle, MD.

CHAPTER 13
Ultrasound-Guided Procedures

VASCULAR ACCESS

▶ CLINICAL CONSIDERATIONS

- Evidence supporting the use of ultrasound for vascular access has become overwhelming.
- The Agency for Healthcare Research and Quality recommends ultrasound guidance for all central venous catheterization.

▶ CLINICAL INDICATIONS

- All central venous catheters
- Difficult peripheral access because of obesity, intravenous drug abuse, or challenging anatomy

▶ ANATOMIC CONSIDERATIONS

- The internal jugular and femoral veins are the most commonly used access sites for ultrasound-guided central cannulation.
- The basilic, cephalic, and external jugular veins are common sites for ultrasound-guided peripheral access.

► TECHNIQUES

- Transverse approach (Figure 13-1A)
- Longitudinal approach (Figure 13-1B)

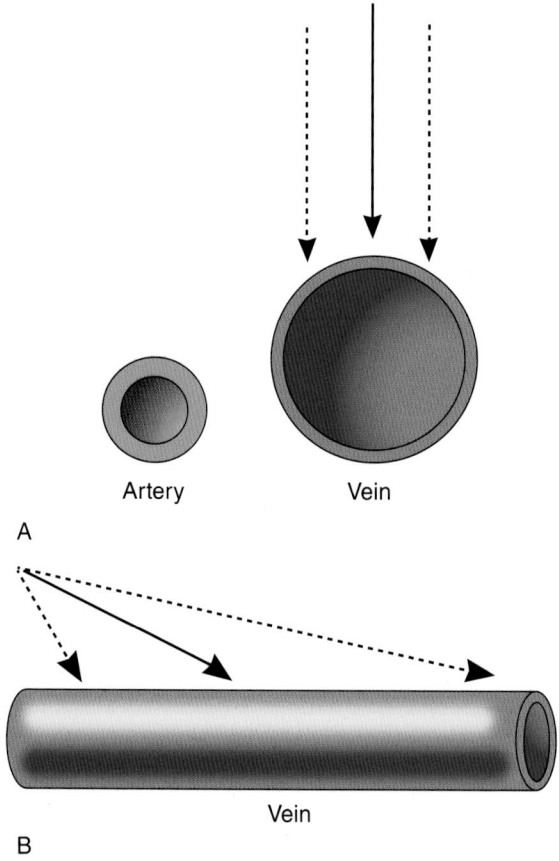

Figure 13–1. Diagram illustrating transverse and longitudinal orientations. **A.** The transverse orientation gives better lateral/medial positioning. **B.** The longitudinal orientation gives better slope and depth positioning.

▶ TIPS TO IMPROVE PROCEDURE SUCCESS

- Position the machine optimally, prescan, and adjust before sterile prep (Figure 13-2).
- Use a steeper needle angle for the transverse approach.
- Look for needle artifact when using the transverse approach (Figure 13-3).
- Bounce the needle to visualize the movement of adjacent soft tissues when using the transverse approach (Figure 13-4).
- The longitudinal approach is more difficult, so practice on an ultrasound simulation phantom before attempting on a patient (Figure 13-5).

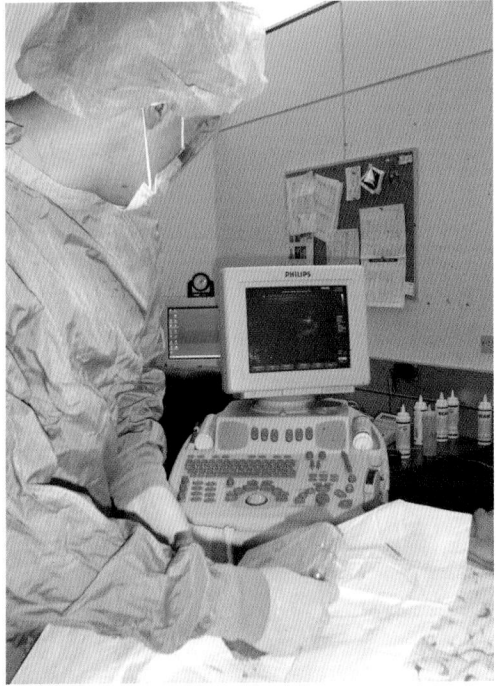

Figure 13–2. Inappropriately positioned equipment. Note that the operator has to turn his head to see the screen.

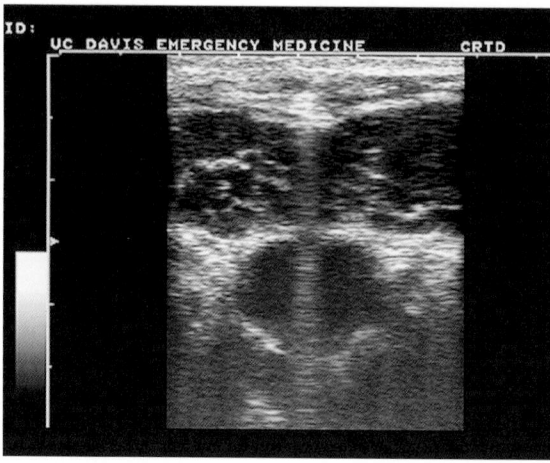

Figure 13–3. Ring-down artifact of the needle after the initial puncture. This is used to localize the needle before advancing.

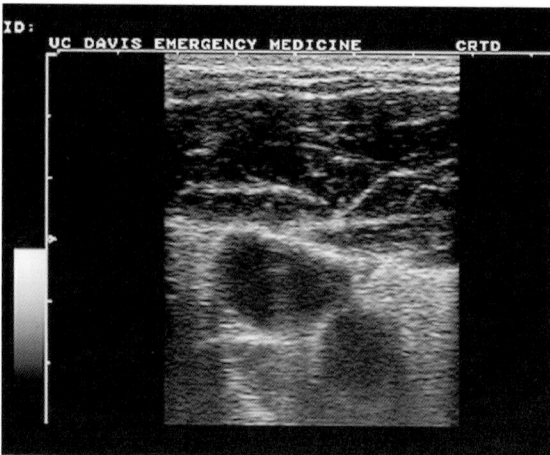

Figure 13–4. Tenting or deformity of the vessel occurs before needle penetration. In this example, the vessel is slightly collapsed. In real time, the vessel wall may briefly indent and then quickly rebound as the needle enters.

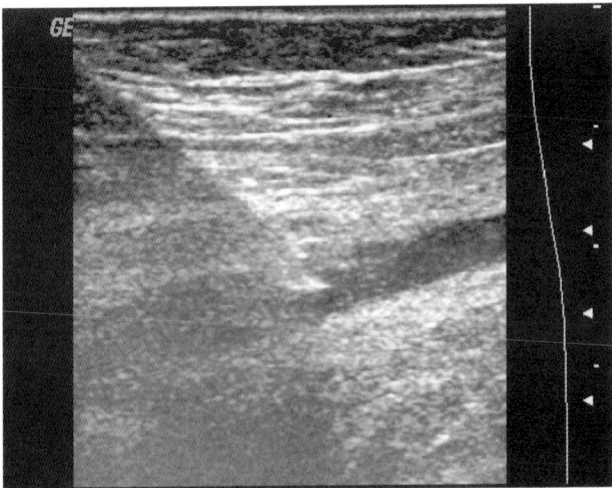

Figure 13–5. Long-axis approach with the needle tip visualized within the vessel lumen.

► COMMON PROCEDURES

- Internal jugular vein cannulation (Figures 13-6 and 13-7)
- Femoral vein cannulation (Figure 13-8)
- Peripheral vein cannulation (Figure 13-9)

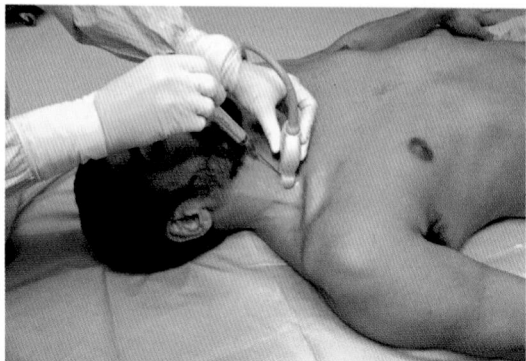

A

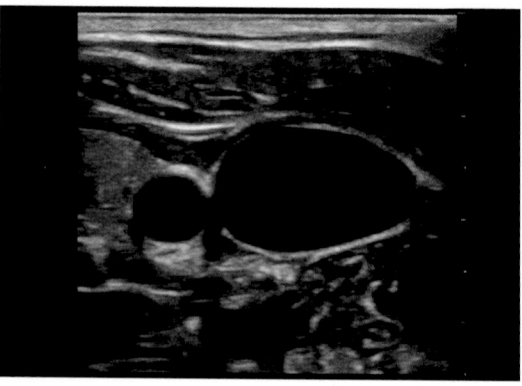

B

Figure 13–6. Transverse approach to the internal jugular (IJ) vein. **A.** Transducer placement. **B.** Ultrasound image.

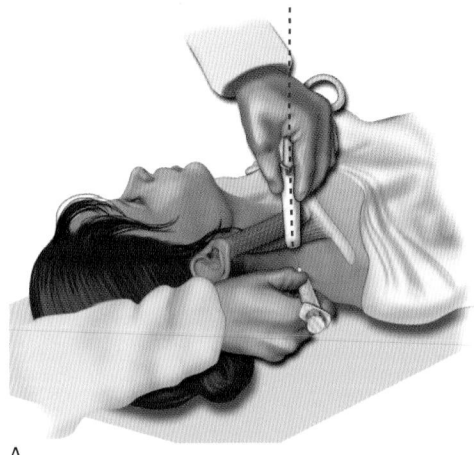

A

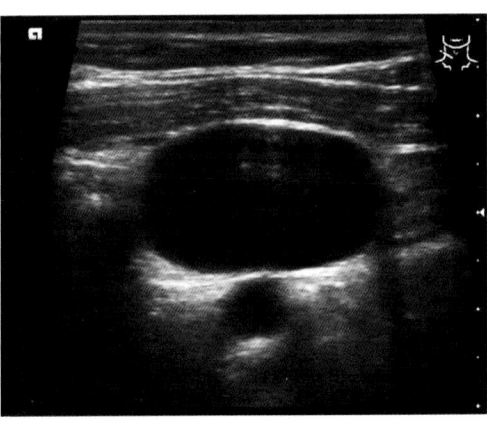

B

Figure 13–7. **A.** Diagram illustrating orientation and approach for the oblique view of the internal jugular vein. The ultrasound probe indicator is pointed toward the patient's left side. **B.** Oblique approach to the internal jugular vein. When the transducer is rotated approximately 45 degrees to the internal jugular vein, the vessel appears larger and oval shaped. The carotid artery is noted directly posterior to the internal jugular vein in this case, so an anterior transverse approach may not be optimal.

(Figure 13-7C continued on next page)

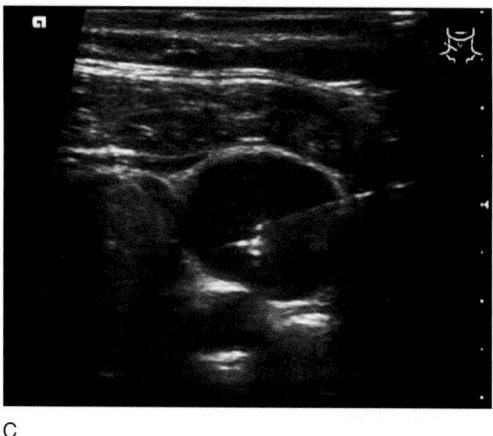

C

Figure 13–7. **C.** The needle approach is in-plane, tracking just below the sternocleidomastoid (SCM) muscle, and is directed above the carotid artery. (Courtesy of James Mateer, MD.)

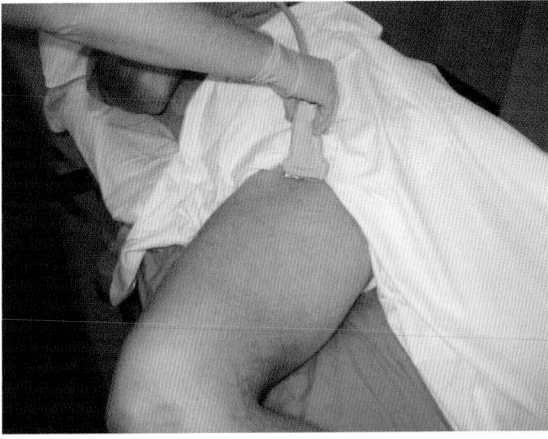

Figure 13–8. Transverse approach to the femoral vein.
A. Transducer position. (Photo contributed by Stephen J. Leech, MD, RDMS.) **B.** Ultrasound images of the femoral vein (FV) and femoral artery (FA) with the hip in the neutral position (*left frame*) and with the hip abducted and externally rotated (*right frame*).

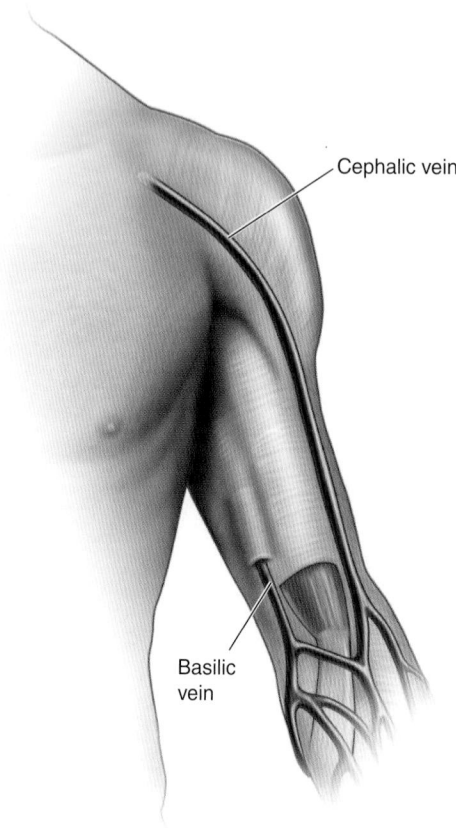

A

Figure 13–9. **A.** The superficial veins of the proximal upper extremity.

(Figures 13-9B and C continued on next page)

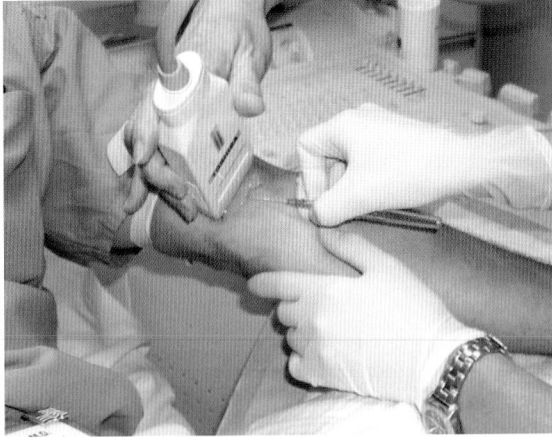

B

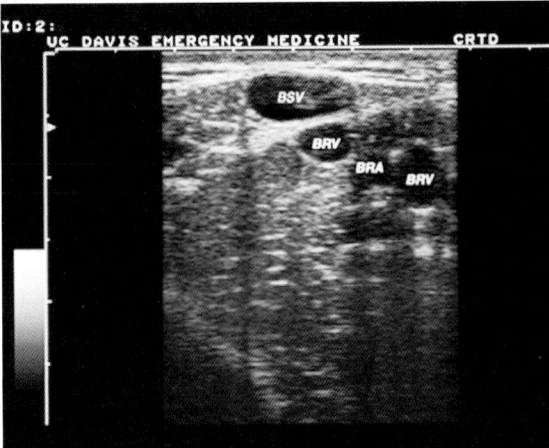

C

Figure 13–9. **B.** Transducer placement for ultrasound-guided cannulation of the basilic or brachial veins, transverse orientation. **C.** Ultrasound image showing the normal relationship and relative sizes of the basilic vein (BSV), brachial artery (BRA) and paired brachial veins (BRV) on either side of the artery.

▶ ADDITIONAL PROCEDURE

- Subclavian vein cannulation

▶ PITFALLS

- Advancing the needle when the practitioner does not know where the tip is (Figure 13-10)
- Failure to appreciate that the needle tip is already posterior to the vessel
- Failure to identify the needle in the tissue
- Failure to angle the transducer into the needle puncture area when using the transverse approach (Figure 13-11)
- Failure to clearly visualize the needle tip when using the longitudinal approach
- Failure to distinguish between a vein and an artery using compression (Figure 13-12)
- Causing injury by advancing the needle too deeply during ultrasound-guided line placement

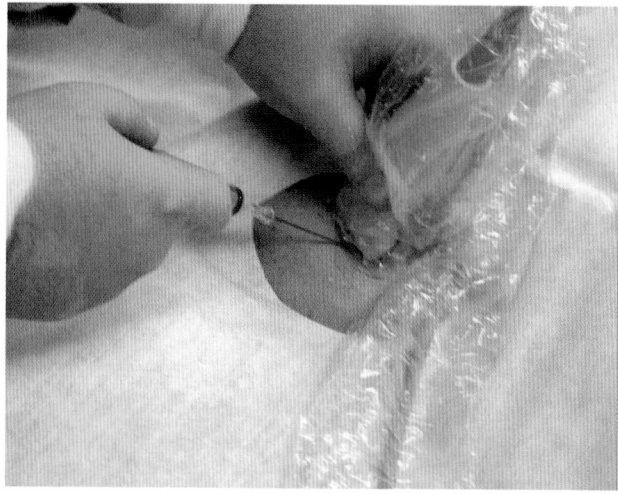

Figure 13–10. The needle must be close to the transducer to locate the needle tip immediately after the puncture.

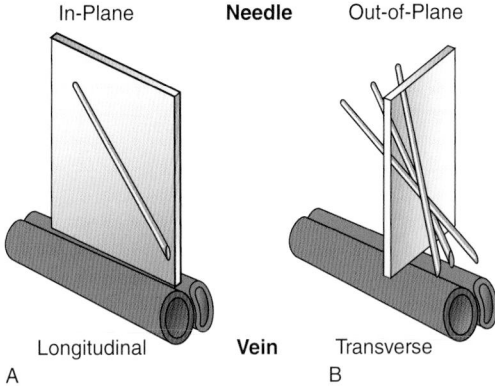

Figure 13–11. Longitudinal and transverse approaches. **A.** With the longitudinal (in-plane) approach, the entire shaft and tip of the needle can be seen simultaneously on the ultrasound image, but only if the needle path is perfectly aligned with the scanning plane, which is can be challenging. Also, only one of the two vessels can be in the scanning plane, so it is important to assure that it is the correct vessel. **B.** With the transverse (out-of-plane) approach, the needle will always pass through the scanning plane, but only at a single point, so it will appear as just a bright dot. It is important to realize that the bright dot may be difficult to recognize and it is not necessarily the tip of the needle, so the tip may be much deeper than recognized.

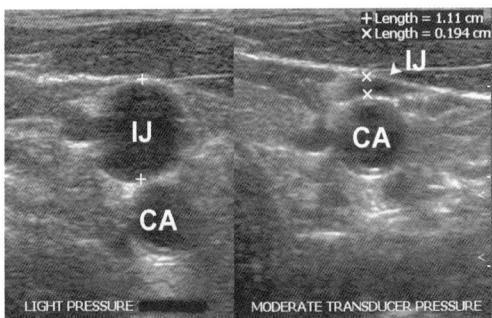

Figure 13–12. Split-screen image demonstrating the effect of compression of the internal jugular vein (*arrowhead*) by heavy transducer pressure. CA = carotid artery; IJ = internal jugular vein.

ARTHROCENTESIS

▶ CLINICAL CONSIDERATION

- Ultrasound guidance makes it possible to aspirate nearly any joint and decreases the chance of a "dry tap".

▶ CLINICAL INDICATIONS

- Diagnostic fluid sampling of a painful or swollen joint
- Therapeutic drainage of a joint effusion

▶ ANATOMIC CONSIDERATIONS

- A joint can be aspirated wherever a fluid collection is visualized.
- Adjacent structures, such as blood vessels, can be located and avoided when using ultrasound guidance.
- Simple effusions are anechoic; chronic effusions or hematomas are more echogenic.

▶ TECHNIQUES

- Static technique: Ultrasound evaluation of anatomy before the procedure but no ultrasound during the procedure.
- Dynamic technique: Real-time ultrasound guidance during the procedure.
- Use a high-frequency (7–10 MHz) linear transducer for most joints.
- Use a lower-frequency curved transducer for identifying hip effusions.
- Orientation is longitudinal or transverse to the joint.

▶ TIPS TO IMPROVE PROCEDURE SUCCESS

- Obtain comparison images from joints on the normal extremity.
- Range the joint while scanning to better appreciate the anatomy.

▶ COMMON PROCEDURES

- Knee (Figures 13-13 and 13-14)
- Hip (Figures 13-15 to 13-17)
- Ankle (Figures 13-18 to 13-20)
- Elbow (Figures 13-21 and 13-22)
- Shoulder (Figures 13-23 to 13-26)

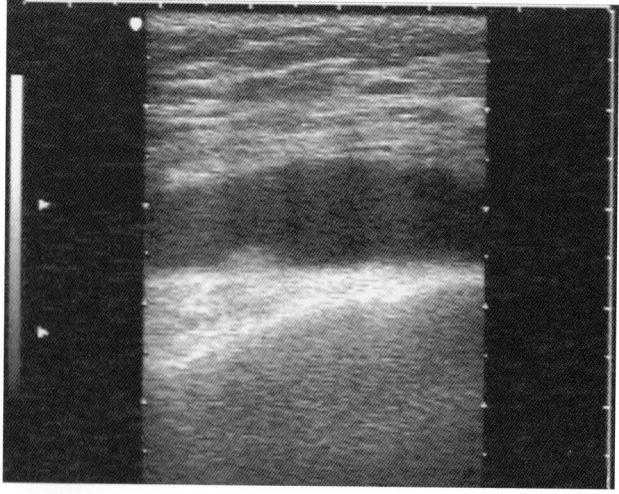

Figure 13–13. Transverse sonogram of a knee effusion at the lateral suprapatellar recess. Hyperechoic prefemoral fat is seen just below the hypoechoic effusion.

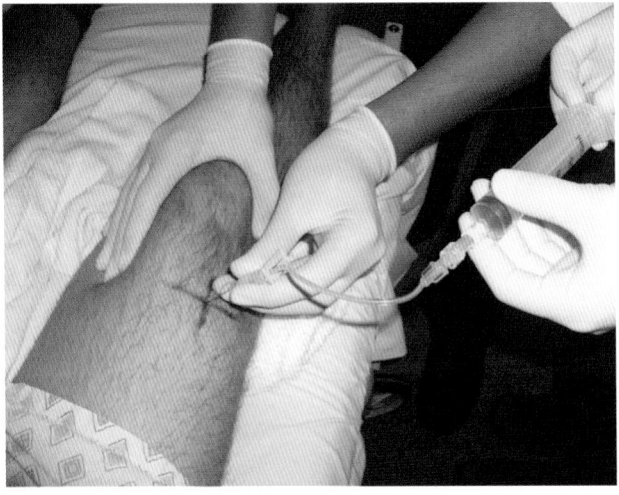

Figure 13–14. Knee aspiration technique at the lateral supra-patellar recess. This is a two-person technique during which pressure is applied to the contralateral recess for maximal joint cavity distension. The sterile drape was omitted for purposes of illustration.

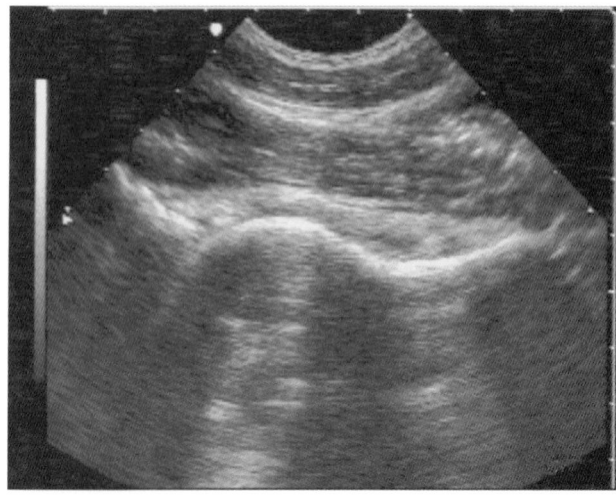

Figure 13–15. Ventral oblique sonogram of the hip. The joint capsule is seen as a hyperechoic, horizontally oriented layer extending from the acetabular labrum to the femoral neck. A small amount of joint fluid is noted below the joint capsule.

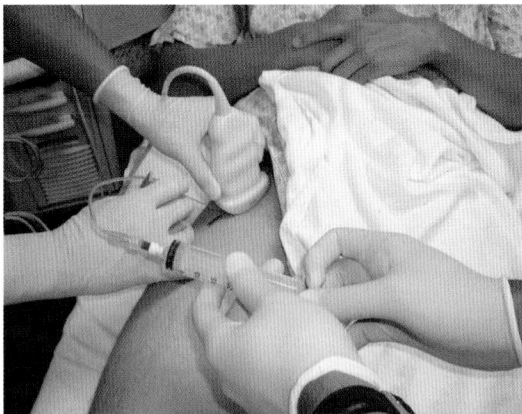

Figure 13–16. Ultrasound-guided hip aspiration technique. The needle is advanced in line within the long-axis scan plane of the transducer, and its characteristic reverberation artifact is used to guide the needle tip into the effusion. For purposes of illustration, the sterile drape and probe cover are not shown.

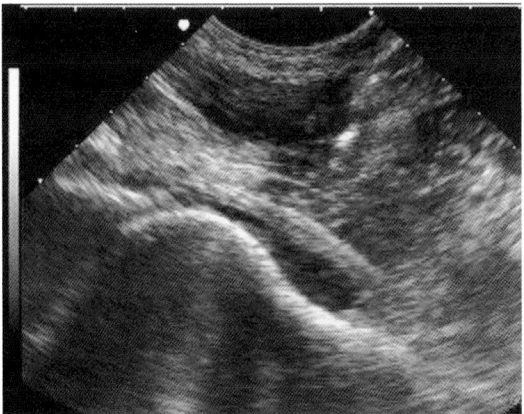

Figure 13–17. The anterior synovial recess is distended with fluid, and the capsule is seen to bulge anteriorly. The hyperechoic echo from the aspirating needle is seen in the upper right of the image.

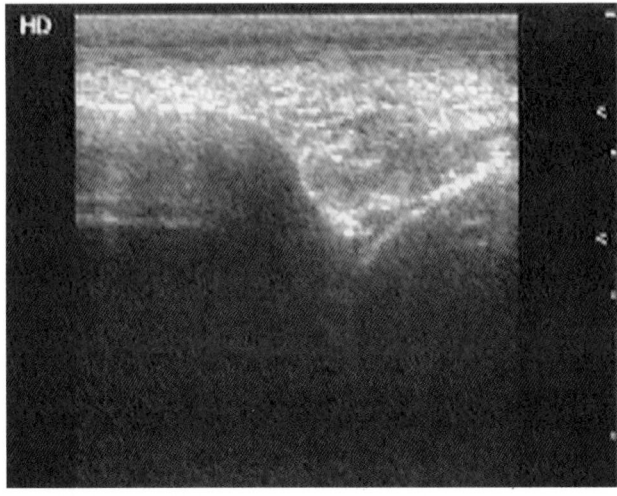

Figure 13–18. Sagittal midline sonogram of a normal ankle joint. The V-shaped recess is formed by the distal tibia on left and the talar dome on the right and is filled by the anterior intracapsular fat pad. No fluid is seen in this example.

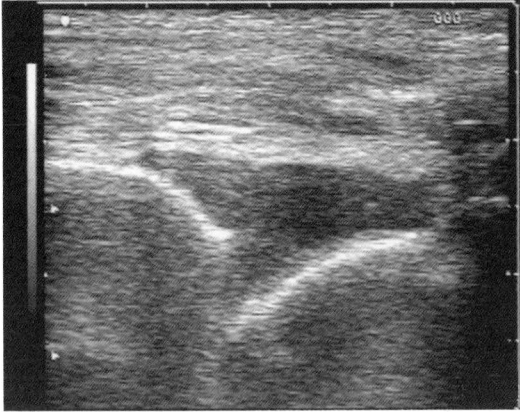

Figure 13–19. The joint capsule is seen as somewhat echogenic structure just above the hypoechoic effusion. The cortical echoes from the distal tibia and talar dome outline the posterior surface of the triangular effusion.

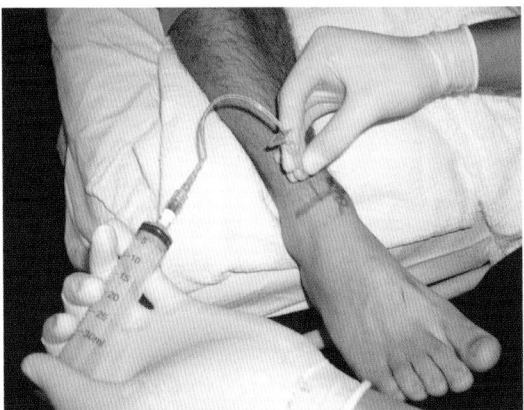

Figure 13–20. The location of both the deepest portion of the anterior recess and the anterior tibial/dorsalis pedis artery has been marked on the skin. Needle entry is lateral to the artery. The sterile drape was omitted for purposes of illustration.

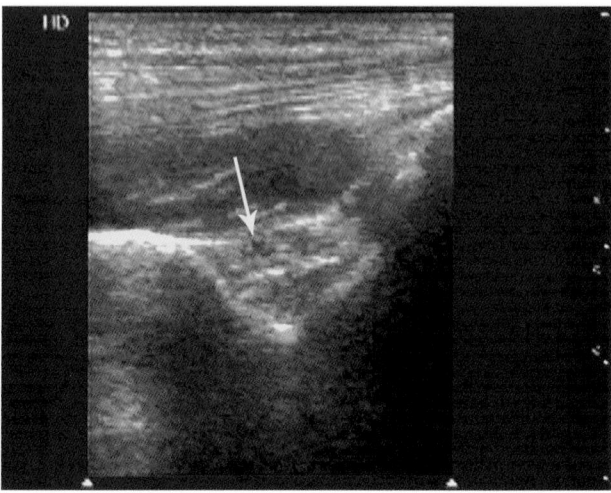

Figure 13–21. Sagittal sonogram of the normal posterior elbow. The humerus is to the left, and the olecranon process is to the right. The olecranon fossa is V-shaped in this orientation, and the somewhat echogenic posterior fat pad is seen filling the recess (*arrow*). The fibrillar triceps tendon is seen just below the skin, and it inserts on the echogenic olecranon on the right of the image. The hypoechoic region below the tendon is a portion of the triceps muscle.

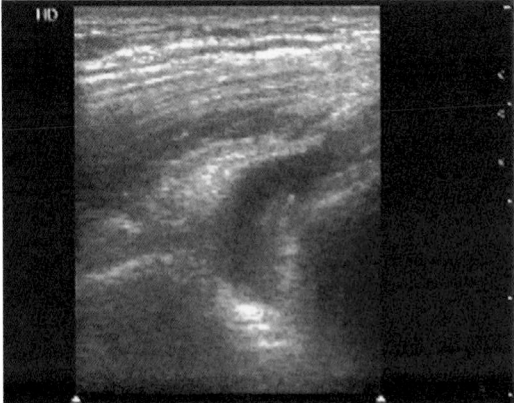

A

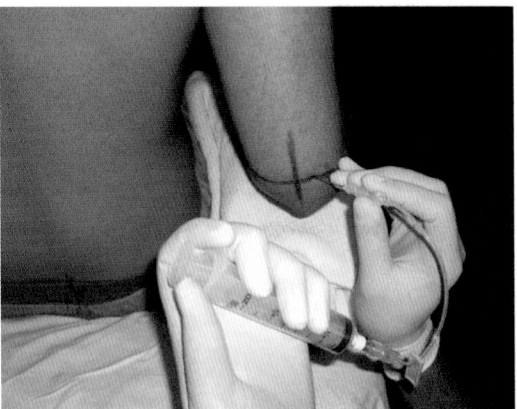

B

Figure 13–22. **A.** Sagittal sonogram of the posterior elbow in a patient with an anechoic effusion. The echogenic fat pad has been pushed superiorly, and the joint capsule bulges posteriorly. **B.** Elbow arthrocentesis technique, posterior approach. The effusion has been mapped and marked. Needle insertion is lateral to the midline to avoid the triceps tendon and to stay well remote from the ulnar nerve. The needle should be medially angulated so it will reach the deepest portion of the centrally located recess.

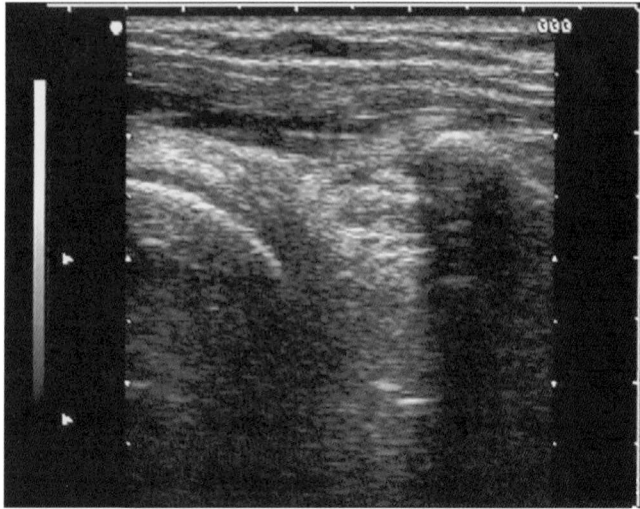

Figure 13–23. Transverse sonogram of right anterior shoulder. The deltoid muscle is seen as a thin hypoechoic layer just below the skin. The curved medial humeral head appears on the left, and the coracoid process with its pronounced posterior acoustic shadow appears on the right. The midline between these two structures represents the sagittal plane where the aspiration should occur (several centimeters below the level of the coracoid process, however).

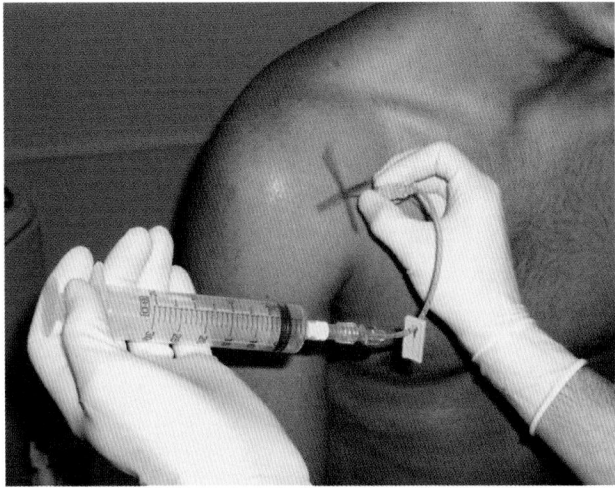

Figure 13-24. Shoulder anterior approach. The space midway between with coracoid process and the medial humeral head has been mapped and marked with a vertical line. The aspiration should occur perpendicular to the skin, several centimeters below the level of the coracoid (at the horizontal line), and the needle should always remain lateral to the coracoid process.

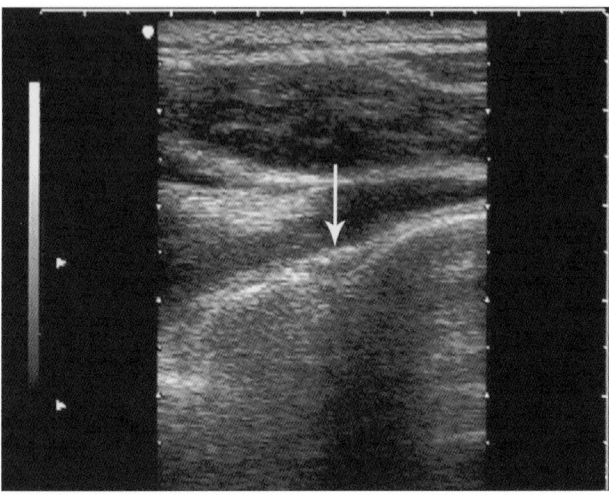

Figure 13–25. Transverse sonogram of right posterior shoulder. In this example, the infraspinatus tendon is noted to be brightly echogenic on the left of the image, but hypoechoic on the right; this is because of tendon anisotropy. With slight movement of the transducer, the entire tendon could be visualized. The glenoid rim is seen as a more distinct curved structure just medial to the larger curve of the head of the humerus. The site for the aspiration will be between the glenoid rim and the medial humeral head (*arrow*). The flatter echo to the left of the glenoid emanates from the surface of the scapula.

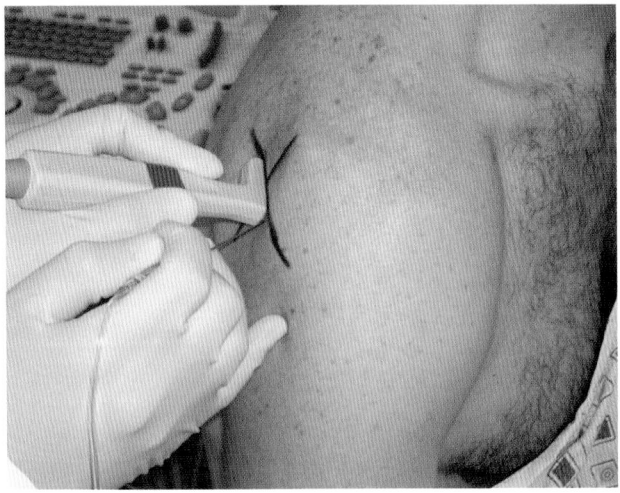

Figure 13–26. Shoulder approach. The effusion is mapped and marked several centimeters inferior and medial to the bulge of the posterior angle of the acromion. The aspiration needle is guided to the space between the glenoid rim and the medial humeral head under ultrasound guidance. The sterile drape and probe cover are omitted for purposes of illustration.

▶ ADDITIONAL PROCEDURE

- Acromioclavicular joint (Figure 13-27)

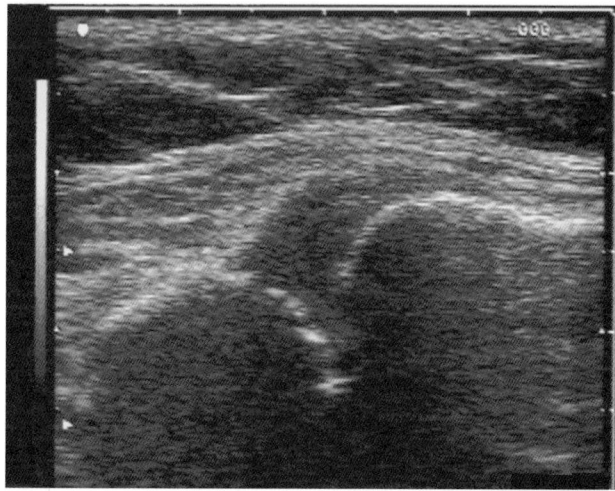

Figure 13–27. Longitudinal sonogram across the right acromioclavicular joint in a patient with gout. The hypoechoic V-shaped recess between the acromion on the left and the clavicle on the right represents the site where an aspiration or steroid injection would be directed.

▶ PITFALLS

- Puncture of adjacent vessels or nerves
- Iatrogenic joint infection
- Failure to aspirate fluid

LUMBAR PUNCTURE

▶ CLINICAL CONSIDERATIONS

- Lumbar puncture can be difficult if anatomic landmarks are not apparent.
- Ultrasound can be used to find basic anatomic landmarks.

▶ CLINICAL INDICATION

- When no anatomic landmarks are visible or palpable

▶ ANATOMIC CONSIDERATIONS

- The interspinous spaces and the midline are the most basic anatomic structures that must be identified before a lumbar puncture is attempted.
- The spinous processes are the most superficial structures of the lumbar spine and are usually the easiest structures to identify (Figure 13-28).
- Identification of the lamina can also be used to locate the interspinous spaces.
- Identifying deeper structures such as the ligamentum flavum and dura mater can allow determination of the distance from the skin to the dural sac.

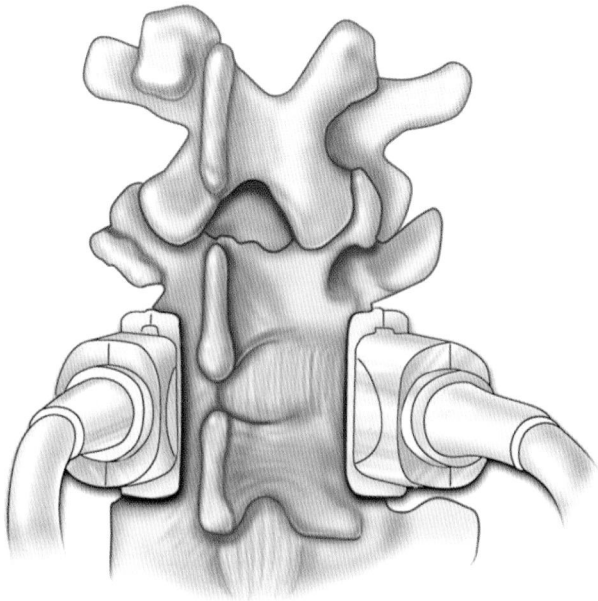

A

Figure 13–28. Sagittal (A) and transverse (B, next page) diagrams of the lumbar spine demonstrating the relationship of the spinous processes, laminate, ligamentum flavin, and dura mater as well as the recommended transducer positions for imaging the lumbar spine from both midline and paramedian locations.

(Figure 13-28B continued on next page)

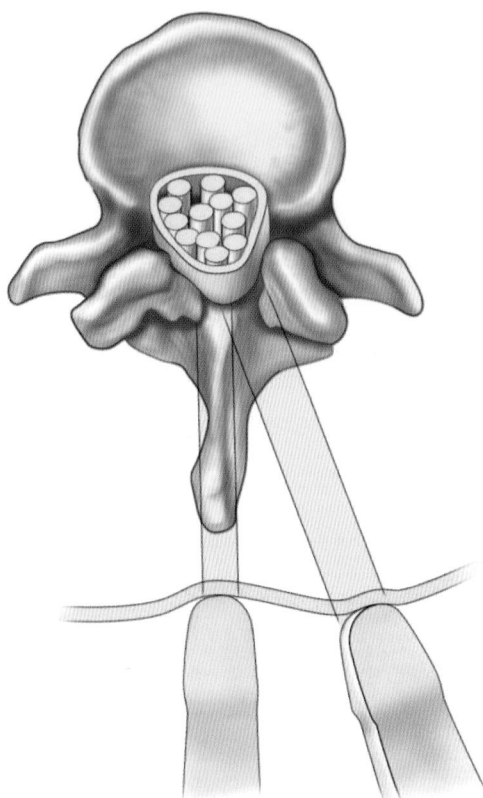

B

Figure 13–28. Sagittal (A, previous page) and transverse (B) diagrams of the lumbar spine demonstrating the relationship of the spinous processes, laminate, ligamentum flavin, and dura mater as well as the recommended transducer positions for imaging the lumbar spine from both midline and paramedian locations.

▶ TECHNIQUES

- Start with the transducer in the midline sagittal position and find the bony cortex of the lumbar spinous processes (Figure 13-29) and the interspinous spaces (Figure 13-30).

- If more information is needed, obtain paramedian sagittal views. (Figure 13-31 shows an image in a thin patient, and Figure 13-32 shows an image in a thicker patient, 3.5-MHz to 5-MHz probe.)

- Midline transverse views are more difficult to interpret but may help to identify the midline, interspinous spaces, and deeper structures (Figure 13-33).

- The needle entry is in the lower half of the interspace with the needle angled cephalad (Figure 13-34).

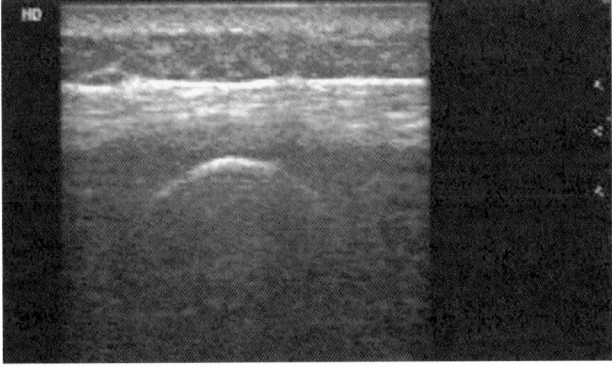

Figure 13–29. Midline sagittal linear array image of a lumbar spinous process in a patient in whom the spinous processes were not palpable. The skin appears hyperechoic, the subcutaneous tissue appears hypoechoic, and the thoracolumbar fascia and supraspinal ligament appear as a hyperechoic layer above the contour of the hyperechoic spinous process.

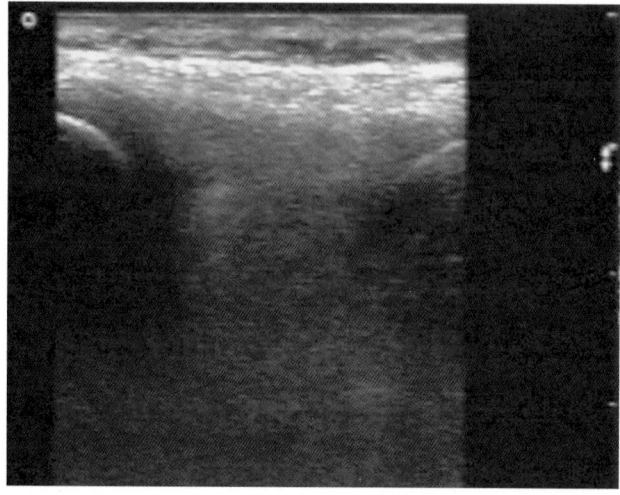

Figure 13–30. Midline sagittal linear array image of the interspinous space. The hyperechoic convexities of adjacent spinous processes are seen in the lateral portions of the image.

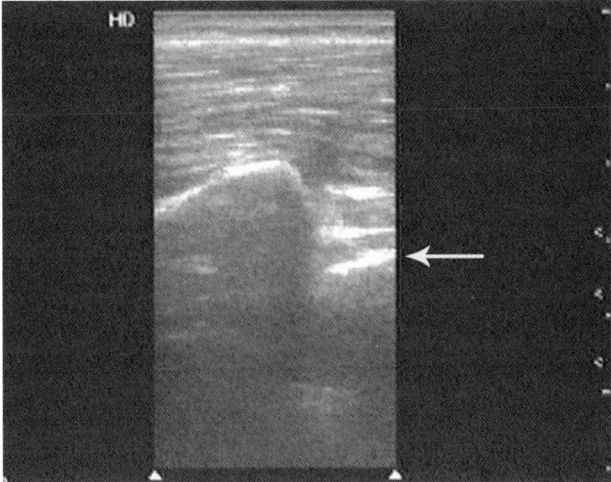

Figure 13–31. Paramedian sagittal linear array image. The echogenic posterior-facing surface of the lamina is seen to the left of the image, and a prominent posterior acoustic shadow is noted. The first two horizontal lines to the right of the lamina represent the two surfaces of the ligamentum flavum. Immediately below lies the epidural space, followed by another usually somewhat more echogenic horizontal line that represents the posterior wall of the dural sac (*arrow*). The distance from the posterior facing surface of the ligamentum flavum and the posterior-facing wall of the dural sac is usually about 8 to 10 mm.

360 POCKET ATLAS OF EMERGENCY ULTRASOUND

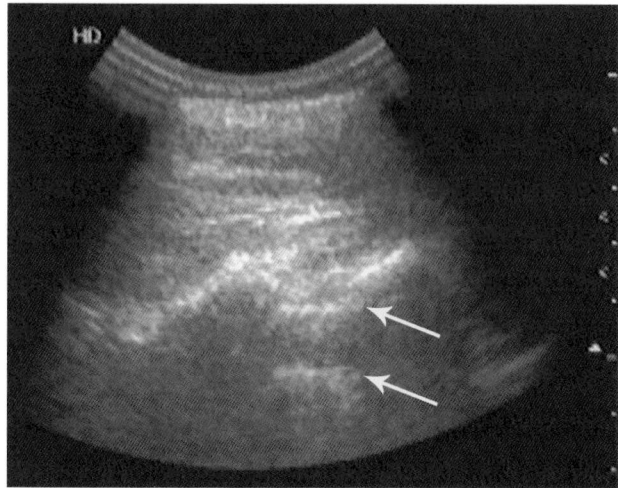

Figure 13-32. Paramedian sagittal curved array image. Laminae of adjacent vertebra are seen as brightly echogenic angulated lines with prominent posterior acoustic shadowing. The ligamentum flavum no longer appears as a distinct structure. Both walls of the dural sac (*arrows*) are apparent as horizontal echogenic lines in the space between and deep to the adjacent laminae.

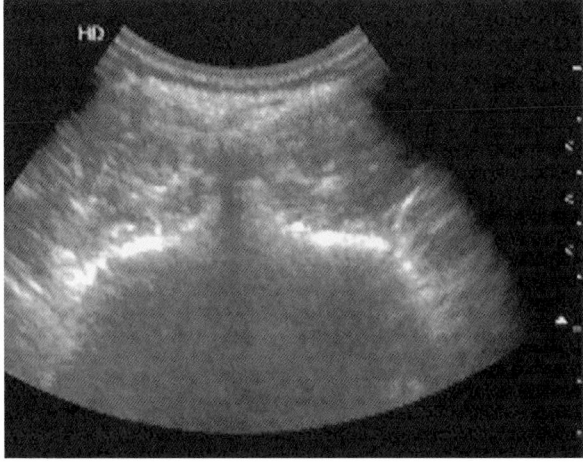

A

Figure 13–33. **A.** In this transverse curved array image, the lumbar spinous process is best found by following its midline posterior acoustic shadow up to the near field of the image. The paraspinal muscles appear as symmetric circular bundles on either side of the spinous process. The echogenic posterior-facing surfaces of the laminae appear as a cape-like structure with dense posterior acoustic shadowing below.

(Figure 13-33B continued on next page)

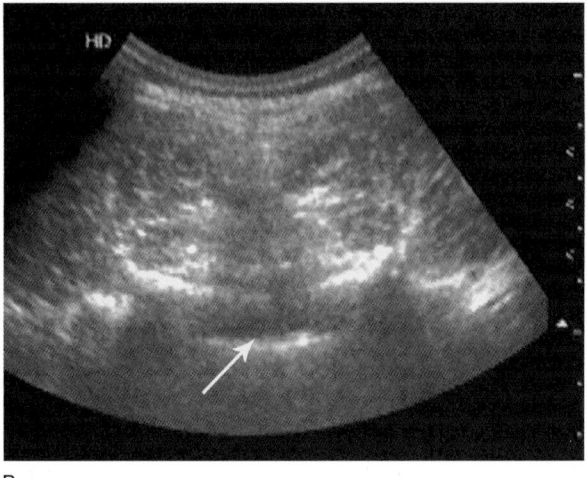

B

Figure 13–33. B. In this somewhat more cephalad transverse curved array image, a series of echogenic lines is seen that corresponds to the articular and transverse processes and the posterior-facing surface of the vertebral body. The paired articular processes appear brightly echogenic and exhibit prominent posterior acoustic shadowing. To their immediate right and somewhat deeper are a pair of echogenic lines that correspond to the transverse processes. The bright echo from the posterior-facing surface of the vertebral body lies somewhat deeper in the midline of the image. The spinal canal appears as the hypoechoic region just anterior to this vertebral body echo (*arrow*).

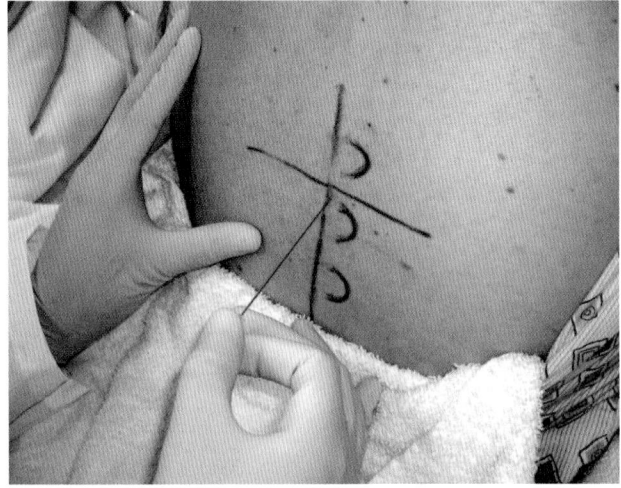

Figure 13–34. The precise location of the lumbar midline and the relative location of the curved spinous processes have been mapped and marked with an indelible marker. A horizontal line is used to indicate the L3–L4 interspace. Needle entry begins in the lower half of the interspace, and the needle is angled cephalad both to avoid the spinous process above and to follow the cranial slanting path to the dural sac. For purposes of illustration, the sterile drape is not shown.

▶ TIPS TO IMPROVE PROCEDURE SUCCESS

- A high-frequency linear probe can be used on a child or a thin adult, but a lower-frequency (abdominal) curved transducer is best for very obese patients.
- Most lumbar punctures can be successfully performed if the spinous processes can be identified.
- Practice image acquisition initially using thin subjects with normal anatomy.

▶ PITFALLS

- The spinous processes and other structures may be very deep in morbidly obese patients.
- Overreliance on ultrasound when anatomic landmarks can be identified by simple palpation.

NERVE BLOCKS

▶ CLINICAL CONSIDERATIONS

- The ability to deposit anesthetic very close to the nerve under direct vision leads to high success rates (>95%) and a much lower risk of complications.
- Patients with acute hip fractures need significantly less parenteral narcotics if a femoral nerve block is performed in the emergency department.

▶ CLINICAL INDICATION

- Regional nerve blocks may be used before painful procedures or after painful extremity injuries.

▶ ANATOMIC CONSIDERATIONS

- Peripheral nerves tend to be found adjacent to arteries and veins, so it is critically important to identify the nerves, arteries, and veins before proceeding.
- Generally, it is easiest to identify nerves (and vessels) in the transverse orientation.

► TECHNIQUES

- The basic technique is the same for all nerve blocks—hold the probe transverse to the nerve and advance the needle in the plane of the ultrasound image.

- Supraclavicular brachial plexus block (Figures 13-35 and 13-36).

- Axillary perivascular brachial plexus block (Figures 13-37 and 13-38).

- Femoral nerve block (Figures 13-39 and 13-40).

- "Three-in-one" block: Apply and hold firm pressure over the femoral nerve just distal to the injection site during the femoral nerve block; this forces the anesthetic to spread cephalad and blocks the lateral femoral cutaneous and obturator nerves.

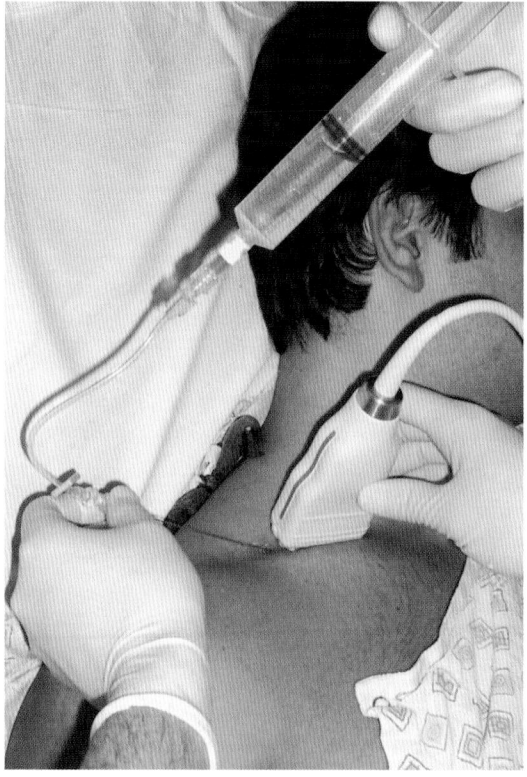

Figure 13–35. Supraclavicular brachial plexus technique. The patient's head is turned to the opposite side, and the transducer is held in an oblique coronal plane just behind the clavicle. The anesthetic delivery needle is inserted on the lateral aspect of the transducer and positioned under direct ultrasound guidance. When the needle tip reaches the desired location, the operator can hold it in a fixed position while an assistant delivers a test dose (1–2 cc) of the anesthetic solution to confirm adequate needle tip placement. For purposes of illustration, the sterile drape and probe cover are not shown.

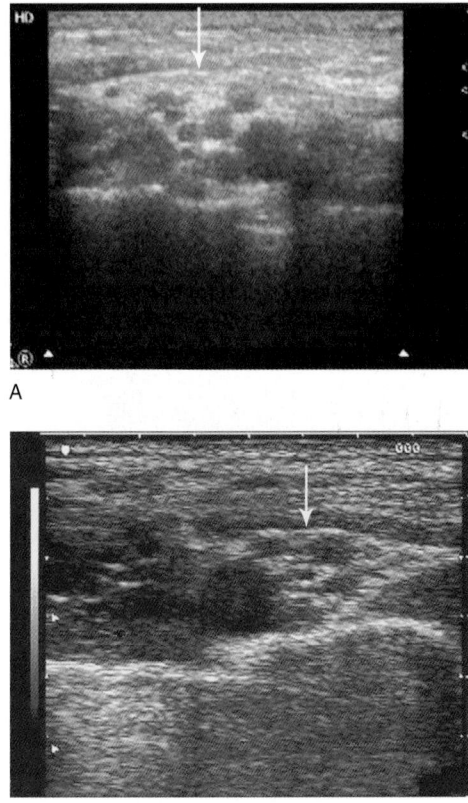

Figure 13–36. Supraclavicular brachial plexus. **A.** Right supraclavicular brachial plexus with the nerve trunks and divisions
appearing as a cluster of superficial hypoechoic circles within
a more hyperechoic fascial sheath (*arrow*). The middle scalene
muscle appears as a hypoechoic structure just lateral to the
plexus (to the left in this image), the subclavian artery is seen as
the largest and most hypoechoic circle near the center of the
image, and the anterior scalene muscle appears as a somewhat
indistinct hypoechoic structure just medial to the subclavian artery
(to the right in this image). **B.** Left supraclavicular brachial plexus.
The subclavian artery and brachial plexus (*arrow*) are seen
overlying the brightly echogenic superior surface of the first rib.

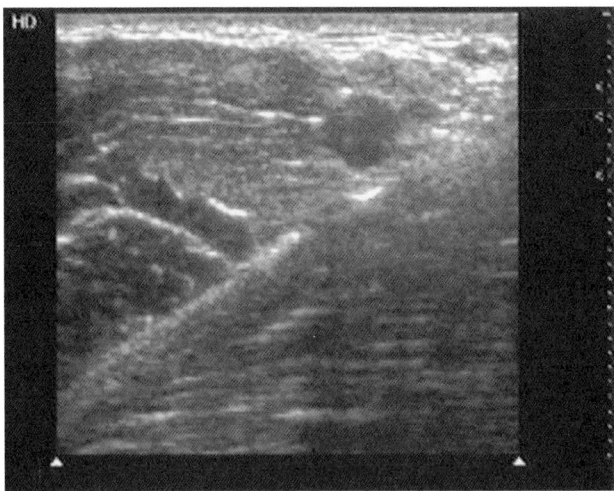

Figure 13–37. Right axillary brachial plexus. Typically, only the axillary artery will be apparent because even light probe pressure will collapse the superficially located axillary vein. The echogenic fascial plane on which the vessels and plexus rest (the medial brachial intermuscular septum) separates the arm extensors above from flexors below. This septum may be obliquely or horizontally situated in the image.

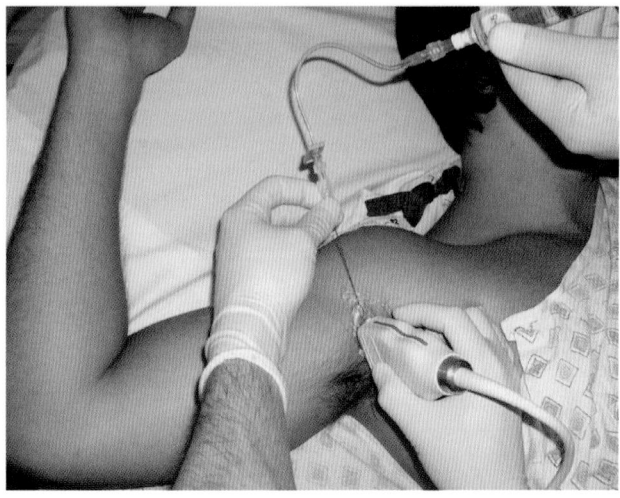

Figure 13–38. Axillary brachial plexus technique. The patient is in the "high-5" position with transducer placed high in the anterior axilla at the level of the anterior axillary crease (at the border between the biceps and deltoid muscles). The transducer is oriented vertically, perpendicular to the long axis of the humerus. The anesthetic delivery needle is inserted from the superior aspect of the transducer and positioned under direct ultrasound guidance. When the needle tip reaches the desired location, the operator can hold it in a fixed position while an assistant delivers a test dose (1–2 cc) of the anesthetic solution to confirm adequate needle tip placement. For purposes of illustration, the sterile drape and probe cover are not shown.

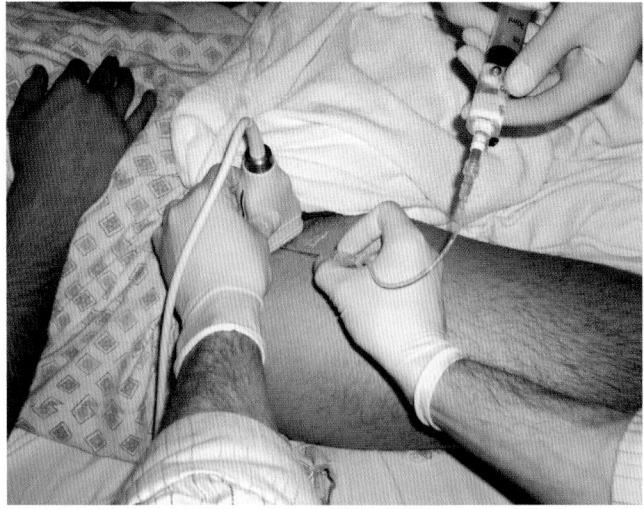

Figure 13–39. Femoral nerve block technique. The transducer is placed in an oblique transverse orientation at the level of and in line with the inguinal crease with the orientation marker facing left. The femoral nerve is positioned in the center of the image, and the anesthetic delivery needle is inserted below the center of the transducer in an out-of-plane approach. Under ultrasound guidance, the needle tip is positioned below the iliopectineal fascia as close to the femoral nerve as possible. When the needle tip reaches the desired location, the operator can hold it in a fixed position while an assistant delivers a test dose (1–2 cc) of the anesthetic solution to confirm adequate needle tip placement. For purposes of illustration, the sterile drape and probe cover are not shown.

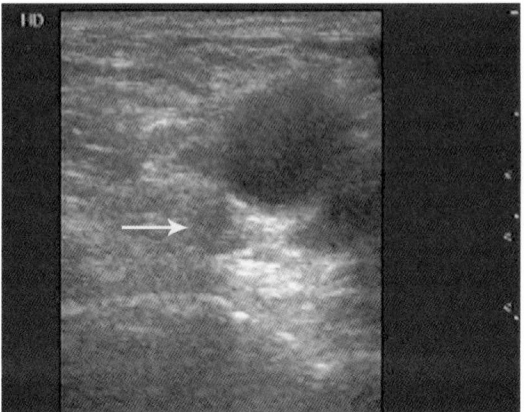

A

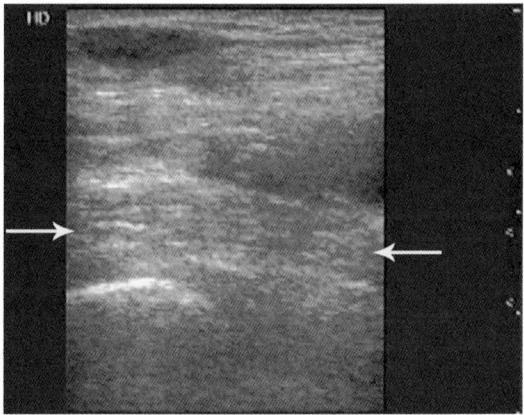

B

Figure 13–40. A. The right femoral nerve is seen in this short-axis image as an ovoid hypoechoic circle (*arrow*) that lies just deep and slightly lateral to the common femoral artery. The somewhat deeper echogenic curve below the nerve represents the iliopubic eminence of the acetabulum. **B.** In a long-axis view of this same femoral nerve, the subtle fibrillar echotexture of the nerve is apparent as it courses approximately 5 mm above the echogenic iliopubic eminence (*arrows*).

► TIPS TO IMPROVE PROCEDURE SUCCESS

- Use a high-frequency linear transducer (7–10 MHz).
- Introduce the needle along the long axis of the ultrasound plane and advance it using real-time guidance (never advance the needle if you cannot see the tip).
- Practice hand–eye skills of nerve and vessel imaging and needle placement using an ultrasound simulation phantom.
- Practice identifying selected nerves in volunteers before attempting to identify them in patients.

► PITFALLS

- Vascular puncture or intravascular injection of local anesthetic.
- Avoid performing a regional nerve block before the physical exam or when anesthesia may mask complications (eg, compartment syndrome).
- Educate patients that they will not be able to use the extremity until the anesthesia resolves.
- Nerve damage: Use a noncutting needle (22-gauge spinal needle) and only move the needle straight in and out; avoid "waving" the tip after insertion.

PERICARDIOCENTESIS

▶ CLINICAL CONSIDERATIONS

- Ultrasound-guided pericardiocentesis is safer and more effective than the blind approach.

- A study of 1127 consecutive ultrasound-guided pericardiocenteses demonstrated a 97% success rate and 4.7% complication rate.

▶ CLINICAL INDICATIONS

- Moderate or large pericardial effusion with symptoms of tamponade or cardiac arrest (Figure 13-41).

▶ ANATOMIC CONSIDERATIONS

- The parasternal/apical views usually provide the best approach when using ultrasound guidance. Imaging and fluid localization are facilitated by left lateral decubitus positioning.

- The best location for needle entry is the point on the chest wall closest to the largest collection of pericardial fluid.

- Visualization of fluid ensures that the lung is not in the pathway of the needle.

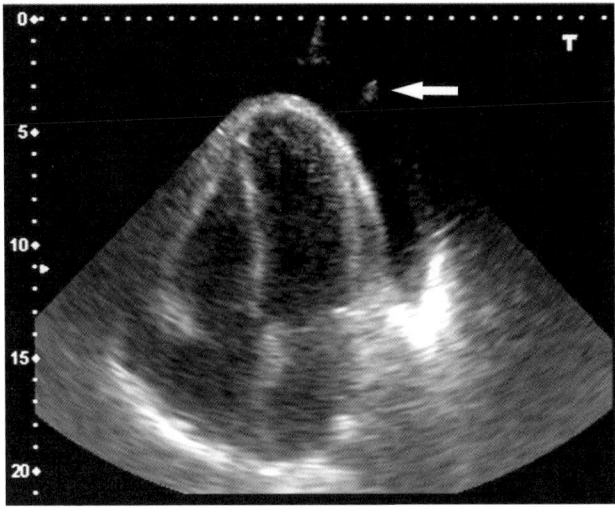

A

Figure 13–41. Cardiac tamponade. Apical (A) and subcostal four-chamber views (B, next page). **A.** Pericardiocentesis in a patient with a large pericardial effusion and tamponade. The tip of the needle is entering the effusion at about the 2 o'clock position (*arrow*). A catheter was placed using the Seldinger technique after a bubble test confirmed the location of the needle tip inside the effusion. A total of 500 mL of straw-colored fluid was removed.

(Figure 13-41B continued on next page)

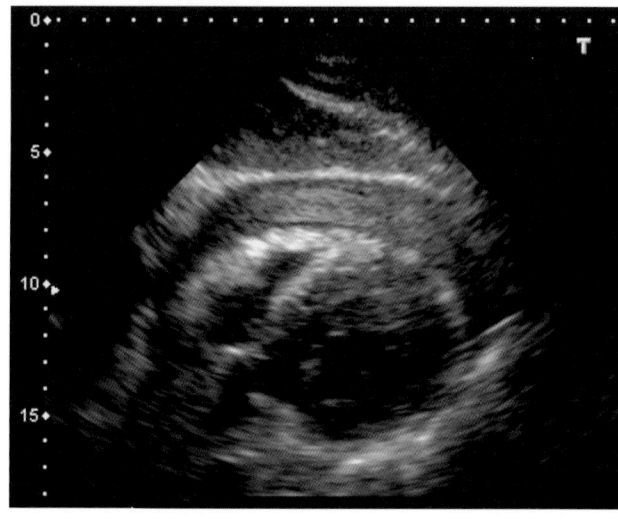

B

Figure 13–41. **B.** Tamponade from a pericardial clot secondary to an acute myocardial infarction and ventricular free wall rupture. This is not a good candidate for a pericardiocentesis and needs a thoracotomy.

▶ TECHNIQUES

- Use a long 18-gauge or 19-gauge needle from a pericardiocentesis or central line kit.

- With the static technique, the skin entry site and needle trajectory are preplanned using ultrasound guidance, but needle advancement is not observed in real time. The patient's position should not change between imaging and needle entry!

- To use the dynamic technique, it is usually best to obtain a parasternal long-axis view, enter the skin over the cardiac apex, and then advance the needle in the long axis of the ultrasound beam while directly watching the needle tip as it is advanced.

- Withdraw pericardial fluid and consider placing a catheter (pigtail or central line catheter) using the Seldinger technique.

- When uncertain, the needle tip location can be confirmed by an injection of agitated saline (Figure 13-42).

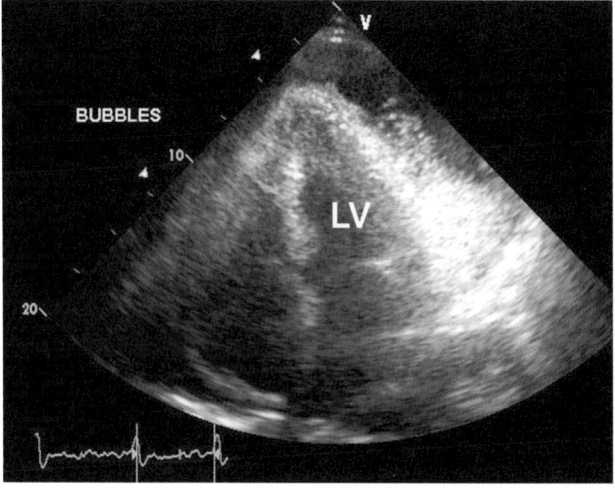

Figure 13–42. Apical four-chamber view with bubbles from agitated saline injection into the pericardial fluid. LV = left ventricle.

▶ TIPS TO IMPROVE PROCEDURE SUCCESS

- The static technique is easier to perform.
- In most cases, the effusion is only a few centimeters deep to the skin entry point, so stop advancing the needle as soon as pericardial fluid is aspirated.
- Most effusions that need to be emergently drained are large.

▶ PITFALLS

- Injury to the internal mammary artery (3–5 cm lateral to the sternal border)
- Injury to an intercostal artery
- Failure to confirm the location of the needle tip within the pericardium, especially when there is a bloody effusion or a pericardial catheter is going to be placed
- Patient movement between imaging and needle entry (static method)

THORACENTESIS

► CLINICAL CONSIDERATIONS

- Ultrasound-guided thoracentesis is safer and more effective than the blind approach.
- The risk of iatrogenic pneumothorax with ultrasound guidance is close to zero; the risk is about 20% without ultrasound guidance.

► CLINICAL INDICATIONS

- Sampling of pleural fluid for diagnostic reasons
- Therapeutic drainage for pleural effusion with respiratory compromise

► ANATOMIC CONSIDERATIONS

- Pleural fluid initially collects in the potential space called the costodiaphragmatic recess.
- The size of the pleural effusion and the respiratory cycle may determine how the effusion is drained.
- Care must be taken not to damage the intercostal artery, vein, or nerve.

► TECHNIQUES

- The most common location for thoracentesis is the mid to lateral back with the patient in a sitting position (Figure 13-43).
- Alternatively, thoracentesis can be performed in the midaxillary line with the patient supine and the head of the bed elevated to 30 to 45 degrees.
- A low-frequency transducer with a small footprint works best for intercostal imaging (Figures 13-44 and 13-45).

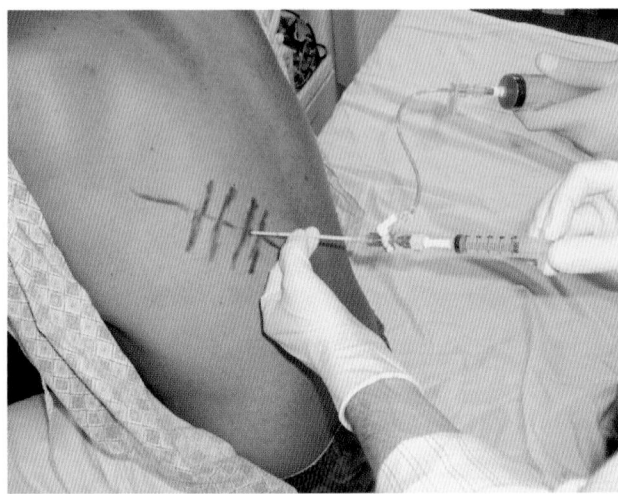

Figure 13–43. Thoracentesis procedural technique, dorsal approach. The rib interspace for the aspiration has been marked and mapped. Needle insertion is over the center of the rib; the aspirating needle is then moved to a point immediately above the superior border of the rib into the interspace. A commercially available self-sealing thoracentesis needle is used, and an assistant is available to aspirate the pleural fluid sample or connect the side port to a drainage bag.

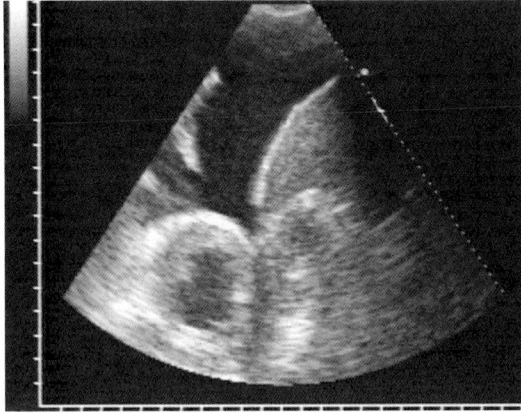

Figure 13–44. A longitudinal view of a left pleural effusion from the posterior chest. The heart is seen in short axis in the far field, the spleen is seen to the right, and the inferior lung border is seen to the left, with the posterior chest wall closest to the transducer.

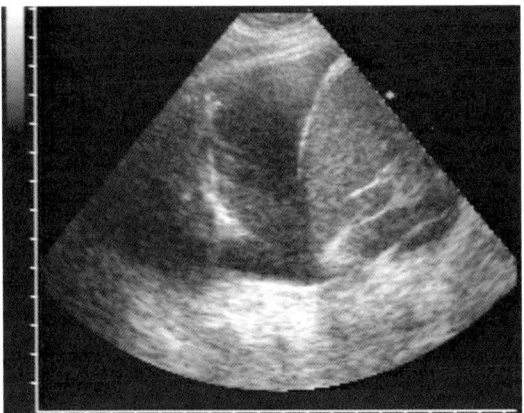

Figure 13–45. A large pleural effusion with somewhat increased fluid echogenicity; the echogenic inferior lung border is seen in the effusion on the left side of the image.

▶ TIPS TO IMPROVE PROCEDURE SUCCESS

- Scan the chest from the intended needle entry point just before starting the procedure.
- Tilt the probe in many different directions to plan the best needle trajectory and to identify nearby anatomic structures.

▶ PITFALLS

- Changes in patient position or respiratory cycle may change the position of the effusion relative to skin markings
- Penetrating too deeply
- Morbid obesity

PARACENTESIS

▶ CLINICAL CONSIDERATIONS

- Bedside ultrasound can be used to confirm the diagnosis of ascites.
- Ultrasound-guided paracentesis is safer and has a higher success rate than the blind technique.

▶ CLINICAL INDICATIONS

- Diagnostic: Suspected cancer, bacterial peritonitis, or hemorrhage into ascites
- Therapeutic: Discomfort or respiratory compromise

▶ ANATOMIC CONSIDERATIONS

- Ultrasound guidance allows for paracentesis at nontraditional sites.
- It is still important to stay away from the rectus muscles to avoid puncture of the epigastric vessels.
- The abdominal wall is usually thinnest in the lower quadrants, but a midline infraumbilical approach is also acceptable (locate the bladder and avoid it).

▶ TECHNIQUES

- Use a 3-MHz to 5-MHz abdominal transducer.
- Start in the suprapubic region and obtain a midline sagittal view (Figure 13-46).
- To choose the best site for paracentesis, find the largest (and deepest) fluid pocket as far as possible from any floating loops of bowel (Figure 13-47).
- Mark the intended skin penetration site with indelible ink and then advance the needle on the predetermined trajectory (Figures 13-48 and 13-49).

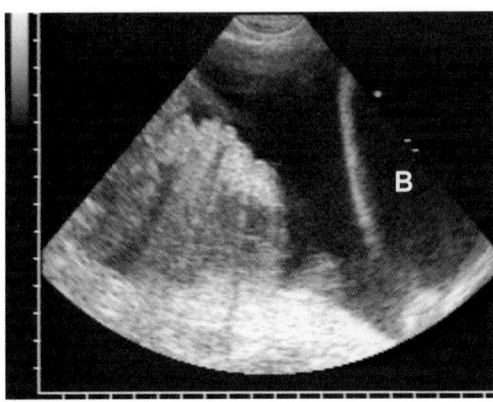

Figure 13–46. Midline sagittal view of a patient with a large amount of simple ascites. The echogenic bladder (B) dome appears to the right of the image. Both urine and simple ascites appear similarly hypoechoic. Echogenic loops of bowel with "dirty" shadowing from intraluminal bowel gas are seen to the left of the image.

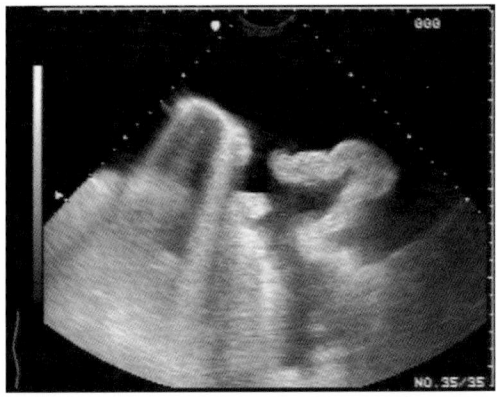

Figure 13–47. Large-volume simple ascites with hyperechoic loops of small bowel. Some "dirty" shadowing and hyperechoic reverberation artifacts from intraluminal bowel gas are noted. Gain settings have been adjusted to make the simple fluid appear uniformly black.

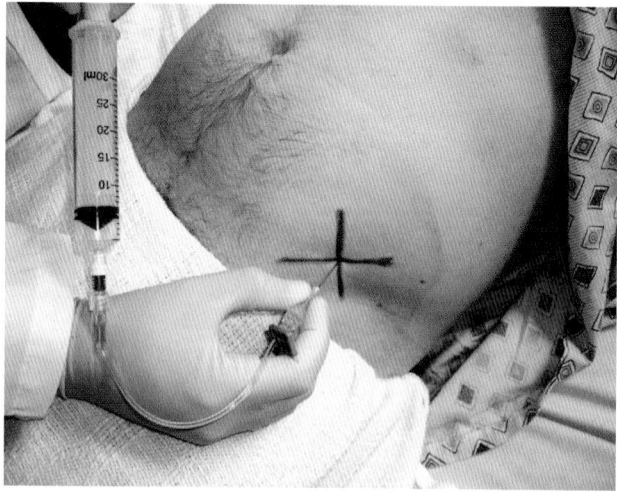

Figure 13–48. Paracentesis: Small-volume aspiration technique. The fluid pocket has been mapped and marked in two orthogonal planes, and the skin has been prepped in and anesthetized down to the peritoneum. The patient remains in the same position for the aspiration as when mapped and is asked to protrude the abdomen during the procedure to facilitate needle insertion and prevent inadvertent puncture of deeper structures. The extension tubing allows for manipulation of the syringe while the needle is held fixed in place. For purposes of illustration, the sterile drape is not shown.

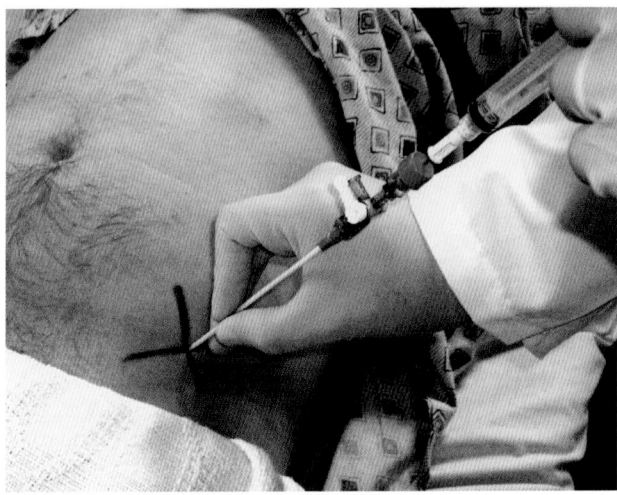

Figure 13–49. Paracentesis: Large-volume aspiration technique. Procedural details are similar to the small-volume aspiration technique but with several additions. A skin stab wound is made to the beveled edge of the scalpel blade included in the centesis kit; this facilitates passage of the 8-French catheter. After ascitic fluid has been aspirated, the catheter needle is held fixed while the catheter is advanced several centimeters. The large-gauge needle is then withdrawn from the catheter assembly, and connector tubing may then be attached to the side port of the stopcock. Drainage may be passive into a collection bag included in the kit or vacuum assisted into evacuated glass containers. For purposes of illustration, the sterile drape is not shown.

► TIPS TO IMPROVE PROCEDURE SUCCESS

- Ultrasound imaging should be performed during or immediately before the procedure.
- Avoid moving the patient after imaging because doing so may reposition the fluid, bowel, or both.

► PITFALL

- Mistaking other fluid-filled structures (bladder, bowel) for intraperitoneal fluid

ABSCESS LOCALIZATION

▶ CLINICAL CONSIDERATIONS

- The physical exam is poor for differentiating cellulitis from abscess.
- Occult abscesses are common.
- Ultrasound significantly improves the positive and negative predictive value for the diagnosis of abscesses.

▶ CLINICAL INDICATIONS

- Detection of occult abscess
- Localization of the optimal site for incision and drainage

▶ ANATOMIC CONSIDERATIONS

- Subcutaneous abscesses can occur nearly anywhere.
- Common sites are the hand, face, forearm, groin, legs, buttocks, and perianal region.
- Peritonsillar abscesses are the most common deep space infection of the neck.
- Ultrasound allows identification of nearby structures such as arteries and veins.

▶ TECHNIQUES AND FINDINGS

- Use a 5-MHz to 10-MHz linear or annular array transducer for subcutaneous abscesses.

- Evaluate all structures in two orthogonal planes.

- Cellulitis causes increased echogenicity compared to the surrounding soft tissue (Figure 13-50).

- Abscesses are usually hypoechoic and surrounded by hyperechoic soft tissue (Figure 13-51).

- Abscesses have well-demarcated borders and exhibit "ultrasonic fluctuance" (Figures 13-52 to 13-56). ("Ultrasonic fluctuance" is visualization of fluid or debris moving inside the abscess cavity when the tip of the transducer is pressed against the abscess.)

- Use an endocavitary transducer to evaluate for peritonsillar abscess (Figures 13-57 and 13-58).

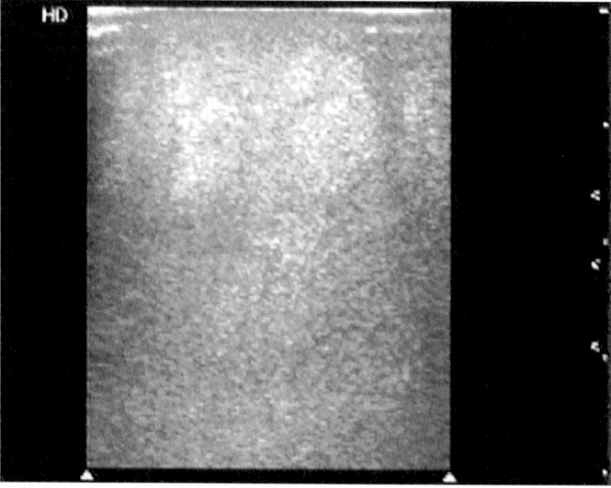

Figure 13–50. Sonogram of a region of cellulitis on a buttock. The skin and subcutaneous tissues appear diffusely hyperechoic, and no soft tissue detail is appreciated. Some fine reticular areas of hypoechoic stranding are seen and are likely attributable to edema within the tissue.

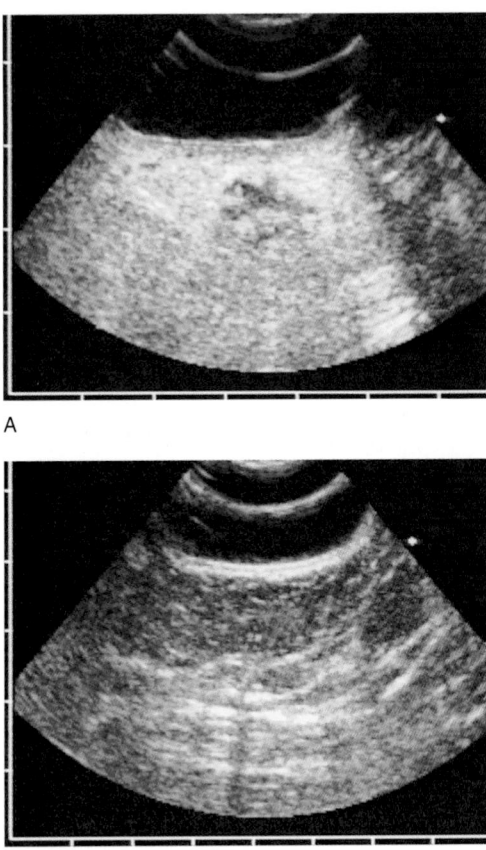

A

B

Figure 13–51. **A.** Sonogram of a patient with cellulitis of the lateral chest wall. The image was taken with an annular array transducer and an acoustic stand-off. The tissues are diffusely hyperechoic with little detail resolution. A small region of hypoechogenicity is seen in the center of the image and represents early abscess formation. **B.** Sonogram of the contralateral normal chest wall of the same patient. The skin layer is hyperechoic, and the subcutaneous tissue is relatively hypoechoic with much greater detail resolution than on the abnormal side.

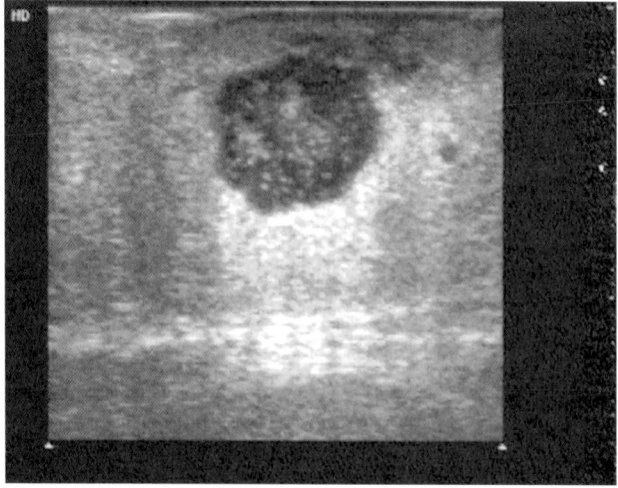

Figure 13–52. Typical appearance of a subcutaneous abscess on a thigh. The abscess cavity is rounded and hypoechoic with mixed internal echogenicity. Posterior acoustic enhancement reflects the liquid nature of the abscess contents. The surrounding skin is hyperechoic because of adjacent tissue edema and possibly cellulitis.

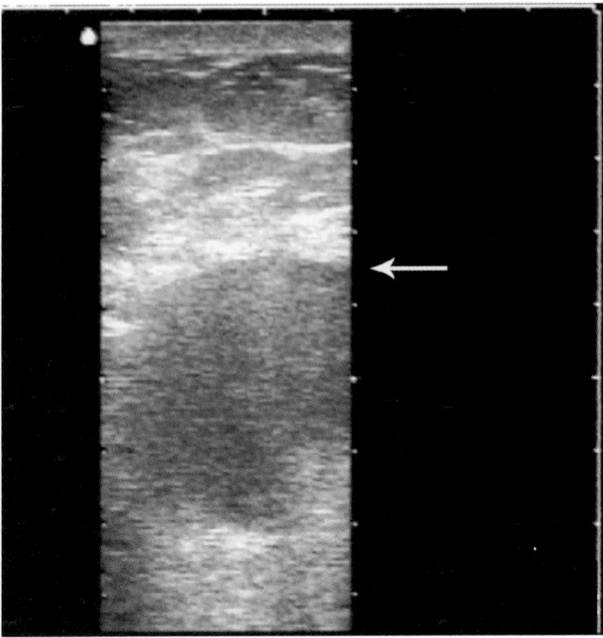

Figure 13–53. Long-axis sonogram of a deep midline buttock abscess in the region of the gluteal fold. The skin and immediate subcutaneous tissue appear to be of relatively normal echogenicity. The deeper tissues surrounding the rounded abscess cavity appear more hyperechoic and edematous. Note that the superior edge of this large abscess cavity is 3.5 cm from the skin surface (*arrow*). Knowledge of the depth of this abscess cavity is crucial to the individual performing the drainage procedure.

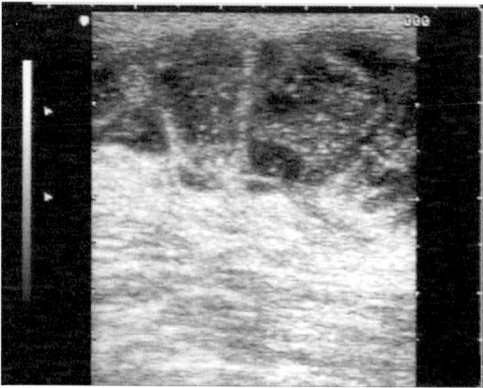

Figure 13–54. Sonogram of a postoperative abdominal wall wound infection. Multiple septae are seen in the hypoechoic collection immediately beneath the skin. Motion of the abscess contents was seen with gentle transducer pressure on real-time scanning. Posterior acoustic enhancement is also present.

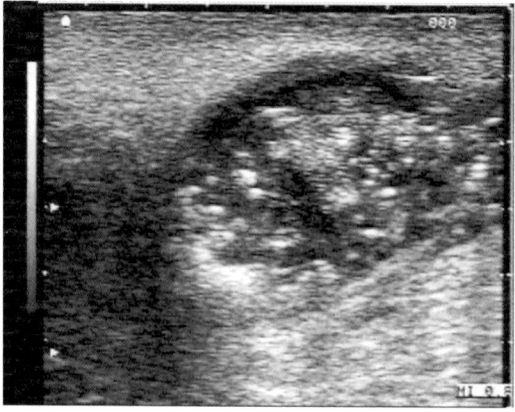

Figure 13–55. Hyperechoic foci with some associated ring-down artifact are seen within the mixed echogenicity contents of this abscess cavity. These hyperechoic regions on this sonogram correspond to small gas pockets within the abscess cavity.

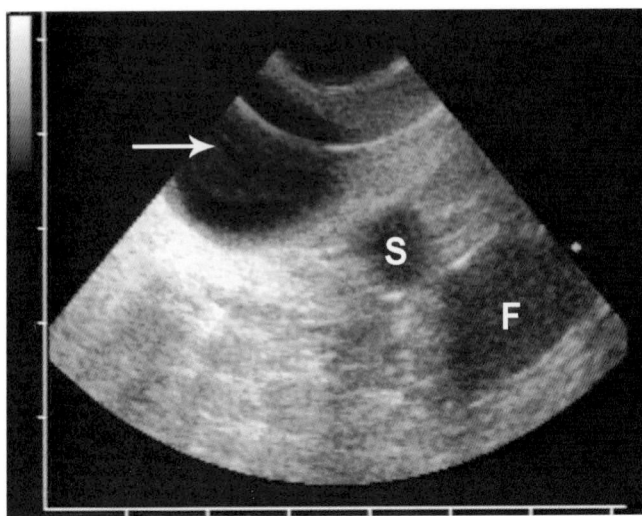

Figure 13–56. Short-axis sonogram of an abscess cavity in the left groin of an injection drug user. The thick-walled hypoechoic abscess cavity (*arrow*) is seen on the left of the image; adjacent are the hypoechoic saphenous (S) and common femoral veins (F). Careful preprocedure ultrasound mapping provided useful information to guide the incision.

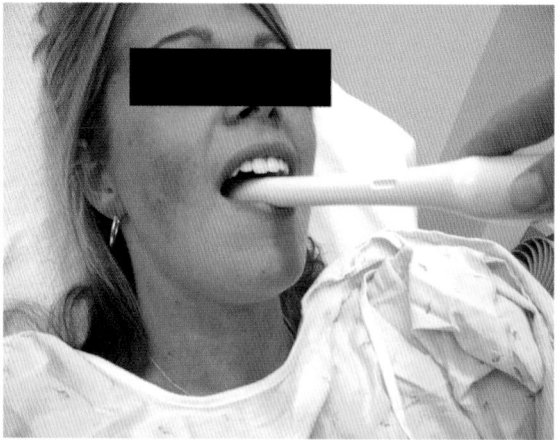

Figure 13–57. Intraoral transducer insertion for peritonsillar evaluation.

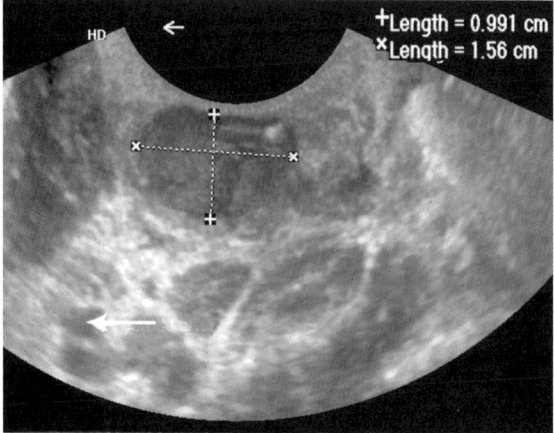

Figure 13–58. Right peritonsillar abscess. Note the presence of the hypoechoic, purulent fluid collection within the abscess cavity (*cursors*) and the proximity of the carotid artery (*arrow*).

▶ TIPS TO IMPROVE IMAGE ACQUISITION AND INTERPRETATION

- As you face the monitor, orient the transducer so structures on the left of the image are to the operator's left and structures on the right of the image are to the operator's right.

- Scanning normal structures on the patient's opposite side can help sonographers differentiate normal anatomy from pathology.

▶ PITFALLS

- Failure to differentiate an abscess from cellulitis
- Failure to consider the diagnosis of necrotizing fasciitis
- Failure to identify adjacent structures such as nerves, arteries, and veins

DIAGNOSIS OF TESTICULAR TORSION AND MANUAL DETORSION

► CLINICAL CONSIDERATIONS

- Diagnosis and management of testicular torsion are time-sensitive if the testicle is to be salvaged.
- Point-of-care ultrasound can decrease the time to diagnosis and bedside management of testicular torsion.

► CLINICAL INDICATIONS

- Acute testicular pain

► ANATOMIC CONSIDERATIONS

- Left-sided torsion is more common than the right because of the greater length of the spermatic cord on the left.
- In early torsion, the venous blood supply may be the only thing compromised as it is a lower pressure system.
- In about 60% of cases, the testicle will be twisted in the medial direction; therefore, the initial attempt at detorsion is by "opening the book."

► TECHNIQUES

- Select a linear transducer and use the testicular preset on the machine.
- Scan the normal contralateral testicle to adjust the color Doppler scale and gain.
- Use color Doppler to identify blood flow within the painful testicle, and pulsed-wave Doppler to demonstrate both venous and arterial waveforms.
- If blood flow is decreased or absent (compared to the other testicle), perform manual detorsion at the bedside. This often requires some type of procedural sedation.
- Begin by trying to twist the affected testicle laterally. If this is making the testicle rise higher in the scrotum or causing significant pain, then try twisting in the opposite direction.

▶ TIPS TO IMPROVE SUCCESS

- Scan the unaffected testicle so that the color Doppler can be adjusted on a normal testicle.

- Once the color Doppler is set, obtain a view of the testicles side-by-side (Figure 13-59). This alone can often make the diagnosis of torsion.

- Scan through the affected testicle with color Doppler (Figure 13-60).

- Sometimes a testicle is twisted multiple times around the spermatic cord. Continue to manually twist the testicle until blood flow has returned and can be confirmed by ultrasound.

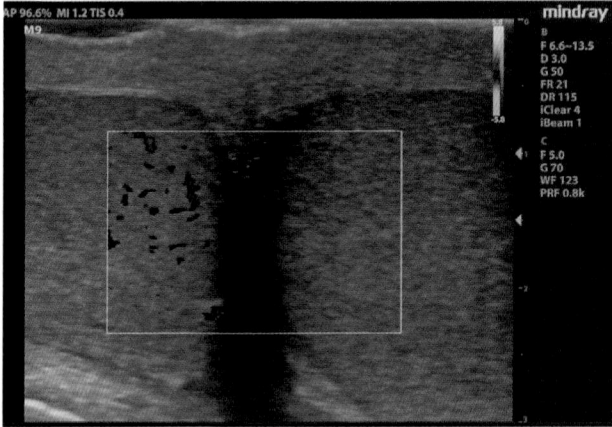

Figure 13–59. Side-by-side color Doppler imaging of both testicles. There is no color flow in the left testicle. This is the simplest way to demonstrate absent or decreased flow in a painful testicle.

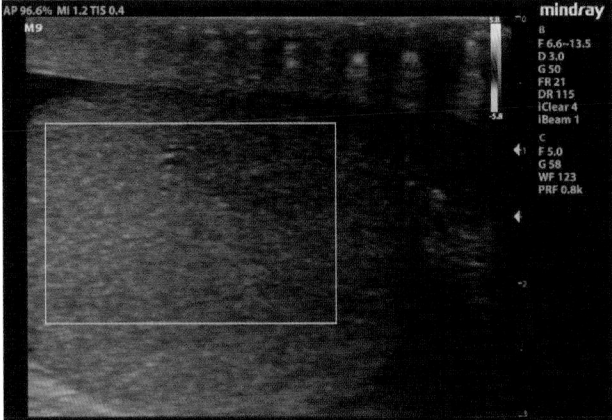

Figure 13–60. Testicular torsion. Absent blood flow, by color Doppler exam, in the center of the testicle. Note that the color Doppler scale (set at 5.8 cm/s) has been properly adjusted by first scanning the unaffected testicle.

▶ PITFALLS

- Inexperienced operators could miss early torsion with only venous obstruction, but complete torsion is straightforward to diagnose.

- If pain is resolved at the time of the ultrasound exam, spontaneous detorsion may have occurred and this may be undetectable by ultrasound.

For more detailed information go to the comprehensive textbook Ma and Mateer's Emergency Ultrasound, 3rd edition, Chapter 18 "Musculoskeletal, Soft Tissue, and Miscellaneous Applications" by Andreas Dewitz, MD; Chapter 21 "Vascular Access" by John Rose, MD, Aaron Blair, MD and Aman Parikh, MD; and Chapter 22 "Additional Ultrasound-Guided Procedures" by Andreas Dewitz, MD, Robert Jones, MD, Jessica Resnick, MD and Michael Stone, MD.

Index

Page numbers followed by *f* indicate figures; *t* indicate tables.